Children and Violence

Children and Violence
The World of the Defenceless

Einar A. Helander

Forewords by

Halfdan Mahler
Former Director-General of the World Health Organization

and

H.D. Deve Gowda
Former Prime Minister of India

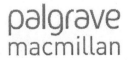

First published 2008 by
PALGRAVE MACMILLAN
Houndmills, Basingstoke, Hampshire RG21 6XS and
175 Fifth Avenue, New York, N.Y. 10010
Companies and representatives throughout the world

PALGRAVE MACMILLAN is the global academic imprint of the Palgrave
Macmillan division of St. Martin's Press, LLC and of Palgrave Macmillan Ltd.
Macmillan® is a registered trademark in the United States, United Kingdom
and other countries. Palgrave is a registered trademark in the European
Union and other countries.

ISBN-13: 978–0–230–57394–9   hardback
ISBN-10: 0–230–57394–0   hardback

This book is printed on paper suitable for recycling and made from fully
managed and sustained forest sources. Logging, pulping and manufacturing
processes are expected to conform to the environmental regulations of the
country of origin.

A catalogue record for this book is available from the British Library.

Library of Congress Cataloging-in-Publication Data

Helander, Einar.
    Children and violence : the world of the defenceless / Einar
    Helander.
        p. cm.
    Includes bibliographical references and index.
    ISBN 0–230–57394–0 (alk. paper)
    1. Child abuse. 2. Children—Violence against. 3. Children—
    Institutional care. I. Title.
    HV6626.5.H375 2008
    362.76—dc22

                                                        2008015138

10   9   8   7   6   5   4   3   2   1
17 16 15 14 13 12 11 10 09 08

Printed and bound in Great Britain by
CPI Antony Rowe, Chippenham and Eastbourne

All that is necessary for evil to triumph is for good men to do nothing.

Edmund Burke (1729–1797)

The world has slowly grown accustomed to the symptoms of moral decay. One misses the elementary reaction against injustice and for justice – that reaction which in the end represents man's only protection against a relapse into barbarism. I am firmly convinced that the passion for justice and truth has done more to improve man's condition than calculating political shrewdness, which in the end only breeds distrust ... Let us not shun the fight when it is unavoidable to preserve the right and the dignity of man.

Albert Einstein (1879–1955)

It is my firm conviction that nothing enduring can be built on violence.

Mohandas Karamchand Gandhi (1869–1948)

Contents

List of Photographs

Jacket photograph: Ten-year-old girl straitjacketed to the bed and drugged 'because of overactivity'. She receives no training or daily activities, is doubly incontinent and unable to walk and speak. She is unable to distinguish night from day, underweight and malnourished. She was a healthy infant abandoned by her poor mother to the 'protection of the state', but she has suffered years of abuse and neglect from indifferent staff and because of insufficient government funding. © P. O. Sjöberg, Sweden.

List of Tables

List of Figures

List of Boxes

Foreword (1)

Dr Einar Helander came to the headquarters of the World Health Organization in 1974 to participate in the Organization's development of the rehabilitation component of the new primary health care strategy. During fourteen of my fifteen years as Director-General of WHO, I followed his work. In 1974, in a WHO document he summarized the challenge related to the unmet needs of persons with disabilities: 'We have in our hands a growing moral, social, health and economic problem of vast proportions, which we are incapable of dealing with by using the conventional system.' As a response to that challenge, he first developed the disability prevention programme and then the community-based rehabilitation (CBR) strategy. His approaches were always innovative, but also practical and cost-effective. Many were very unconventional – the CBR technology was based on observations of indigenous spontaneous methods and a thorough knowledge of the living conditions in poor villages and marginal urban areas in the developing countries where he spent most of his time. He realized that managerial capacity building was crucial and devoted many years to the teaching of CBR policies, planning, programme design, service delivery systems, quality/cost control methods and human rights in courses for participants from ninety countries. The CBR is now implanted in some 100 nations; the WHO technology manual has been translated into more than fifty languages.

In this new book Dr Helander follows up his thirty years of field experience by outlining first the cruel, inhuman and degrading treatment to which some ten million abandoned children in residential institutions are currently subjected. He then continues with a thorough analysis of the global extent and consequences of child abuse and neglect. His descriptions are shocking, and so are his conclusions about the moral vacuum that seems to be a common feature among the perpetrators.

This book is carefully researched. Building on the vast published evidence and on his own observations, the author describes some of the most important features of the 'world of the defenceless', one of the most visible of which is its pervasive violence. It is cautiously estimated that over three billion people – half of the world's population – are the traumatized victims of childhood sexual, physical, psychological and other forms of abuse and that over one billion become disabled or meet a premature death as a consequence.

Dr Helander's criticism of 140 governments' attitudes to human rights application is very frank. These governments represent five billion citizens, and they will not allow any outside, independent and unfettered inspections of what takes place in their 'orphanages' and other services for children. Another of his conclusions is that the present level of development aid – a few US dollars per person per year – is totally insufficient to bring about any significant reduction of global poverty, which now leaves over one billion children severely neglected. Helander points out that with the present negative environment, it is not easy to mobilize true enthusiasm for assistance for human and economic development. For the time being, poor nations will have to rely mainly on what can be achieved by mobilizing their own national resources. He finally outlines a community-based primary prevention programme to reduce the global level of child violence.

I recommend this powerful book for reading and serious reflection: what is the future for a world where its people find themselves surrounded by oceans of contagious violence, immoral behaviour, lack of compassion, and unwillingness to change?

Halfdan Mahler, MD
Director-General of the World
Health Organization, 1973–1988

Foreword (2)

Children and Violence: the World of the Defenceless exposes a number of large-scale problems in the human environment. The author is well known for his ground-breaking work to improve the quality of life and the independence of disabled persons. I met Dr Einar Helander for the first time over fifteen years ago in Bangalore. He worked closely with my Karnataka state administration for several years and with several local organizations to successfully prepare a state-wide community-based programme. In this book he draws from experience of thirty years of fieldwork in many developing countries.

Dr Helander has widened the perspective of the disabled defenceless to analyse the basic conditions of abused and neglected children. He has always been a strong spokesman for human rights and solidarity and points out the many weaknesses in our nations: the widespread violence against children, the inadequate education systems and the lack of security and justice in a world where most people struggle to escape poverty. He strongly criticizes the attitudes of many donor agencies and the futility of official external aid. The very small amounts of such aid that reach the poor appear to be used more and more as an instrument for the globalization of power in the hands of the few and the rich. He points to national mobilization for community development using grassroots resources as the tool for success.

The development of democratic, people-oriented decision-making and decentralization of financing – changes that took place in India in the 1990s – are factors of immense importance for poverty alleviation and progress.

I recommend all those concerned with development to read this frank and sincere analysis of the human condition, learning from the past and planning for a better future.

Rt. Hon H.D. Deve Gowda
Prime Minister of India 1996–1997
Chief Minister of the State of Karnataka 1994–1996

Preface

This global analysis of childhood violence builds on my experience of over thirty years of international work, most of the time as a staff member of the World Health Organization (WHO) and of the United Nations Development Programme (UNDP), and in co-operation with many bilateral governmental and non-governmental organizations. My first international observations go back to 1974, when I saw three women, all dressed in black, just leaving the office of a doctor in a small town in a Middle East country. He told me that they were a mother and two daughters who had been raped during the previous night by the father when he was drunk. Such sexual abuse was common. The doctor was instructed to report such crimes to the police, but could not, as the girls refused to be examined, and under an Islamic ordinance, a woman had to present four male, Muslim witnesses in order to prove a case of sexual assault. Abortions were forbidden and any children in that country issuing from incest usually perished soon after birth.

During my career I have worked in ninety-four countries[1] and I have personally examined thousands of children, at home, in health centres or institutions, and observed them at play, in the streets, in schools and as underage workers. Main sources have been interviews with parents, local families, teachers and the leaders in poor villages and marginal urban areas where I have stayed long enough to win the confidence of the local population. In each country, there have been official meetings with several ministries – mostly Health and Social Welfare – to discuss child maltreatment problems, approaches, planning, technical assistance, training programmes, financing, management and the environmental political and cultural aspects.

Information given in this book has also originated from the professional staff of headquarters, regional and country offices of various organizations, including WHO, UNDP, the World Bank, the High Commission of Human Rights, the High Commission for Refugees, ILO, UNICEF, UNESCO, the UN Population Fund, the UN Institute for Social Research, and the UN Conference on Trade and Development. I have met with colleagues with long experience in their own countries: diplomats, social anthropologists, economists, criminologists, schoolteachers, religious leaders, local bankers, agricultural experts and personnel at local health centres, 'orphanages', hospitals, prisons and social programmes.

At the time of the Alma-Ata Declaration on Primary Health Care in 1978 it was obvious that successful delivery of public care was related to the appropriate managerial training of the professionals. To fill this gap I wrote, in 1979, with two co-authors a manual on the technology of community-based rehabilitation – the fourth component of PHC. It has been introduced in more than 100 countries. It was followed by other technical books focused directly on local and country planning, management and evaluation systems. Some thirty national, regional or international specific management courses/seminars have been held, many of these during the last ten years. Some 200 professionals from 90 countries (see note 1) have participated in these courses and they have contributed to the information in this book through an exchange of ideas and experience.

For this book, I have made an extensive study of published scientific literature, seeking confirmation of the field observations. In total, close to 20,000 articles, books and other printed material, originating from 132 countries, have been identified and evaluated. The total information base is reviewed in Chapter 2; it originates from 152 countries (see note 1). The conclusion is that childhood violence has victimized about half of the world's population.

In the text, I have often quoted case studies, statistics, publications and official reports; the literature in this area is virtually inexhaustible. Yet, they often fall short of conveying the impressions of the human condition which can be directly observed. Beyond the descriptions of our asylums and camps and gulags and of the violence on the street and behind the façade at home, there is other evidence that bears witness to the horrors. One of the most shocking initial observations concerned children in residential institutions. The children I have observed – and whenever possible examined – in these asylums amount to several thousands. It was also shocking to realize that some 5–10 million children (less than 5 years old), mainly girls, die annually because of intentional neglect or outright murder.

The text does not allow me to show the reader the glassy stare of the maltreated children who have lost their minds, the desperation of those who have nothing to eat or the fright of those who get beaten up. It will not let you listen to the screams of those who are chained to walls in the mental hospitals' underground cellars and are spitting at visitors, or of the children who in these hospitals receive electro-convulsive treatment (ECT) without anaesthesia as punishment. It is difficult to convey one's anger when you see severely disabled beggars being robbed of their 'daily income' by some young gangsters, armed with knives. It is sad to remember the boy who was in a correction home: he showed me his back that was covered with bloody marks after having been horsewhipped by the sadistic director for being five minutes late for breakfast. Once I sat down in a small African hut with a poor family to examine a boy who had fractures to both arms and both legs. It took me some minutes until I was able to exclude all diagnoses except intentional trauma: the father had in his drunken fits of aggression fractured these bones and disabled his son for life.

It is difficult to explain my feelings of helplessness when I unexpectedly found several thousand people waiting for me at the market place at the end of the day hoping for miracles; or the memories of those who came to the squares or up the hills carrying children who could not walk, of those who invited me home to see family members who were unable to feed themselves or to speak, or who were expecting me to cure children with severe deformities. I remember a long conversation with an African woman, a victim of polio, in a slum area; I met her on a narrow pathway, walking on her knees and elbows to get home through muddy rainwater on the ground. Many times, I have entered the house of a poor family only to find that the child I was going to examine had just died. There were also the odours of the street people, many homeless since childhood, some freezing to death at night; and the touches from those locked up in dilapidated mental wards. I remember the group of Latin American street boys that I used to meet over a period of some weeks: before I left the country the one who always came to chat with me was 'gone'; the police had shot him dead during the night and dumped his body with the garbage.

Who are the defenceless? They are victims or potential victims of violence, of cruel, inhuman and degrading treatment and of injustice, who are unable to find protection because of

- lack of capacity or social recognition to resist such acts, for instance if the victim is a child or a family who lives in poverty;
- lack of anybody willing and capable to help effectively when there are problems;
- a system of impunity that protects the offenders;
- corruption, cover-ups or inaction inside the judicial system (police, prosecutors, judges);
- an uncaring public attitude that leads to lack of pressure on governments to provide sufficient funds for child defence and support;
- non-compliance by governments with their human rights obligations and non-compliance by service providers with their ethical rules.

The main defenceless group and the focus of this book are children under the age of 18; the global child population in 2006 was 2.3 billion. Their parents are the main perpetrators. This book seeks not only to describe the prevalence, manifestations and scope of child violence, but also to assess the disabling life-long consequences which affect over a billion survivors. The results are shocking. Poverty is a main contributor to such violence; an analysis will be made of the efforts to alleviate it.

'Most traditional explanations of violence,' states Barak (2003), 'remain partial and incomplete as they separately emphasize different yet related phenomena of violence, without ever trying to provide a comprehensive explanation or framework that encompasses the full range of interpersonal, institutional, and structural violence. In fact, most of these one-dimensional explanations of violence underscore the violent behaviour of individuals to the relative exclusion of the role of institutions and structures in violence.' This book combines research findings, statistics and personal observations – with focus on children – and uses the human ecology framework. It seeks to present a more inclusive picture of the extent and consequences of the violence in which we are immersed. It also includes explanations of the major role played by the nervous system – even before birth – in every human thought, emotion and action, and how the human and physical environments interact to shape – boost or destroy – a child's development. Any attempts to understand the relations between human cultures and the violence described in this book are incomplete unless related to neurobiology – a mostly unrecognized basic component of human ecology. Limitations of length, however, have prevented a more detailed analysis.

Methods to prevent pervasive childhood violence exist and are analysed here. Such prevention will only be effective, however, if major alterations in human behaviour and in the culture of our societies occur. Our present world is unequal, dangerous, erratic and unsustainable. Consequently, the world of our children is contaminated by a chaotic human environment that seriously harms them; a change of course is urgent.

Acknowledgements

I am most grateful for the considerable help and advice that I received during the long process that resulted in this book. Through my parents, I was at a very early age directly exposed to their social work with the poor and disadvantaged in Sweden to whom they devoted many years of their lives.

Credit for much of the information in this book goes to all my informal contacts during over thirty years of international work: most importantly to the children and their families in poor villages and marginal urban areas in developing countries, to community leaders in these countries, non-governmental organizations, my colleagues, the many expatriates who have spent long years (some as many as fifty years) in the countries visited, anthropologists, local health and social workers, staff of national and community service delivery systems, teachers, legal experts, officials from national administrations and staff from the UN agencies and bilateral donor agencies, and diplomats who have offered me their knowledge and opinions.

My most sincere thanks are due to Dr Vincent Felitti for several years of encouragement, guidance and technical expertise, and for reading and commenting on the entire book. Special thanks go to many of my colleagues in the World Health Organization, especially to Dr Etienne Krug and Dr Alexander Butchart at the Injury and Violence Programme. I have had the advantage of technical expertise from Mr Joerg Mayer, Economist at UNCTAD, Geneva, Switzerland, Mr Stefano Sensi at the Office of the High Commissioner for Human Rights, Geneva, Switzerland and Mr Claes Sandström, Budget Director, WHO, Geneva, Switzerland.

I would also like to mention the assistance and criticisms from Professor Anita Jacobson-Widing and Professor Bernhard Helander, Department of Cultural Anthropology, Uppsala, Sweden; Mr Ture Jönsson, Department of Special Education, University of Gothenburg, Sweden; Mrs Elena Kozhevnikova, Psychologist, St Petersburg, Russia; Dr Padmani Mendis MD, Colombo, Sri Lanka; Mrs Indumathi Rao, Co-ordinator, CBR Network, Bangalore, India; Mr Jorge A. Restrepo, Co-ordinator, International Secretariat, Defence for Children International, Geneva, Switzerland; Professor Gunnar Stangvik, Special Education Department, University, Alta, Norway; and Mrs Maine Viklund-Olofsson, Star of Hope International, Sweden.

The personnel at the WHO Library have given me very valuable guidance and support in my efforts to cover the considerable amount of published literature on child abuse. For the photos and figures, I am obliged to the Archives at WHO; Star of Hope International, Stockholm; Dr Vincent Felitti, La Jolla; Dr Bruce Perry, Houston; Dr James Williams, San Diego; Dr Barton Schmitt, Denver; Dr Céline Rozenblat, Lausanne; The Fordham Institute, Vassar College, Poughkeepsie; and Volcano Press, Volcano. I am also grateful for the assistance with the editing of Mr John Bland and Mrs Hannelore Polanka.

Finally, I am deeply thankful to my wife Margarida for her incalculable source of support and for having endured the sight of her husband sitting at the computer for years on end. She has read it all and engaged in hours of discussions, based on her own experience of social community work with children in Portugal, and on what she has seen in the many villages and slums to which she has accompanied me.

List of Abbreviations

AB	antisocial behaviour
ACE	adverse childhood experiences
ACTH	adrenocorticotropic hormone
ADHD	attention deficit hyperactivity disorder
AIDS	acquired immuno-deficiency syndrome
APA	American Psychiatric Association
ASD	acute stress disorder
ASPD	antisocial personality disorder
CAT	Convention Against Torture and other Cruel, Inhuman or Degrading Treatment or Punishment
CBR	community-based rehabilitation
CDC	Centers of Disease Control, Atlanta, Georgia
CIDI	Composite International Diagnostic Interview
CRC	Convention on the Rights of the Child
CSA	child sexual abuse
CU	callous unemotional traits
DD	development disability
DNA	deoxyribonucleic acid
DQ	development quotient
DSM-IV	*Diagnostic and Statistical Manual of Mental Disorders*, 4th edition 1993 by the APA
ECT	electro-convulsive treatment
EEG	electroencephalogram
EU	European Union
FAO	United Nations Food and Agricultural Organization
GABA	γ-aminobutyric acid
GDP	gross domestic product
GNI	gross national income
HIV	human immunodeficiency virus
ICCPR	International Covenant on Civil and Political Rights
ICD-X	*International Classification of Diseases*, 10th edition 1993, by WHO
ICESCR	International Covenant on Economic, Social and Cultural Rights
ICF	*International Classification of Functioning, Disability and Health*, by WHO

ILO	International Labour Organization
IMF	International Monetary Fund
IQ	intelligence quotient
JAMA	*Journal of the American Medical Association*
LWOP	life without parole (prison sentence)
MAO-A	monoaminooxidase A
MDG	Millennium Development Goals
MDRI	Mental Disability Rights International
M/m	age in months
MR	mental retardation
MRI	magnetic resonance imaging
n.a.	not annotated
NGO	non-governmental organization
OCHR	Office of the UN High Commissioner for Human Rights
OECD	Organization for Economic Co-operation and Development
OFC	orbitofrontal cortex
OT	oxytocin
PET	positron emission tomography
PHC	primary health care
POW	prisoner of war
PPP	purchasing power parity
PTSD	post-traumatic stress disorder
RAD	reactive attachment disorder
SD	standard deviation
UDHR	Universal Declaration on Human Rights
UN	United Nations
UNAIDS	United Nations Agency for AIDS
UNCTAD	United Nations Conference on Trade and Development
UNDP	United Nations Development Programme
UNESCO	United Nations Educational, Scientific and Cultural Organization
UNHCR	United Nations High Commission for Refugees
UNICEF	United Nations International Children's Emergency Fund
UNRISD	United Nations Research Institute for Social Development
USAID	United States Agency for International Development
WB	World Bank
WFP	World Food Programme
WGI	worldwide governance indicators
WHO	World Health Organization
WMA	World Medical Association
WPA	World Psychiatric Association
WTO	World Trade Organization

Part I
Introduction

1
You Cut a Rose and Release a Tornado

A stone thrown into the water creates circles on the surface; these last for a few minutes: the circles of childhood abuse may last for a lifetime. The calamitous consequences of such abuse may not be immediately visible or easy to detect; to adapt a meteorological explanation of how natural disasters may start: 'you cut a rose and release a tornado'.[2]

A person who starts to study what at first appears to be a limited problem opens a keyhole to the world, trying to learn, to define problems, to find explanations, and to act. Looking through the next keyhole will provide a contrasting perspective, and teach the viewer another lesson about the difference between appearance and reality. With growing knowledge, more opportunities to observe and a great deal of patience, the mists surrounding the obscurities and complexities of the violence-saturated human ecology will start to dispel. Eventually, the time will come when one will be able to fuse multiple, limited observations into a broader vision that exposes the dark corners of reality. The reality is that abusing, abandoning, neglecting and assassinating defenceless children are merely the symptoms of a much wider, unresolved predicament: that of an uncaring and cruel world. Large-scale interpersonal violence – a drastic mass-destruction of human lives – has existed since time immemorial. Human history reveals the heritage of thousands of years of killings and abuse of millions of children that have taken place without much public reaction. Not until the 1960s was child abuse recognized by the medical establishment as a diagnostic entity and since then major research has finally created an awareness of its role in people's lives.

The following pages serve to guide the reader through the book's main contents. Its starting point – after the Introduction (materials, methods, definitions and short history) in Part I – is the abuse and neglect experienced by some ten million children presently confined – hidden, incarcerated and silenced – in residential institutions (Part II, Chapter 4). The practices in many thousands of these amount to 'cruel, inhuman and degrading treatment' defined by international law as equivalent to torture. Chapter 5 describes the abuse and neglect of some 400 million uprooted children who live without parents as biological or social orphans, forced to be soldiers, as labourers 'in the worst conditions', in refugee camps, as prostitutes or who are trafficked. Chapter 6 reviews the consequences of parent deprivation and the alternatives for substitute parents and providing care, education and shelter for the homeless.

Part III presents a comprehensive, global account of the prevalence of childhood violence experienced by those who have grown up with their birth parents (Chapter 7). It is based in information from 152 countries (see note 1); the conclusion is that half of the world's population have been victims of childhood violence before the age of 18. Also, half of the world's children experience serious structural neglect. In Chapter 8 the serious, long-term health and social consequences of the violence that has already occurred are assessed. There are also major judicial and economic effects, yet to be fully understood.

Part IV describes the most frequently used methods through which child violence can be prevented and treated. It includes a review of the explanations of why people become perpetrators (Chapter 9). Twelve major causes of and contributors to childhood violence are reviewed. These include: pregnancy and delivery complications, conduct disorder, genetic factors, antisocial personality disorder, paedophilia, maladaptive alcohol use, mental disorders among care-givers, family malfunction, domestic violence, violence in the society, lack of child support and services, and poverty. On the basis of present knowledge of the extent of the problem, and of the potential effectiveness of the interventions, the conclusion is that priority should be given to primary prevention. The availability and efficacy of existing care and rehabilitation services for abused and neglected children are reviewed in Chapter 10.

Part V reviews the influence of the global systems in childhood violence, starting with international law. Many nations are embarrassed by references to and discussions about the lack of observance of the United Nations treaties on human rights in their countries (Chapter 11). A large majority of all United Nations member states have opted out of core parts of the international law. Children in these countries who are victims of 'cruel, inhuman or degrading treatment' and their representatives are not even allowed to communicate their problems to the Human Rights Council in Geneva.

The situation of the world's poor people is analysed in Chapter 12. Poverty is widespread: close to 3,600 million people (well over half of the world's population, 40 per cent of them children) continue to be deprived of their necessities in spite of fifty years of international aid. The economic inequalities are large and growing and for children this means that for very large proportions of them, quality education, food, clean water, decent housing and protection against violence are unavailable. Poverty-related structural neglect affects over one billion children. There then follows an analysis of the international assistance programmes. Present official aid after subtraction of delivery and administrative costs amounts to a few US dollars per poor person per year and even that has never been shown to trickle down to the poor. These poor children cannot count on more than token assistance from rich donors.

Chapter 13 reviews the current United Nations Millennium Development Programme. This programme mentions neither community and interpersonal violence, nor the need to protect children. Many of the goals of the Millennium Programme concern children. The Millennium Programme set a twenty-five-year period (1990–2015) for completion of these goals: two-thirds of that period has passed. A review of the present outcomes is made for each of the targets that apply to children (poverty, hunger, schooling, gender disparity, under-5 mortality, maternal mortality, spread of infectious diseases, access to clean water and sanitation, decent and productive work for youth, and commitment to good governance).

There are very serious problems with the implementation of these targets, and most countries will not reach them by 2015. It is concluded that to progress – to give their children better life and to prevent childhood violence – poor nations have to build on their own strengths and learn how to mobilize their populations for progress, beginning during their childhood. Governments and people can co-operate: phasing out indifferent, uncaring and immobile bureaucracy; combating corruption and incompetence wherever it appears; supporting the local mobilization of their communities by increasing self-rule and decentralization; phasing in a modernized, socially oriented education system; and promoting justice, peace and human rights of the poor. The present promotion of global 'crash' programmes based on dreams at the top of the global system should with few exceptions (such as the immunization projects) be changed. A new entry point for development is proposed: to work directly with people, build on what they have and do, and assist communities to take gradual steps forward. To the extent that international aid is available it should be redirected to the civil society which is better placed for a role in these more humble, gradual approaches.

Finally, Part VI presents an analysis of methods for a universal, community-based primary prevention of childhood violence. The reason for preferring universal prevention of violence is its high prevalence and global presence. Abuse of children takes place across all cultures, societies, economic, social and religious strata. It is not just a problem seen in a few disadvantaged families. Four different strategies for coping with the problem of child violence are analysed: family life education; community child watch; use of media for information about the consequences of childhood violence; and legislation. Because of the high prevalence of violence towards children, no country will have sufficient professional personnel to conduct a universal prevention programme. Consequently, ordinary people in the community need to be mobilized and trained (Chapter 14). Once in place, the positive results of an effective universal, community-based programme will be important: it will decrease social and health problems that now affect people on a massive scale and are the known outcomes of childhood violence – alcohol and drug addiction, criminality, chronic mental and physical disorders, decrease of productivity and creativity in the workforce, and fear. Chapter 15 contains the conclusions of the book.

The human ecology of childhood violence

To better organize all the materials in this book I have applied the human ecology system. 'Ecology' as a term was proposed in 1866 by Ernst Haeckel. Ecological scientists study *all levels of the organization of life on earth and the interrelations between organisms and their environment*. Most ecology has focused on the physical environment, but eventually has come to include research on the social environment: human ecology.

This book describes the global, human-ecology context in which childhood violence takes place. This approach provides a broader, cross-disciplinary perspective, explaining how human–environment relations are influenced by a combination of environmental, political, economic, legal, psychological, physical, cultural and societal forces, and the quality of basic human relationships. A well-known theoretical system has been developed by Urie Bronfenbrenner (1979, 2004), a leading American psychologist. He seeks to explain the biological, environmental, demographic and technical conditions of the life of all individuals as determined by an interactive and interrelated series of systems that begin to have an influence in early childhood.

James Garbarino (1995) points out that:

> Applying a human ecology perspective to the issue will help us to see
> the wider aspects: it forces us to consider the concept of risk beyond
> the narrow confines of individual personality and family dynamics. In
> the ecological approach, both are 'causes' of parenting patterns and
> 'reflections' of broader sociocultural forces. The social environment
> can become poisonous to the development of children and youth
> much as the physical environment can undermine their physical well-
> being. The term *social* toxicity parallels the concept of *physical* toxicity
> as a threat to human well-being and survival. A socially toxic envi-
> ronment contains widespread threats to the development of identity,
> competence, moral reasoning, trust, hope, and the other features of
> social maps that make for success in school, family, work, and the
> community.

To better understand human behavioural development Bronfenbrenner proposed the use of the functions and influences of four layers of
environment systems; for this book some adaptations have been made
to his system:

1. The *micro-system*: the child has his/her own micro-system: the body
   with its cognitive, emotional and physiological components. The
   micro-system encompasses the relationships and interactions a child
   has with his/her immediate surroundings; major parts of these influences such as beliefs and behaviour are affected by the parents.
   Children are cognitively, emotionally and physiologically influenced
   by violence and maltreatment; it affects their present and future
   behaviour, social functions and health.
2. The *meso-system* comprises relations among the major settings next
   to the person: the family, the school, friends and peers. Meso-systems
   make inputs into the child's micro-system, for instance by transfers
   of the parents', teachers' and peers' attitudes and behaviour. The
   influence is bi-directional; the child's behaviour also influences the
   parents, the teachers and its peers.
3. The *exo-system* is the environment (mainly in the community) in
   which a child may or may not be directly involved, but which
   nonetheless indirectly affects him or her. Examples include: the parents' workplace experiences and local inter-family relationships, and
   their reactions related to poverty, frustration and powerlessness. The

quality of the exo-system is related to community leadership and performance, the presence of services and utilities, the efforts to alleviate poverty, the reliability of the legal system and the behaviour environment, for instance community violence, racism and women's status.

4. The *macro-system* (e.g. represented by the nation) includes a larger institutional context of culture, religion and politics; how the UN human rights obligations and national laws are implemented; and the function and fairness of the national legal system. The quality of the performance of the government and its handling of the economy and of poor people's needs are important issues when it comes to preventing violence. Abject poverty is a reality for close to half of the world's population; it is one of the most important predictors for family violence against children.

5. To these a fifth level is proposed: the *global system*. Children's lives are influenced by many global factors such as: the development and follow-up of governments' compliance with the United Nations Human Rights Covenants and Conventions; the global economy; trade regulations; international health campaigns; educational programmes; and foreign media penetration leading to increasing pollution of national cultures. Among these factors, the rich countries' attitudes and actions (or lack of actions) related to poverty alleviation and respect of foreign cultures stand out.

Figure 1.1 presents a schema showing the interactions between the different systems. The thicker arrow from the global to the meso-system reflects the view that the global influences on the economy dominate. The thinner arrows at that level indicate that the expressed needs of poor nations have an insufficient influence.

With the adaptations to this system, one will be able to describe: (a) *upstream*, (b) *downstream* and (c) *parallel interactions*. For example:

(a) The knowledge of the extent of childhood violence (experienced at the level of the micro-system) may lead to *upstream* realization of the needs to strengthen: health services (provided at the level of the exo-system), government programmes for prevention (through the macro-system), and initiatives to provide grants from donor nations for such programmes (global system).

(b) *Downstream* interaction by the global system may include assistance to governments or regions (macro-systems) to eradicate poverty, as this is a main factor causing childhood maltreatment; knowing

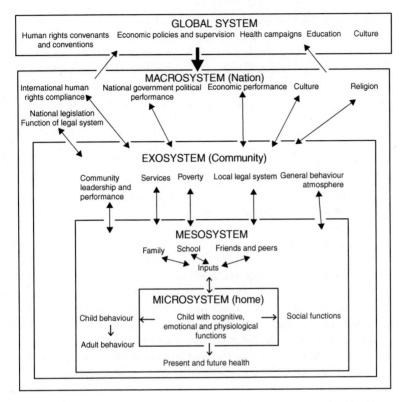

Figure 1.1 Human ecology systems, schema of interactions (based on Bronfenbrenner)

the global extent of such violence governments (macro-systems) may include pre-parent training programmes (proposed by a global agency, such as UNESCO) in the national school curriculum. Downstream interaction may also involve enforcing the implementation of global level human rights laws, leading to their integration in national constitutions and laws (by the meso-system) to be applied by the judicial system at the community (exo-system) and by legal referral levels;

(c) *Parallel* interactions might include the inter-exo-systems, such as transfers of knowledge and skills needed for the setting up of community mobilization programmes, or international co-operation between neighbour countries to develop jointly technical personnel (inter-macro-systems).

The five ecological systems mentioned above all affect our children directly or indirectly: their behaviour, their social functions and health. They are the determinants of the form, function and future of human cultures and social systems.

The micro- and meso-systems – child, home, family, school, friends

(a) The evidence is that about half of all children living in their immediate 'toxic' human environment become victims of sexual and/or physical and/or emotional abuse. Moreover, millions are neglected, abandoned or assassinated. The main perpetrators are the parents; most of this violence occurs in the developing countries. Can this be explained?

We need to open our minds to see the extent of frustration in the parents' human and physical environment: their poverty and hunger (most poor people own no land; many have just seasonal work), the lack of help when they are sick, their grief when close relatives and friends suddenly die from unexplained causes, and the miserable quality of education they have received. Women are often overburdened by work and frequent childbirths; they also have many chronic health conditions: recurrent fevers, anaemia, back and joint pains, toothache, gynaecological problems, depression and general tiredness. These factors influence their interaction with their children. We need to appreciate what it means to live in an environment of general violence and insecurity where many (sometimes even women and children) carry a knife ready for attack or defence. Millions of people in small communities are raided repeatedly by armies and vigilantes. They passively watch the arriving fighters burning their houses, raping the women, killing the men and kidnapping the children. Furthermore, we need to recognize their feelings of powerlessness in the face of an inactive and corrupted – if it exists at all – judicial system. We need to comprehend the long-term effects of their failing struggle to keep hope alive, as they cannot see any signs of a better future.

Many parents live in loveless marriages or partnerships (a large proportion are consanguineous) arranged by others. This is one more explanation for the very high frequency of partner and child abuse, of prostitution and promiscuity. When poor people's debts to moneylenders and gamblers reach insurmountable levels, each year over a million of them sell their children to traffickers; these parents can have no illusions about their fates. When the man – frustrated by so many worries: lack of income, no food for the family, no money for his children to go to school – has lost his self-respect, he may seek to drown his sorrows in alcohol (often brewed by the women) or drugs. Then what we see is a vicious circle, further increasing the violence.

Knowing these features of the human ecology, we may perhaps better understand – although not excuse – the extent of aggression towards defenceless children by their parents. Less understandable is the fact that frustrated abusers are also from better-educated upper and middle classes, and may live in the economically more developed regions. These parents may have been abused during their childhood; there may be conflicts at their place of work, marital problems, and alcohol and drug abuse. Both victims and perpetrators hide most child maltreatment; when revealed, it is a cause for denial, embarrassment and disbelief.

The children's friends and peers play a role in inspiring the abuse carried out by underage perpetrators. Some of this abuse is homosexual, especially when premarital contacts between boys and girls are forbidden and severely punished. Many schoolteachers in the developing countries are physically, sexually and emotionally abusive of their pupils. Several millions of especially vulnerable children exist: those with disabilities and those who live without parents, outside the 'normal' meso-system: in residential institutions, as child soldiers, on the street, working in the worst labour conditions, in refugee camps, in prisons and as prostitutes. They are targets for very extensive abuse. Gendercide is common in some countries.

(b) The chronic consequences for the victims of childhood violence are extensive; affecting over a billion surviving children and adults in the world. The most common mental disorders are post-traumatic stress disorder, anxiety, depression, phobias, conduct disorder, borderline personality disorders and cognitive impairments. Victims adopt health-risk behaviours (alcohol, tobacco and illicit drugs), show antisocial behaviour (aggression and delinquency) and promiscuity; they experience poor self-esteem, fear, nightmares, and some attempt or commit suicide. Their behaviour often leads to social ostracism; thus, they often choose to join groups or gangs outside the 'normal' environment, or just run away. Many victims have somatic consequences: fractures, head injuries, burns, bleedings, spinal cord injury and, the cruellest: 135 million women are sexually mutilated.

When they reach adulthood, the childhood victims have an increased risk for many common somatic diseases: ischaemic heart disease, stroke, chronic obstructive pulmonary disease, hepatitis, gastro-intestinal and gynaecological disorders, chronic headache, obesity and so on. Their mortality rates are higher than those of non-abused people. Most of them remain in their meso- and exo-system with little or no health care or social support. Their impaired work capacity has serious economic consequences.

The health and social consequences for the victims have large-scale secondary effects on the family members: for example, anxiety, depression, fatigue, role impairments, increased workload at home, decreases in productivity and creativity, decreased incomes, social isolation, and/or family disruption. In a study of US residents by Kessler et al. (1995) 61 per cent of men and 51 per cent of women had experienced some traumatic event, including rape, molestation, physical attacks, combat, shock, threat with a weapon, accident, natural disaster with fire, witnessing gross violence, neglect, physical abuse and other qualifying trauma. For about half of those, there had been more than one such trauma. Although there appear to be few published studies on the secondary effects for families (meso-system), one gets the impression that most families in the world have to cope with some of these secondary effects.

(c) Violence not only brings suffering to all its victims; it also creates feelings of helplessness, because others control one's destiny and the victim is often unable to escape from the continuation of maltreatment. It creates normlessness, because of distrust in the legal system when perpetrators enjoy impunity. Violence creates social isolation, because often it is taboo to mention one's violent experiences to others; and when nobody knows, nobody helps. Moreover, violence causes loss of faith in people in positions of trust or responsibility who are supposed to offer protection. For these reasons, action to prevent violence should be given high priority and visibility in all development programmes. Most people will be shocked to learn that childhood violence is so frequent, that it has such severe consequences, and that so little has been, and is being, done to prevent it.

(d) Let us now look at the parallel ecological interactions taking place at the micro- and meso-systems. Do other people, networks of friends, neighbour families, schoolmates or teachers have knowledge of the existing abuse, and will they help? Mostly not, because the truth remains hidden, and most victims do not tell anything until they are adults. The willingness to help is certainly there. Resilience exists, mostly when the victims have found confidants.

(e) The knowledge of the extent of childhood violence (experienced in micro-systems) could lead to upstream realization of the need to strengthen health services (provided at the level of the exo-system), government programmes for prevention (through the macro-system), and initiatives to provide grants from donor nations for such programmes (global system).

However, upstream communications are mostly thin. Community leaders and local organizations for health, social support and schools do not initiate sufficient action, as they are unaware of the real extent of violence against children. Macro-systems do not react, as they should, for several reasons: they accept physical and emotional abuse as part of 'normal education' (and it is legal in most countries), and they hear little about sexual abuse and neglect. In addition, their direct contacts with the realities of 'ordinary people' are often restricted or superficial.

(f) Hundreds of books have been published about and by child abusers and their victims: from Mark Twain, Charles Dickens, André Gide, Thomas Mann and Stephen King, to Jan Guillou and Carylon Lehman. These authors have contributed to create upstream consciousness about the anguish of maltreated children and about the indifference of the meso- or exo-systems in which they are abused. Analyses in such books have thrown light on the background of cruel dictators such as Adolf Hitler, Joseph Stalin and Mao Zedong (Miller, 2002).[3]

The exo-system – the community

The abuse and neglect of children at the micro- and meso-systems do not take place in a vacuum. In many countries, they often exist together with a pattern of incompetence, chaos and non-action by exo-system leaders facing and not knowing how to cope with a socially toxic society. The performance of the community leaders is sometimes excellent, but many exhibit indifference, obstruction, nepotism and corruption. Many human ecological, unresolved deficiencies of the exo-system directly or indirectly contribute to the continuation of childhood violence. There is not enough interaction between the grassroots and the exo-system for a number of reasons:

(a) Effective, community-based violence prevention is lacking.
(b) The exo-systems' health services are insufficient, inaccessible or unavailable to assist the victims: between 36 per cent and 50 per cent of even serious cases of mental disorder (such as psychoses) do

not now receive treatment even in the developed countries; for the developing ones, the rates are 77–85 per cent. Treatments and reha-bilitation of the victims are insufficient everywhere in the developing countries. This ecological problem further impairs the health of the victims.

(c) Community social personnel who intervene in cases of child abuse or neglect are often perceived as exercising impersonal police control rather than trying to help in a friendly way.

(d) Many of the poor live in exo-systems with major unresolved prob-lems: lack of food, clean water, sewers, rubbish disposal, proper roads, electricity, communication and so on. Among them are many fam-ilies who have used land for centuries but do not have a legal title to it, and thus cannot get bank loans to increase the agricultural production. Banks (if they exist at all in developing countries' com-munities) have little or no venture capital for the poor. The – mostly unchecked – population growth adds to the lack of land, to the poverty and to the high mortality and morbidity rates among infants and pregnant mothers. It also adds to the pressure of urbanization (50 per cent of the world's population now live in cities), moving people into extremely poor, unhygienic, highly polluted, crowded and unsafe marginal environments. These factors contribute to peo-ple's frustration, leading to community aggression and to child violence, abandonment and assassination.

(e) The education provided by the exo-system in developing countries is of poor quality. Instead of being a tool for liberation, enlightenment and consciousness-raising, it has often remained as an instrument of oppression by the elite leading to the creation of a caste of obedient serfs. Parents and teachers – unaware of the damage they cause – commonly resort to severe physical and psychological punishment to instil obedience.

(f) The judicial exo-system – the police, the prosecutors, the judges – often malfunctions and there are few advocates to assist the poor. For the poor the neglect of their lawful rights is a clear reality. Their experience of seeking justice often leads them to resignation; those in power will 'always win', by corruption or by the use of personal influence. This explains, among other things, the impunity enjoyed by those who are trusted by the defenceless children and who misuse their authority.

(g) Local leaders in the developing countries often fail to react in an appropriate manner to child violence in their communities, for instance, by introducing child watch schemes, improving the 'social components' of education or by reining in the local production of alcohol and the use of illicit drugs.

(h) Successful development is generated in exo-systems (communities), which benefit from local mobilization programmes, especially when they are part of a macro-system (national) policy. The legal rights to raise and spend local taxes are of the utmost importance for the economic, educational and social development of communities. These rights transfer the initiatives, legal responsibility, decision-making and ownership of the development programmes to local people. However, most countries have a long way to go to ensure the degree of independence that allows community leaders and councils to take their own action to meet the expressed needs of their people. The few examples set up to prevent childhood violence through adequate pre-parent education and home visits have been very successful.

(i) Parallel interactions could include the inter-exo-systems, such as transfers of knowledge and skills needed for modernizing education, the setting up of community mobilization programmes, and judicial systems.

The macro-system – national level

The macro-system has many functions and its leaders have vast responsibilities, some of them directly related to the human ecology of childhood violence. These functions are impeded by a host of problems, especially visible in the developing regions.

(a) The quality of governance in the developing countries is low and in most of them is decreasing. In 1996 the World Bank (Kaufmann and Kraay, 2007) introduced a scale rated from 0–100 to measure six dimensions showing the quality of governance. Individual assessments were made every other year individually for some 200 countries and territories. The World Bank's calculations indicate that from 1996–2006 the quality of governance – which at the start of the project was already very low – declined or halted for 80 per cent of all people in the developing countries. Such nation-building can hardly be rated as a success, and failure in the quality of governance negatively influences the quality of children's lives.

(b) The national politicians' and bureaucrats' dialogue with people at the grassroots is meagre.

(c) Poverty is the overriding, mainly unsolved problem. Economic performance has been impressive in some countries, among them China and India (which together have one-third of the world's population). Still, the added income has mainly benefited the growing upper and middle classes; many poor are still left well behind. The economic inequalities are growing. Governments' budgets to cope with social issues are insufficient. Child neglect is everywhere accompanying poverty, corrective action is totally insufficient and the future consequences are grave.

(d) There are many visible and many hidden ecological society problems in countries composed of several ethnic, religious and political groups, tribes, clans and castes. There are often large economic, educational, social and political differences between them. The real or perceived lack of equality and the quest for power leads to hostilities, armed conflicts, religious persecution and racism. 'Vigilantes' and organized rebel armies (such as those in Algeria, Angola, Bosnia, Colombia, Congo, Ecuador, Guatemala, Guinea-Bissau, Iraq, Kenya, Kosovo, Lebanon, Mozambique, Nepal, Nicaragua, Nigeria, Northern Ireland, Peru, the Philippines, Russia, Rwanda, Sierra Leone, Somalia, Sri Lanka, South Africa, Tanzania, Timor Leste and Uganda) have caused violent intra-national conflicts. Several hundred 'wars' have taken place since the 1950s, creating a widespread atmosphere of terror, violence and insecurity: overall half of the dead and injured victims are children.

(e) Macro-systems have been largely unsuccessful in dealing with child prostitution, street children, beggars, child labour, abandonment of children, trafficking of children, people smuggling, crime, alcoholism and substance abuse, reducing the access to weapons, coping with cruel, inhuman and degrading treatment and the continuing abuse of illicit drugs even in closed residential institutions and prisons.

(f) The national legal systems continue to be afflicted by slowness and corruption. Self-amnesty and impunity are troubling confirmations of the power that the elite exercises over justice at the expense of the poor. The compliance is low or non-existent when it comes to important human rights, such as those related to the UN Child and Torture Conventions.

(g) The national education systems are in crisis. Although there have been some increases in primary school attendance, many children still do not complete the legal minimum of schooling. The training of teachers is insufficient. Secondary and tertiary education needs new direction; there is a lack of co-operation with national enterprises and the civil society.

(h) Health policies are not yet fully developed in many countries. Services are under-budgeted and according to WHO, a quarter of the poor in developing countries still lack primary health care.

(i) Cultural and religious forces in all countries should be mobilized to prevent childhood violence, but not much is seen of them. Non-governmental organizations are active, but their funds or personnel only allow them to scratch the surface. In some countries, they are unwelcome.

(j) Preserving the national culture from foreign and national pollution with media violence is important, but appears hard to resist because of the money involved.

(k) Parallel international co-operation between neighbour countries (inter-macro-systems) to develop jointly technical and managerial personnel is taking place, but needs expansion. Economic co-operation is developing fast in many regions; trade is growing and could lead to increases of the national resources to deal with the problems mentioned above.

The global system

Many important international policies and programmes aimed at improving the human ecology are mediated through the United Nations organizations. They were designed to have important downstream effects.

(a) The first act of the UN was to formulate the Universal Declaration on Human Rights. It then took twenty years (until 1966) of heated disputes, watering down and wrangles over the formulations before the ratification of detailed legal treaties could even begin. The implementation of the treaties has been only partly successful. States known for their non-compliance with the international law have for years paralyzed decision-making in the Geneva-based Human Rights Commission, resulting in a 'credibility deficit . . . which casts a shadow on the reputation of the UN system as a whole' (UN Secretary-General, 2005).

Such a massive failure has downstream human ecological effects – it cast shadows directly over the judicial macro-system and indirectly over the exo-system. The experience that international laws do not have to be followed has a toxic influence over the application of national laws. Eighty per cent of all children are now denied the protection against abuse offered by international inspections. It strengthens the view that childhood violence may continue with impunity. Political leaders – role models for whole countries – are allowed to declare their non-adherence to core parts of the international law and act as they see useful for their own careers. There are no adverse consequences for them.

There is no doubt that had the UN human rights covenants and conventions been adopted with sincerity everywhere they would have prevented a major proportion of the abuse that victimizes children today. Compliance with these laws would have reduced the arrogance and indifference shown by many political leaders to the victimization of the defenceless. The failures of the human rights system have large downstream effects, including for the environment of the children – the micro-system. It is urgent to better integrate the international law system in national constitutions and laws (by the macro-system) to be applied by the judicial system at the community (exo-system) and legal referral levels.

(b) Another global system initiative has been to provide funds for economic development: to 'eradicate poverty'. However, the conclusion by the World Bank's economists is that there is 'no evidence that aid promotes growth even in good policy environments' (Burnside and Dollar, 2000; Easterly et al., 2004). The reason for this international failure is above all that the funds provided by the rich countries have been too small to make any significant results. In spite of fifty years of international grants and loans amounting to US$2.3 trillion (Easterly, 2005), over 3,500 million poor people continue to be deprived of the bare necessities of life. 'Structural neglect', which is not caused by care-givers but results from poverty (see p. 21), still concerns over one billion children. It does not seem realistic to believe that the failed global policies and programmes will change in the near future. The responsible organizations are seen to constantly increase their staffs and budgets, although the evidence – carefully managed by the stakeholders, so that it will appear undisputed and optimistic – would indicate that the programmes built on the chosen unique orthodox economic model for development do not and will not work.

One favourite idea is that a major poverty reduction will result from fair trade (as defined by WTO). Firstly, the economic gains were initially overestimated; secondly, the gains of increased trade are unlikely to reach the poor directly; thirdly, the trade negotiations have reached a dead end.

Another feature of global influence is the institutional control (the International Monetary Fund, the World Bank and the World Trade

Organization) of economic development dominated by the rich countries. This has been severely criticized by many economists and by many developing countries, and has had damaging downstream effects (Stiglitz, 2002).

(c) International health campaigns have had several great successes, among them the eradication of smallpox and polio. These have been helpful examples of how countries can manage large-scale preventive systems. Further efforts are taking place for AIDS, malaria and tuberculosis. General health service development has, however, been slow – a reflection of lack of funds.

(d) Education needs much more support through international aid. It is unlikely that we will see much community development as long as education in the developing countries focuses on the primary level and does not send more students to the secondary and tertiary levels.

(e) The question of culture preservation is important. By exportation, the rich countries influence many aspects of daily life and culture in the poor and dependent countries: what people eat and drink, how they dress, the amounts of violence and sex they see on television and at the cinema, the music they listen to, the software they use, the toys and games that children have, and so forth. Poor and proud nations see their own language and traditions being submerged under the threats of an ever expanding and superior selling of imitations of foreign culture. Certainly, these transfers influence all the human ecology systems down to the micro level.

(f) Downstream interaction by the global system may include help to governments or regions (macro-systems) to eradicate poverty, as this is a main factor causing childhood violence. Knowing the global extent of such violence, global efforts should help governments (macro-systems) to set up and maintain pre-parent training programmes and other child defence and support programmes in the national school curriculum. The necessity of improving the management competence in the recipient countries has not received enough attention.

Before presenting the evidence, a review will be made in Chapter 2 of the materials and methods of the published and informal information, on which the conclusions of this book are based. Chapter 3 will provide a short historical background.

2
Definitions, Materials and Methods

Definitions of violence and related behaviours

The definition of violence in this book is that of article 19 of the UN Convention on the Rights of the Child: 'all forms of physical or mental violence, injury and abuse, neglect or negligent treatment, maltreatment or exploitation, including sexual abuse'.

The following detailed definitions are by WHO (2002) and represent the international consensus for their use:

- Child sexual abuse (CSA) as the involvement of a child in sexual activity that he or she does not fully comprehend, is unable to give informed consent to, or for which the child is not developmentally prepared and cannot give consent, or that violates the laws or social taboos of society. Child sexual abuse is evidenced by the activity between a child and an adult or another child who by age or development is in a relationship of responsibility, trust or power, the activity being intended to gratify or satisfy the needs of the other person. This may include but is not limited to: (a) the inducement or coercion of a child to engage in any unlawful sexual activity; (b) the exploitative use of a child in prostitution or other unlawful sexual practices; (c) the exploitative use of children in pornographic performances and materials.
- Physical abuse in children is that which results in actual not potential physical harm from an interaction or lack of interaction which is reasonably within the control of a parent or in a position of responsibility, power or trust. There may be single or repeated incidents.
- Emotional/psychological abuse includes the failure to provide a developmentally appropriate, supportive environment,

including...a primary attachment figure, so that the child can develop a stable and full range of emotional and social competencies commensurate with her or his personal potentials and in the context of the society in which the child dwells...acts towards the child [may] cause...harm to the child's health or physical, mental, spiritual, moral or social development. These acts must be reasonably within the control of the parent or person in a relationship of responsibility, trust or power. Acts include restriction of movement, patterns of belittling, denigrating, scapegoating, threatening, scaring, discriminating, ridiculing or other forms of hostile and rejecting treatment.

- Commercial or other exploitation of a child refers to the use of the child in work, or other activities for the benefit of others. This includes, but is not limited to, child labour and child prostitution. These activities are to the detriment of the child's physical and mental health, education, or spiritual, moral or social-emotional development.
- Care neglect is the failure of an adult care-giver to provide for the development of the child in terms of health, nutrition, shelter and safe living conditions, nurturing and emotional attachments, education and the opportunity for self-actualization, in the presence of available and adequate resources.
- To this the author has added 'structural neglect', which is the failure of the society (macro- and global systems) to provide health care, nutrition, education, shelter, safe living and other conditions necessary for the development of the child. Most of this is related to poverty.

Some comments about the cultural aspects of these definitions follow. Children live in micro-systems with rules dictated by cultures. For example, the perception of sexual abuse is very different in Western societies compared to many developing countries, where men and women, and indeed boys and girls, never touch anyone of the other gender, unless it is a member of the same family. Verbal sexual harassment has recently become criminal in some Western societies, but has for many years been a taboo in less developed regions. The author has followed the WHO definition and in the prevalence estimates accepted definitions which mirror the local perceptions and cultural taboos. Peer abuse is in some cultures very common; it has not received enough attention (see Box 7.1, p. 91). Contact abusive incidents are by many researchers regularly seen as more severe than those with no contact. However, the latter may be highly terrifying; for instance, if a child was chased by a threatening exhibitionist, or witnessed the father severely assaulting the mother, or saw a classmate being viciously and unfairly humiliated by a teacher, or witnessed how a friend was beaten up and then sexually abused. Classifications need to be complemented with an assessment of how traumatic the incident was to the child.

Definitions of mental disorders

In this book, many mental disorders will be discussed. Diagnoses of mental disorders are frequently ascertained using standardized, thoroughly tested questionnaires such as CIDI (the Composite International Diagnostic Interview, Robins et al., 1988). Most results quoted are based on these techniques. The diagnoses of these disorders are universally standardized and appear in the *Diagnostic and Statistical Manual of Mental Disorders* published by the American Psychiatric Association (APA; its latest version appeared in 1994 (DSM-IV)), and in the *International Classification of Diseases* (ICD-X), by the World Health Organization. The system represented by these two repositories is not definitive and has been criticized for being neither exclusive nor exhaustive. It does not sufficiently recognize that illness is a quantitative problem; there might be no clear break-off point between disorder and no disorder. A description of an 'unusual' behaviour or cluster of such behaviours should preferably not be labelled with a diagnosis without being anchored in an organic/somatic context. DSM-IV diagnoses appear to focus on antisocial behaviours rather than personality traits central to traditional conceptions. The *British Medical Journal* (13(4), 2002) states in an editorial: 'the concept of what is and what is not a disease is extremely slippery', and we should be aware of the risk of over-medicalization. Some symptoms seen as mental disorders, such as anxiety and depression, may be completely normal reactions to frustrating life events.

Definition of disability

According to WHO (2001b) disability is 'an umbrella term for impairments, activity limitations and participation restrictions. It denotes the negative aspects of the interaction between an individual (with a health condition) and that individual's contextual factors (environment and personal factors).' Definitions of disability are not globally standardized; neither are they – using WHO's system – straightforward to define; thus conclusions on prevalence are not easy. The WHO system claims 'to provide a scientific basis for understanding and studying health and health-related states, outcomes and determinants' on a 'universal' scale (it includes a selection of environmental factors) but does not mention childhood violence, abuse, neglect, criminal behaviour, poverty or hunger; and malnutrition receives just three words under 'weight maintenance functions'.

Many disabilities relate to environmental factors, of which poverty and hunger are the most important. For over 1 billion children these are combined with poor health; and about one-quarter of them still lack primary health care. Hunger affects over 300 million children every day; many more if droughts or floods or pests destroy their crops. 170 million children are underweight at the age of 5 and many suffer from stunted growth and reduced physical fitness. Poverty and hunger are traumatic and contribute to reduced capacity at school and work: impairments leading to functional limitations. Other environmental constraints – participation restrictions – may contribute to disability: gender bias, cultural and social status systems, lack of physical access and access to opportunities, ethnic differences and, finally, the political and judicial power structures over which the 'defenceless' have no influence.

Very large numbers of people underachieve because of a health condition. Some persons with 'hidden' disabilities may appear, superficially, to function normally at work, in their families and in social contacts. However, on using deeper analysis, they may be found with significant role impairments (such as decreased quality and creativity at work, disturbed relations with their family members and friends, and so on) caused by mental and somatic disorders; for others the causes may be related to daily frustrations, poverty and hunger. The global estimates of the disabling consequences of childhood violence appear in Chapter 8.

Socio-economic definitions

The operational definitions used in this book are as follows:

- *Evolution* is the process of observed change in single sectors such as the macro-economy, industrial innovations, communication networks, agriculture yields per hectare, and polio eradication.
- *Development* means the combined results – both positive and negative – of all evolutions, including, for instance, economic outcomes for the poor, human and physical ecological consequences, and social restructuring.
- *Progress* means advancement towards a set of desirable goals, such as quality of life or happiness. Such goals are mainly seen as non-monetary. Do I as a person have opportunities for self-realization? Are my opinions, rights and freedoms respected? Are the members of my family and my friends getting on well; are they healthy and secure?

Are we happier? Evaluating global progress includes analysing the human perceptions of the totality of development effects resulting from all evolutions, including the quality of governance. Were my goals and those of others met? Did humanity as a whole benefit or lose? Some people perceive progress during their lifetime as a zero-sum game, with losses in human dignity and a combination of decreasing compliance with human rights and escalating violence and terrorism outweighing the evolution in technology and economic growth.

Materials and methods

The information in this book of the prevalence of abuse, neglect and violence has been collected from a large number of sources in 152 countries from 1974–2007 (see note 1). The main difficulty from the beginning was to find reliable information in the developing countries. In many developing countries, surveys on childhood violence are still limited and not always built on representative samples. Published papers are mostly from countries with a tradition of research grants, and the recipient of a grant will seek publicity in one of the many journals which have developed as a 'service' for the 'research industry'. But, in the developing countries, there are few such grants, and even specialists with a solid knowledge do not publish much. Also, publications from developing countries are not always included in the literature databases.

In the Preface, I recorded some personal observations from visits to 94 countries during the period 1974–2007. These were complemented with direct information from the participants from 90 countries who attended special management courses. Specific information about prevalence and other related subjects was collected by screening *PubMed* articles from October 1963 to January 2008 on 'child abuse'. The search yielded over 19,000 publications. From this 'primary' group of identified articles, cross-references were researched. Other sources are anthropological, economic, ecological, human rights, legal, psychological (psycINF), counselling, health care, educational (ERIC database), diplomatic, newspapers, political and social books, articles and reports. Several important ones originate from the Injuries and Violence Prevention (WHO, 2002, 2004a, 2004b) and the Global Burden of Disease Programmes at WHO (Lopez et al., 2006). Many unpublished reports from developing countries have been screened. Altogether close to 20,000 publications and reports have been reviewed (most of them published in peer-reviewed journals). Most of these originated in the USA. In some there are only indicative data; others represent carefully designed and analysed scientific contributions. I have not sought to give a full presentation of all information, methods, or problems of coding in each of these documents: there are just too many. The trend in published data during the last forty years is that reported prevalence rates of childhood violence have mostly been increasing, especially in the developing countries. When choosing which data to include, I considered the methods used, the size of the sample and the response rate.

There are also official sources of population data, special surveys (such as on poverty, health, education, disability, macro-economic reports and other statistics) provided by many countries and by international organizations. Some child protection agencies, health services, institutions and hospitals and school health personnel keep records of child health, maltreatment, social and family problems. Alleged crimes against children are reported to the police. Some offenders are punished; such crimes are in many countries accounted for in their annual Justice Department statistics. Some such services do publish reports from which information can be retrieved. Many of these reports, however, are not easily available, especially in developing countries, and knowledge about them can sometimes only be collected through country visits and personal contacts.

The primary purposes of the search related to childhood violence were to

- identify information that would lead to an assessment of the global number of victims;
- estimate the resulting health, social and economic consequences;
- analyse its causes and contributors;
- review interventions, actions and programmes for prevention and care.

Reliability of information

The texts contain many estimates, based on published data. There are several methodological issues regarding the reliability of the results presented.

Official reports

Violence occurs everywhere: in the home, in schools, working environments, day-care or residential institutions, and public places; few of these possible sources collect and present data. Thus, country studies, patient files from hospitals, school reviews of violence, police reports, court records about convictions, and criminological research do reflect part of the reality, but these sources commonly under-report. In Ireland, for example, in 1996, only two cases of child cruelty and neglect were reported to the police. In comparison, the Department of Health in Ireland received 903 such reports during the same year (European Forum for Child Welfare, 1998). In Canada (Macmillan et al., 2003), a study was made of a random sample of 9,953 children to record their histories of maltreatment and contacts with the Child Protection Services in Ontario. Only 5.1 per cent of those with a history of physical abuse and 8.7 per cent of those with a history of sexual abuse were known to the Child Protection Agency. Some violent acts are not criminal everywhere, hence they are not reported in some countries. For instance, physical abuse of family members (beating wives and children) is not routinely considered a crime or even disapproved of. In Nigeria (Ovediran and Isiugo-Abanihe, 2005), for example, a large survey of married women found 66 per cent of them expressing approval of wife beating (including punishment for burning food and not cooking on time).

The underestimations depend partly on the taboos; the truth is hidden and uncomfortable. Most survivors do not want to disclose the abuse to anybody because a member of their family was involved. Any reference to haunting memories is for them traumatic and increases the survivor's feelings of anxiety, stigma, shame and fear and may upset other people important to the survivor. These factors lead to drop-outs from study cohorts; almost all published articles have a relatively high frequency of non-responders.

Surveys: representativeness

It is common to find that most surveys have been carried out on non-institutionalized persons. In many developed countries, however, large numbers of persons are in institutions: prisons, special treatment institutions for alcoholics and drug addicts, nursing homes, shelters for those who have lived off the street or for abused women, special boarding schools for children with behaviour problems, and residential homes for children who have been removed from the custody of the biological parents or have a disability. In developing countries, especially in large cities, it is common to find thousands of people sleeping on the streets, in railway and metro stations, in parks and in other public places – they are unlikely to be included in 'ordinary' surveys, as they have no fixed address and no telephone. If the purpose of the surveys is to identify health and social problems in order to design interventions, these groups should not be excluded.

One conclusion in this book is that every other person now living has been a victim of childhood violence. In most surveys, comparisons are made between a group of victims and a control group of non-victims. As denial of childhood abuse is so common, there is a risk that control groups may be 'contaminated' and include persons with undeclared, hidden adverse childhood experiences.

Surveys: validity of techniques

Survey techniques mostly consist of interviews, telephone contacts, or requests to fill out questionnaires. The latter are often very well developed and tested in North America and Western Europe. We must realize, however, that what are measured are admissions of child abuse and not the incidents themselves. Some of these surveys are to be filled out in front of the surveyor (I have observed instances when the surveyor was a care-giver in a residential institution, in which case the children would not mention any of the institution's personnel among the abusers); others are self-administered, or they may be sent by mail with a response envelope enclosed. In the rush to get results many standardized questionnaires are translated literally and used with a minimum of preparation in the developing countries. This leads to many problems of misunderstanding. Abuse is never even mentioned by most people in the developing countries. Questionnaires should not be used without careful testing and analysis of every word. It is common to see Western scientists going to a developing country with one or several questionnaires and then discussing them with a local 'expert'. I have extensive experience of such discussions. The final impression is that in these countries, even university professors seldom question anything that is proposed by Western scientists, and will rarely come up with any suggestions for change. The developing country counterpart will be happy just to get a chance to co-author a publication.

Some questionnaires undergo 'improvements' from time to time, so one cannot always compare the results of studies spaced several years apart. Also, similar questionnaires may be used with a change of interview techniques. One such example can be found in two studies by Straus and Gelles (1986). In 1975, they conducted the National Family Violence Survey to determine the incidence of child abuse and spousal abuse in the United States. The results were based on one-hour-long face-to-face interviews of parents in 1,146 households; the response rate was 65 per cent. In 1985, they conducted a second survey (the National Family Violence Re-Survey) to update their findings. This time the results were based on 35-minute telephone interviews of parents in 1,428 households; the response rate was 85 per cent. Their most striking discovery was that child abuse (which they defined as kicking, biting, punching, beating, threatening with a gun or knife, or using a gun or knife) had declined by 47 per cent among two-parent families with at least one child aged 3 to 17. There were thirty-six incidents of child abuse per thousand children in 1975, but only nineteen per thousand children in 1985. Straus and Gelles had two alternatives for interpretation: (a) child abuse had decreased over that ten-year period, or (b) respondents were more reluctant to admit to child abuse in 1985 than in 1975. Interestingly, the authors stated that 'the differences in methodology should have led to higher, not lower, rates of reported violence, because (a) a telephone interview offers more anonymity and "leads to more truthfulness", and (b) the response rate was higher and "a higher response rate tends to produce a higher rate of violence"' (Straus and Gelles, 1986). Their study is an interesting example of the methodological difficulties. One cannot compare face-to-face interviews with telephone calls (with the calls lasting 35 minutes while the interviews were for 60 minutes). Many poor and marginal people do not have a telephone and so the second sample may be biased. The belief that 'anonymous' telephone calls would extract more of the truth may not always be based on proper evidence. First, none of these calls is anonymous; the interviewer has the telephone number and name of the family contacted, and may even tape record the conversation. Second, as a counterweight to truthfulness during the period 1975–85, it had become more commonly known in the USA that many professionals are by law obliged to report crimes to the police; thus some respondents who feel uncomfortable with the police will not disclose criminal incidents of abuse.

Regarding the veracity of retrospective reporting there are different opinions, but it appears unlikely that any significant proportion of violent incidences is invented; denial is more common than fabrication. A discussion on memory accuracy appears in Chapter 8.

Surveys: non-response rates

It is important to know all the consequences of childhood abuse and violence. The results published have several problems, increasing the likelihood of a high non-response rate. Among them are:

1. Mortality (suicides, accidents, murder, diseases, alcoholism and drug abuse).
2. Social and economic situation (poverty, unemployment, homeless, in institutions, prisoners, low literacy, intimidation, alcohol and substance abusers) may diminish the likelihood of response.

3. The subject may be seen as too sensitive or taboo.
4. Attempts or threats of abuse are not always taken seriously, and there-fore not considered worth mentioning or not identified by people as relevant.
5. A large proportion of the victims never mention the abuse to anybody. A Swedish study (Swedin and Back, 2003) reports on thirty children who had been exploited in the production of child pornography films. The average duration of the abusive acts was twenty-two months. Five children were drugged at the time of victimization, two were too young to understand what happened, but twenty-three were old enough and fully capable of describing the crime in detail. None of them spontaneously told anybody.

These factors influence the prevalence estimates in child violence surveys. Most experts agree that over-reporting of sexual abuse in developing countries is very uncommon, because of the resulting stigmatization.

It is common to find high attrition rates. Some studies show 50 per cent non-responders or more. An example of the difficulties can be seen in Dunne et al.'s Australian study (2003) in which 4,449 adults aged 18–59 were drawn from the electoral roll (which itself may not be complete). For 69 per cent (=3,070) of them there was a valid telephone number. These persons were contacted and 61 per cent (=1,873) agreed to participate in the interviews. Finally, after even more attrition 1,784 persons took part in the interviews. Thus, the drop-out was 60 per cent (2,665 of 4,449) of the original sample. Dunne et al. (2003) state: 'the volunteers are broadly representative; of course it is not possible to know whether the sexual experience of the participants differed from the global population'. When there is attrition, most scientists just look at the non-responders' age, gender and racial distribution, but do not screen school, social and criminal records, or try again. In spite of this important attrition rate, Dunne et al. reported 19.6 per cent of the men and 25 per cent of the women had experienced at least one incidence of non-penetrative, sexual body contact, and 4 per cent of the men and 12 per cent of the women a penetrative experience. Supplementary studies of non-responders are needed.

It is well known that drop-outs from statistical samples – especially those who do not have a telephone or a permanent address – are over-represented by persons who have previous criminal records and/or ongoing social problems with high prevalence of alcohol and substance abuse, unemployment and permanent homelessness. A United States economic long-term study (Fitzgerald et al., 1998) showed that attrition is highly selective and is concentrated among those with unstable earnings, marriage and migration histories.

Many victims are afraid to report sexual assault to the police. In a US study, Fitzgerald et al. (1998) noted the following reasons for this:

- further victimization by the offender;
- other forms of retribution by the offender or by the offender's friends or family;
- arrest, prosecution and incarceration of an offender who may be a family member or friend and on whom the victim or others may depend;
- others finding out about the sexual assault (friends, family members, media, and the public);
- not being believed; and
- being traumatized by the criminal justice system response.

When studies with high attrition rates are presented, the data may seriously underestimate the prevalence of a health condition. When attrition rates are zero or very low, many studies reveal higher prevalence rates of childhood violence as shown in Box 2.1.

Socio-economic and cultural factors influencing what is perceived as abuse and neglect

For the reader unaccustomed to the situations in the developing countries, a few general descriptions follow. Of course, these conditions are very varied. Typically, poor people have a combination of serious problems. One will, however, often find that programmes to assist them have single components only, such as immunization or distribution of vitamin A.

Living conditions

Many children in developing countries live in extended families (with up to fifty members). The surroundings are often poor and contaminated with filth. Some 2 billion people lack basic sanitation and 1.5 billion have no access to clean and safe water. Electricity is rare in most rural areas, but may be available in marginal urban areas. The houses are often small, crowded and poorly constructed; they offer little protection against rain and storms. Most people sleep on the floor close to each other, perhaps on a thin mat. There may be lots of mosquitoes, flies, grasshoppers, stray dogs, cats, and large rats around. Winter heating in cold climates is very uncommon. The houses are sparsely furnished; kitchen equipment may consist of a few pots and pans; most people eat

---

Box 2.1:   Results of reported childhood violence when there are no or very low numbers of non-responders

Many studies reviewed in this book report abuse rates around 15–20 per cent (for each of sexual and physical abuse). When the attrition is low, reporting rates of abuse are often substantially higher than the 15–20 per cent range. Himelein and McElrath (1996), who had a response rate of 97 per cent, found that 26 per cent of college women reported a history of contact child sexual abuse (CSA) ranging from fondling to rape. In the Cáceres et al. (2000) study in Peru, where the supervisors (using a questionnaire) pointed out missing and contradictory answers to participants for revision, there was 98 per cent participation in one group and 82 per cent in the second group. Among those who had at least one sexual experience, males reported a 20 per cent experience of heterosexual lifetime coercion and the females a prevalence of 46 per cent; for the group with homosexual experience, coercion was 48 per cent for the males and 41 per cent for the females. In the Chen et al. (2004) study in Beijing there were no drop-outs: 26 per cent of the all-female participants had experienced sexual abuse before the age of 16 (at the median age of 12). High prevalence rates emerged from the Kim et al. (2000) study in China and the Republic of Korea. The group interviewed consisted of 4–6 grade (aged about 10–12 years) schoolchildren; there were no drop-outs. Family violence during the last year had been experienced by 71 per cent in China and in 69 per cent of the children in Korea. The rates of corporal punishment by the teachers were 51 per cent in China and 62 per cent in Korea. Qin et al. (2008) studied high school students in China and report an emotional abuse rate of 47 per cent; it had a response rate of 98 per cent. In the Berrien et al. (1995) study (with 91 per cent participation) of Russian schoolchildren severe physical abuse had victimized 29 per cent. Finally, a large-scale Indian study of children aged 5–18 by Kacker (2007) with 96 per cent response rate showed these prevalences: physical abuse experienced by 73 per cent of boys, 65 per cent of girls; sexual abuse by 48 per cent of boys, 39 per cent of girls; and emotional abuse by 50 per cent of boys and 50 per cent of girls.

---

using their hands. Firewood may be in very short supply. One-quarter of all poor people in developing countries do not have access to primary heath care, and the quality of that care – when it exists – varies, with most of the staff concentrating on a short list of preventive measures; curative interventions are limited and rehabilitation virtually non-existent. Half of the world's pregnant women still lack access to skilled care at childbirth (World Health Organization, 2007a).

As regards education, 130 million children do not attend school at all, and for many the drop-out rates are high, the quality of education poor and in some places teachers' absenteeism is high. Books, papers, pens or writing materials at home are rare. School books remain in the school, so no studies can be carried out at home – and besides, a very large proportion of parents in poor countries are functionally illiterate. The family is usually ruled by someone with an iron hand, who makes most of the decisions. Children are brought up to be very obedient and loyal to the family.

Most poor families are very short of food and when eating, males have precedence. What takes place in terms of violence against children and women is known by everybody, and so are the fights between men, women and children. Local alcoholic brews are made almost everywhere – mostly by women, using a variety of products: from bananas to corn to sorghum; local herbs may be added to such brews (containing alkaloids that may cause temporary psychosis and aggression). When men consume these brews the result is increased domestic and community violence. Some 'beers' are distilled; these stronger drinks are often toxic and contain methanol, which causes brain damage and blindness. Maladaptive alcohol use is one of the root causes of domestic violence. Poor people in countries with a culture of opium or cocaine growing are now increasingly using these drugs themselves whereas they were formerly export commodities only. Gambling, and therefore loss of essential family money or assets, is common.

Women's position in society

Most tourists may know that a woman is not allowed to sit next to a Buddhist monk in a bus, and that patting children on the head is in some countries an unforgivable fault. Fewer may be aware of the fact that in many cultures a young girl of 12 who refuses to marry the man chosen by her parents (she may just be part of a business deal) will forever be stigmatized as severely mentally ill (although she is completely healthy) and may be unable to leave the house because other children will throw stones at her.

In most developing countries women are marginalized: many have little or no education, insufficient health care, may be barred from having their own property and inheritance, and play limited roles in politics. In many cultures, men cannot shake hands with women, and forcible kissing of women may be seen as sexual abuse; non-contact sexual abuse is frequently seen as serious sexual abuse (Kacker, 2007; Elbedour et al., 2006). Divorced and widowed women often face an uncertain future: they may lose care of their children and all of their belongings, and many are abused and exploited by their family members.

In countries in the Middle East, Africa and South Asia there is a tradition of arranged marriages to close relatives, most of them to first cousins. The proportion of consanguineous marriages varies from 20 per cent to 60 per cent; it is highest in rural areas. As, in some cultures, young boys' contacts with girls prior to marriage are forbidden, some homosexual pre-marital activities take the place of heterosexual ones; many underage boys are sodomized by their sexually frustrated older peers (Eskin et al., 2005; Jekwes and Abrahams, 2002). In many cultures, homosexual practices are widespread, but their visibility is low. In many developing countries, boys and girls undergo initiation rites including physical, sexual and magic procedures that might be seen as abuse in Europe or North America. A girl who tries to escape from home with a boyfriend and who is caught may in some countries be stoned to death together with the boy, even if there was no sexual intercourse. Members of the families involved may then start revenge killings. It is taken for granted that what happens in the family will never be told to any outsider. Breaking this taboo may have serious consequences. In Turkey, two television series were started in 2004 to give women opportunities to discuss openly their problems of domestic abuse. In March 2005, a woman who had appeared on one of the talk-shows was killed by gunshots by her own son, as she 'had brought shame over the family'. Some of these cultural habits 'travel' with emigrants who settle in developed countries, where the police might intervene when 'honour killings' or sexual mutilation (see below) of young girls take place. Prostitution is widespread and widely used, even in poor areas; sex workers – both male and female – are widely available.

There is a clear tendency to blame any sexually abusive event on the woman, who is in fact the victim. For instance, a woman who is approached by an exhibitionist in a public place may be accused by the village men (even by those who were not present when the abusive event happened) of having provoked the exhibitionist by her 'own indecent behaviour'; she may be publicly stigmatized. Under an Islamic ordinance in force in Pakistan since 1979, a woman had to present four male witnesses in order to prove a case of sexual assault or rape.[4] It is interesting to see how women who go to the well to collect water often go in groups and stay together for a while. With the men absent, this is where they can discuss in confidence their experience of domestic abuse. This is the indigenous equivalent of cognitive group therapy.

About 135 million women have undergone female genital mutilation: the clitoris, most of the outer labia and the inner labia are cut and removed and the remaining outer labia are sutured, leaving a small opening at the posterior part, so urine and menstrual blood can pass. The operation is seldom carried out by anyone with any medical training; sometimes it is the grandmother or a traditional midwife who does it. There is no anaesthesia and dirty knives, scissors or razor blades are used. The little girls (usually under-5) are screaming with pain, all are bleeding, and some die from blood loss or infections. This has been 'obligatory' in some cultures, but it is unrelated to religion, and already existed 1,500 years ago. Unmutilated girls are often perceived as worse than prostitutes. Currently, 2 million girls are at risk of this mutilation annually, an act that should be considered as severe sexual maltreatment. Most sexual mutilations take place in Africa and the Middle East[5] (WHO, 1995). The practice may be forbidden by law but still occurs. Parents born in countries with this 'culture' who have emigrated to Western countries are known to take their daughters 'back home' to have them mutilated, so they can escape prosecution in their adopted countries.

Physical punishment

Physical punishment is seen in many countries as a useful tool for education by both parents and teachers. It is a common part of many children's human ecology. Such punishment unfortunately often causes great damage to the children. To establish a cut-off point between severe physical abuse (such as kicking, biting, punching, beating, threatening with a gun or knife, or using a gun or knife) and so-called lesser physical abuse or slapping children, appears to be unjustified. All forms of physical punishment are associated with increased odds of major depression, alcohol abuse/dependence and externalizing problems in adulthood. The notion that physical punishment by a 'loving parent' does not have any ill consequences remains unproven (Afifi et al., 2006).

Cultural anthropology

Das and co-authors (2000, 2001) have in several books explored the social and cultural anthropological questions about violence. They give many examples of the situation in several different cultures: state terror, local conflicts, threats through narratives of supernatural activities, and the suffering brought upon poor marginalized communities and their efforts to recover from the consequences of violence. Their book entitled *Remaking a World* reflects their perceptions of the seriousness of the present level of violence.

Information problems

Finally, a few words about information problems. Languages are often a barrier to communication. Currently, 6,912 known living human languages have been registered (Gordon, 2007). Even the official language(s) of a country may not be understood by large numbers of its citizens. Translators may be unavailable for this multiplicity of language variations. Difficulties in understanding are obvious, for example, among refugees, and in legal processes. Spoken languages do not always have a written language. Local vocabularies may be small. For example, few people may know that the Somali language has no word for 'bacteria'. Arabic language does not have a proper translation for 'human rights'. Although many poor areas have radios and sometimes television sets screening government programmes, internet access is still uncommon in poor countries, although mobile telephone systems are expanding. Newspapers reach very few people. Most people in developing countries have never heard of international aid or the United Nations, let alone the Human Rights Conventions. If a country receives international criticism for its human rights situation, therefore, most of the population is unlikely to hear about it.

3
Mirrors of the Past

Historically, the situation of children is known less by systematic studies or statistics than by anecdotes, diaries and letters, mostly written by people of the upper classes. By the year AD 1, the world population was just 200 million; by 1000, it had increased to some 300 million. By 1750, the entire world population was estimated at less than 800 million, by 1800 at one billion. One hundred years later (1900), it reached 1.7 billion. In 1945, it was 2.3 billion; the less developed regions then counted for 1.6 billion. By 1960, the world total crossed the 3 billion mark and by 1999, it reached 6 billion; over 80 per cent lived in the less developed regions. It appears that the population might exceed 7 billion by 2015 and 9 billion before 2050. Population growth is concentrated on the developing countries. The more developed countries have shown little growth: between 1950 and 2000, the population only increased from 800,000 to 1,100,000, and will show little growth until 2050. Twenty-eight per cent of the world populations are children aged under 15 (UN Population Division, 2006; Wikipedia, 2007). The world is getting crowded and that affects children.

Children's lives have in the past been influenced by poverty among some 80–90 per cent of them; their education was non-existent or of poor quality; the health services lacked effective interventions; and many infants and women giving birth died early. Infanticide has existed since time immemorial. Religious offerings, especially of the firstborn, are known from the Bible, as well as from the histories of Assyria, Egypt, Greece, Rome and China. Firstborn sacrifice was once common among many peoples; the motive was the offering of one's most precious possession to the deities to make sure, for instance, that the next harvest would be good. Infanticide was common in Europe at least until the end of the nineteenth century. In historic times, child mortality rates were enormous: in 1700, in Finland, children under the age of 10 counted for 76 per cent of all deaths; in 1800 the figure was 61 per cent (Pelo, 2000). The infant mortality rates in the USA were 216 per 1,000 in 1840, 214 in 1880, 116 in 1900, 82 in 1920, and 10 in 1980 (Haines, 2006). By the end of the 1920s, some European countries still had infant mortality rates of 60 per 1,000, which is the average rate for the developing countries at present.

Communicable diseases in the past ravaged whole populations: leprosy, bubonic plague, smallpox, tuberculosis, cholera, scabies, erysipelas, typhoid, anthrax, trachoma, syphilis, gonorrhoea, sleeping sickness, and dancing mania. The Black Death (bubonic plague) during the mid-fourteenth century killed one-third of Europe's population; about 1,000 villages disappeared completely. It took 150 years for the population of Western Europe to reach the pre-plague level.

The growth of population increased urbanization, especially after industrialization started in the early 1800s. People moved to cramped and unhygienic lodgings, infectious diseases were rampant, and as there were no contraceptives many children were born. Poor families abandoned infants by the millions to orphanages.

This book takes a critical view on the performance of many present governments, the institutions of the macro-system. Our history is full of similar observations. This is how the French Revolution leader Brissot (1754–93), described the situation in France – then the country with the highest population in Europe – in the 1790s (Aullard, 1883):

> Laws that are not carried into effect, authorities act without force and are despised, crime remains unpunished, property is attacked, the safety of the individual violated, the morality of the people corrupted, no constitution, no government, no justice functions.

The discovery of child 'battering'

The discovery and description of child abuse as a diagnostic entity did not appear until the second half of the nineteenth century. Then, the French forensic physician Ambroise Tardieu (1818–79) in 1860 described thirty-two battered (severely abused) children, of whom eighteen died, and in 1868 reported his observations on infanticide, built on pathological studies of 555 children. His contemporaries rejected his conclusions that child abuse was a major problem and that preventive measures were needed. His work was consigned to oblivion.

During the times of Tardieu, industrialization and urbanization had led to the establishment of thousands of orphanages for abandoned children in Europe and Northern America. It is estimated that in these orphanages about 100 million children died, from neglect and abuse during the period 1800–1940.[6] This horror has received little publicity. The abuse of children at such institutions and at work became a matter of concern to many new non-governmental organizations. Henry Bergh (1811–88) founded the American Society for the Prevention of Cruelty to Animals in 1866. His attention was drawn in 1874 to the plight of a young abused child called Mary Ellen, and based on this experience he helped to form the Massachusetts Society for the Prevention of Cruelty to Children, followed by the New York Society for the Prevention of Cruelty to Children in 1875. The National Society for the Prevention of Cruelty to Children was set up in the United Kingdom in 1884. Australia followed with the Children's Protection Society in 1896. Today thousands of such NGOs 'to save the children' exist; they carry out a lot of important work.

In 1896[7] Sigmund Freud published articles based on the seduction theory of 'neurosis' (the term then included several mental disorders: depression, post-traumatic stress, phobias, depressive, paranoid, obsessive-compulsive, and personality) built on clinical observations of his patients. Virtually without exception, they recounted experiences of child sexual abuse, usually by the father. He drew the conclusion that childhood sexual abuse was a precondition for their illness. In a letter in the spring of 1896, Freud told his friend Fliess (a doctor who became his confidant) that he was increasingly convinced that there was a great deal of perverse activity involving children, much of it by the fathers. And Freud went on tell Fliess, 'My own father unfortunately was one of these perverts, and is responsible for the neurosis of my brother and that of several of my sisters.' Freud's peers were outraged by his theory, and one of them called it 'a scientific fairy tale'. Under immense pressure, he withdrew it in 1897. Like Tardieu, he did not manage to convince his peers.

These groundbreaking efforts were soon forgotten and the rediscovery of child abuse had to wait until 1962 – 100 years after Tardieu and 65 years after Freud – when Kempe and his colleagues described 'the battered child syndrome' (Kempe et al., 1962). They had surveyed 88 hospitals and identified 302 children who had been 'battered' (the term was later changed to 'abused'). At that time, they concluded that child abuse in USA was a very limited problem for perhaps a few hundred children victimized by a small group of seriously pathological persons. Time would show that these assumptions were gross underestimates. Kempe went on to start an international society for the prevention of child abuse and neglect, an international journal and a research centre, an important legacy.

For thousands of years, children in most countries have been subjected to corporal punishment; it has been the most common method to instil 'discipline'. Many parents believe that it is 'character-building' and there has emerged a culture of parental behaviour that often starts by beating infants for crying and ends with using canes, rods, belts, paddles or whips for teenagers. Already in the eleventh century, Saint Anselm, Archbishop of Canterbury, spoke out against what he saw as the cruel treatment of children (Wicksteed, 1936). The seventeenth-century English philosopher John Locke wrote a number of influential works in which he opposed authoritarianism. In *Some Thoughts Concerning Education* (1692) he explicitly criticized the central role of corporal punishment in education:

> I desire to know what vice can be nam'd, which parents, and those about children, do not season them with, and drop into 'em the seeds of, as soon as they are capable to receive them? I do not mean by the examples they give, and the patterns they set before them, which is encouragement enough; but that which I would take notice of here is, the downright teaching them vice, and actual putting them out of the way of virtue. Before they can go, they principle 'em with violence, revenge, and cruelty. Give me a blow, that I may beat him, is a lesson which most children every day hear; and it is thought nothing, because their hands have not strength to do any mischief. But I ask, does not this corrupt their mind? Is not this the way of force and violence, that they are set in? And if they have been taught when little, to strike and hurt others by proxy, and encouraged to rejoice in the harm they have brought upon them, and see them suffer, are they not prepar'd to do it when they are strong enough to be felt themselves, and can strike to some purpose?

Locke's work was highly influential, and in part influenced Polish legislators to ban corporal punishment from Poland's schools in 1783, the first country to do so. Those countries that followed waited another 200 years before adopting this ban, although they still only number about thirty.

Does child violence increase or decrease?

In 2003 Jones and Finkelhor reported that in the 1990s, the cases of sexual abuse known by child protective agencies in USA declined from about 150,000 in 1992 to 92,000 in 1999. In the Canadian province of Ontario, there was a 49 per cent decline in substantiated sexual abuse from 1993 to 1998, while physical abuse and neglect cases increased during the same period. Jones and Finkelhor write:

> one possible explanation is that it reflects a decline in the incidence of sexual abuse, evidence, perhaps, that the investment by the US ... to protect children from sexual abuse ... can work effectively.

A more long-term review shows that in the United States, total Crime Index Rates (US Justice Department, 2003a) per 100,000 inhabitants rose from 1,888 in 1960 to 5,898 in 1991, and then dropped more than 50 per cent from 1993 to 2004. From 2004–5 they increased again by 1.3 per cent. A similar decrease was seen in the UK: according to the British Crime Survey (2005) violent crime has fallen by 43 per cent since a peak in 1995.

Barclay and Tavares (2003) published international comparisons between violent crime rates from 1997 to 2001 and found the following: those in European countries increased by 22 per cent (the highest increase was 50 per cent in France, 49 per cent in Spain, 35 per cent in the Netherlands, 29 per cent in Portugal, 26 per cent in England and Wales), Australia by 22 per cent, and Japan by 79 per cent, while the USA showed a reduction of 12 per cent. Over this four-year period, police-recorded crimes increased in France by 16 per cent, Spain by 10 per cent, Netherlands by 10 per cent, Portugal by 16 per cent, England and Wales by 22 per cent, Australia by 18 per cent, and Japan by 38 per cent. In these countries, the increase of violent crime was higher than the increase of the total crime rate. The USA showed a decrease of 11 per cent of its total recorded crime rates.

It appears that historically violent crime rates show cyclical trends. Eisner (2003) presents historical trends from the thirteenth to the twentieth century. He states that serious interpersonal violence decreased remarkably between the mid-sixteenth and the early twentieth century in Europe. Various regions differed but the age and sex patterns in serious violent offending changed very little over several centuries. There have been 'bursts' of increases seen after 1850, 1900 and 1960.

The changes noted by Jones and Finkelhor are impressive, but they are not universal, as many other countries show increases; perhaps this confirms that violence follows a globally uneven cyclical pattern.

Garbarino (1998) has made some reflections about what has happened to parenting in over 100 years as he tried to imagine what the problems were in 1893:

1. The problem of substance abuse and addiction was recognized as an insidious and powerful destructive force in family life.
2. There was evidence of a widening gap between rich and poor, and already many voices called for action to improve the conditions of the poor, particularly the 'worthy' poor.
3. Traditional American values and institutions were being challenged by the influx of immigrants who did not speak English and who were perceived to make disproportionate demands on the human service systems, suppressing wages by accepting low pay, long hours, and inferior working conditions.
4. The legacy of slavery and the reality of racism lurked behind the public façade of democracy, and broke out in dramatic incidents from time to time.
5. To their contemporaries, growing numbers of girls and women appeared to be in moral jeopardy due to the frequency of premarital sex and pregnancy, and the sex industry, in fact, flourished.
6. Child abuse was entering the public consciousness and there was a sense that juvenile crime was escalating.
7. Significant numbers of families were not 'intact', as mothers frequently died in childbirth and fathers often abandoned families.

'Does anything ever really change?', asks Garbarino. 'Reading contemporary analyses of parenting issues in the 1990's, we see that there have been changes in the past 100 years: divorce and unmarried teen births have replaced maternal death and paternal separation in the dynamic of "incomplete" families; overtly homosexual adults now assert claims on parental roles publicly; efforts intended to integrate employment and maternity have become common; and, a structural analysis of child abuse as a social problem has arisen. These are real changes, of course, and they demand policy adjustments and innovations at all levels of public life.'

Dube et al. (2001), in another United States study, examined the relationship of the number of adverse childhood experiences (ACE) to six health problems among four successive birth cohorts (born 1900–31, 1932–46, 1947–61, 1962–78) to assess the strength and consistency of these relationships in light of the secular influences that the twentieth century brought to bear in changing health behaviours and conditions. The study concludes that:

> ACEs increased the risk of numerous health behaviours and outcomes for all the 20th century birth cohorts included in the study, suggesting that the effects of ACEs on the risk of various health problems are unaffected by social or secular changes. Research showing detrimental and lasting neurobiological effects of child abuse on the developing brain provides a plausible explanation for the consistency and dose-response relationships found for each health problem across birth cohorts, despite changing secular influences.

Part II

Micro-system Violence towards Biological and Social Orphans

4
Children in Residential Institutions

Some 10 million children are at present estimated to live in residential institutions (University of Stockholm, Sweden, 2003). The four main groups are: (a) healthy infants abandoned by the parents; (b) children with disabilities; (c) children removed from malfunctioning families voluntarily or by legal authorities, or because the child shows behaviour that cannot be controlled by the parents; and (d) children in penal institutions. Such cases are illustrated below.

Most child institutions are inaccessible to outsiders. Modern mass media have played an important role in revealing the realities hidden from the public. Protests against abusive 'care' appeared hundreds of years ago, but change was mostly resisted. Societies have been prejudiced: the role of the 'poorhouse' and other asylums was to 'protect the public' at the expense of the protection of children and other poor residents.

This chapter illustrates the abuse in a variety of residential institutions; the examples are characteristic of what the author has observed in some fifty countries. Some countries have not been identified. Naming a country is not always productive, and – rather than encouraging future co-operation with the visiting professional – it may result in a defensive attitude. The facts from the identified countries are in the public domain.

Disaster in Romania

In December 1989 President Ceauşescu's regime (1965–89) collapsed. There were demonstrations and the army defected. Ceauşescu and his wife were captured, tried and convicted on charges of mass murder and corruption, and executed.

During the days that followed, a large number of television crews and international organizations entered Romania, where they discovered a human disaster of epic proportions. Over 200,000 children and adults lived in some 600 residential institutions under terrible conditions. The author has made eight visits to Romania, the last in late 2006, and can confirm the descriptions given by non-governmental organizations. Below follows an account from a non-governmental organization of their observations of residential institutions during the summer of 1990; with few variations these observations are typical of all the institutions at the time of Ceauşescu's death.

> Children aged 0–4 years were kept in 'child homes'. Their families had faced severe poverty, unemployment, and famine and abandoned these children at birth. The 167 children in this institution were mostly kept in their beds, almost without care, inadequately fed, severely underweight and with stunted growth. Hygienic conditions were abominable: the children lying in their own urine and excrement. The smell was unbearable. The facilities had not been repaired for several years, so the roofs were leaky, sewers and electricity were malfunctioning. Because of the lack of personnel (one 'helper' for 40–50 children), there was no time for human contact; children were left with severe sensory and emotional deprivation, many were intimidated and beaten.
>
> The children were fed with big bottles containing water and milk powder; no other food was available. Because of malnutrition, they looked like 'sacks of bone'. Some of the bigger children who were less affected could eat by themselves in a dining room. Their food was some soup with the appearance of 'pig food'. Many children were on heavy doses of sedatives (to 'protect them'). During the 1980s, medical experiments had been carried out on many of these children. They had been 'treated with micro-transfusions'; and because unchecked HIV-contaminated blood had been used several hundred children died of AIDS in the 1990s.
>
> The outcome of this 'warehousing' – for those who survived – was induced mental retardation and behaviour disturbance. There were no activities, no toys, no training or stimulation of the infants and small children. The children were 'nameless': they had no name on the bed, or any identification tags. There were some records, but they were insufficient to identify any children. Most children were rocking back and forth in their beds, and some were self-aggressive.

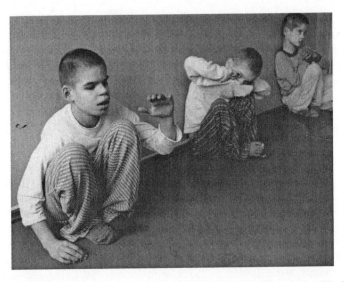

Photo 1. **Residential institution.** *The teenage boy (to the left) was born blind and abandoned by his mother. He sits the whole day long by himself, rocking, is sensorially and emotionally deprived and has 'fled into a world of his own'. The boy (in the centre) was also abandoned by his mother at birth; initially he was healthy. He shows clear signs of being very afraid: the result of abusive beatings and threats by the personnel. The third boy (to the right) is autistic and has no contact with anybody. None of them has proper clothes and shoes. All are incontinent, none can speak, all are malnourished. The 'child home' has no activities, no training in daily activities or any education. The children receive no visits from their families. Credit: Star of Hope, Sweden.*

The personnel were very indifferent to the needs of the children. Everything followed a set time schedule: nappies were changed and food given, but nobody spoke with the children during these procedures. When this work was completed, the personnel spent their remaining time outside the dormitory, with no one looking after the children.

When the children reached the age of 3–4, they were transferred to larger 'placement' centres headed by medical doctors. An example follows of such a centre with 230 children aged 3–18, all of whom were considered 'untreatable'. This centre was in a building with two floors, fenced in, and had no garden. Upon entering, the director-physician explained that because there was no hope for improvement of the 'inmates', the personnel were few and only occupied with 'basic care'. There was one care-provider for each group of 50 children in the daytime and one at night for all the 230 children. Here, the children were in bedrooms several of which were in the windowless cellar. Two to three children often shared a bed. The beds were cage-like and too small even for one child of their ages; the children could not stretch out; their arms and legs had become crooked. The children were in rags or naked; the conditions were the same as in the centre described above. All children had their hair shaved off; several had visible scars on their heads, the result of previous aggression. The water supply was frequently cut, the sewers did not function and very little electricity was available Many children froze to death during the following winter because of lack of heating, food and care.

The children were very frightened by people in white coats, and would try to avoid physical and even eye contact with them because the staff had physically and psychologically abused them. There were no proper records; the names of most children had been lost. Because they sometimes changed beds and institution, at the end nobody knew who they were. The last arrivals, for whom there were no beds available, were hidden in the cellar; they were all soiled and naked – most of them sitting on the potty, rocking all day long. Some of them were eating their own excrement.

(Viklund-Olofsson, 2005)

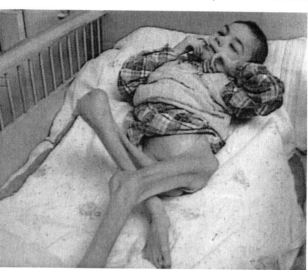

Photo 2.   **Residential institution.** *Abandoned at birth with no disability, this girl has spent more than ten years as a 'resident'. The crookedness of her legs has advanced and is now permanent. She cannot stretch out her body because the bed is too short. She is severely malnourished and doubly incontinent. She has never learnt to speak, because nobody ever spoke to her. Credit: Star of Hope, Sweden.*

There are other problems in the institutions in Romania. Not only did the children become victims of abuse, neglect and intentional killing. Reports have also emerged of organized baby-selling and trafficking by the personnel. This has been possible because of incomplete record-keeping and lack of inspections; hundreds of children in institutions have gone 'missing'.

The new Romanian government reinstated abortion on demand early in 1990 (it had been forbidden by Ceauşescu). This resulted in very high rates (WHO, 2005): 1 million in 1990, 500,000 in 1995, and 250,000 in 2000 (234,521 children born). The 1990 rate is the highest ever recorded in any country (Romania's population in 1990 was 22 million). Although access to contraception was also legalized, only 30 per cent of women were using any. The poverty rate is still very high (the average for the country is 30 per cent; for families with three or more children it is 60

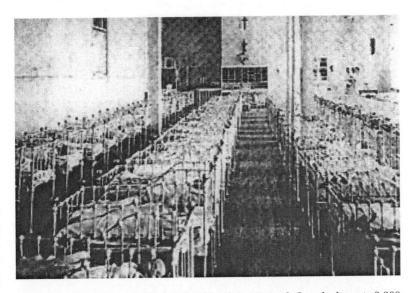

Photo 3. **Orphanage**. *Hôpital de la Miséricorde in Montreal, Canada, home to 3,000 abandoned children from the 1930s into the 1960s. Although most were healthy at arrival, all were classified as mental patients, so the institution could receive federal funding. All boys were christened Joseph by the nuns and monks that ran the hospital and the girls were christened Marie. These children are also known as 'Les enfants de Duplessis' after the Premier of the province. Because of widespread sexual and physical abuse and serious neglect (including slave labour) by the psychiatrists, Roman Catholic priests, nuns and administrators, 5,000 of the surviving orphans pursued a court process in the 1990s for an apology and compensation from the province, but lost. Justice was not done and criminal wrongdoing was allowed to go unpunished (Perry, 2006).*

per cent). In spite of these high rates of free abortion, however, child abandonment continues today.

A major policy change started in 2004: some abandoned infants are now transferred directly from the maternity wards to salaried foster parents. Not all problems have been solved, however: a May 2006 internet report from MDRI describes child institutions with teenagers weighing no more than 27 pounds. Some children were tied down with bed sheets, their arms and legs twisted and left to atrophy.

Controversy in China

I visited China three times in the 1980s and 1990s and became aware of the rumours of violence against children in residential institutions. These institutions mostly received healthy infants (80–90 per cent of whom were girls) abandoned at birth by their mothers. China's Ministry of Civil Affairs in 1989 (*Atlantic Monthly Affairs*, 1996) issued for the first (and last) time an annual report which stated the annual mortality rate in these institutions: the ratio of deaths to admissions in that year was 58 per cent. In four provinces, the death-to-admissions ratio exceeded 90 per cent. A doctor working at one of the institutions in 1996 described what was going on:

> Children were selected for death if they had some deformity, were badly behaved or demanding, or simply not liked. A consultation meeting took place between the staff, at which it was decided to deprive those selected of food and drink. Once the starvation took hold, the child became ill...the orphanage doctors were asked to perform a 'medical consultation', which served as a ritual, marking the child for subsequent termination of care or life-saving intervention. Some children were normal – abandoned for economic reasons. Whatever the condition the children were initially in, they were dying from starvation, diarrhoea and vomiting, and general medical neglect. The dead children were then cremated; the diagnoses were frequently congenital maldevelopment of the brain, or even hare lip and cleft palate.
> (Human Rights Watch, 1996a; Woods, 1996)

These reports were followed up. In 1996, an American film team entered China as tourists, and just walked into several of these institutions, filming what they saw. Nobody hindered them:

> We were able to film infants tied to wicker chairs. In filthy clothes and wearing trousers split wide at the crotch, their legs are held wide.

Beneath some of the chairs, there are potties and old washing bowls. Others simply urinate and defecate straight onto the floor. With no toys or other distractions, they rock back and forth relentlessly. We discovered that, although they were described as orphans, very few were; their parents have abandoned them at birth. Under-staffed and under-funded, these institutions are just not prepared for the relentless tide of rejected babies. These infants lay five to a cot in summer temperatures of over 100°F.

(Woods, 1996)

The film has been screened in thirty-seven countries, with some 100 million viewers. The authorities, embarrassed at what had been discovered, issued several statements denying the descriptions, and later advertised that improvements were taking place. Some of the problems in that country, however, seem to persist. An article in the London *Times* (19 January 2006) describes a Chinese 'boarding school with about 215 boys aged eight to eighteen, who are considered "uneducable" ... compelled to dress in camouflage jackets, sleep in trucks, study in tents'.

The 'Snake Pit': Willowbrook, New York, USA

The Willowbrook State School was an official New York State institution on Staten Island in New York. It had premises of 375 acres with 40–50 low buildings with an initial capacity of about 3,000 beds. In 1947 it started to accommodate children and adults with mental retardation to give them education. The number of residents increased; by 1963 6,000 residents were crammed into a space designed for 4,275. The overcrowding was combined with serious understaffing and an almost complete absence of educational and recreational activities. By 1967, there were 59 nurses for some 6,000 residents. Senator Robert Kennedy, during a visit in 1965, described the hospital as 'less comfortable and cheerful than the cages in which we put animals in a zoo ... a new snake pit'. The descriptions below originate mainly from two books (Rothman and Rothman, 1984; Rivera, 1972) and contain quotes made by witnesses during the court procedures. The scandal finally broke in January 1972, when a TV team filmed one of the wards.

The ward had 60 retarded children with only one attendant to take care of them. Most were naked, lying in their own excrements, some in straitjackets. The TV crew noted the foul air, heard wailing noises and saw distorted bodies and limbs. The walls were full of smeared faeces. Some were in rooms without any furniture lying on the floor.

(Rivera, 1972)

The film was screened several times and was followed by a court process. The general conditions at Willowbrook were as follows:

The residents were either naked or in rags and tags, many toilets could not be flushed, the odours were incredible, flies and other insects abounded. Buildings were un-repaired, roofs leaking, windows broken. There were almost no records of the patients, and medical diagnoses were inaccurate, laboratory and physical evaluations were absent. Proper food was not always available. Willowbrook was a symbol of public abuse against powerless citizens.

(Rothman and Rothman, 1984)

The following are quotes from the court:

Parents reported: We found our daughter with her ear bitten off, part of the nose torn off and her knees completely bruised, black and blue, and scratches on her face and arms . . . cockroaches have taken over the buildings . . . the clients are all undernourished. Residents drink water from toilets. An average 100 violent incidents were reported each month. A nurse testified to the court about a leg plaster of a resident: It was rotten and broken in several places, there was an extremely foul odour from his cast, the odour of urine and faeces . . . before the cast was removed there were maggots crawling out from underneath . . . we picked them off the cast with forceps . . . we picked off 35 or 40 . . . when the cast was off there were numerous maggots in the wound itself and there was a large black bug embedded in the wound. Nudity is commonplace because no clothing is available. The gross disabilities and bizarre behaviour that the visitors saw, legs twisted into brambles and residents banging their heads against the wall, were not the reason for incarceration but the result of incarceration. 75–95% were heavily sedated.

A paediatrician noted: 10.00 p.m. Door of seclusion room opened by request; bare unlighted room, closed screen 2 × 2 inches, mattress and crumpled sheet and single thin blanket on the floor, barefoot 17-year-old girl in dingy loose gown standing by the door – pale pastry appearance, took my hand when offered – responded to questions with gestures and monosyllables. Had been in seclusion for

7 years; heavily tranquillized, teeth extracted long ago because 'she bit someone' – no signs of aggressive behaviour during our visit. Residents had their names written on their legs with indelible ink. A doctor told the court: Willowbrook is dangerous for children. It breeds more than disease. It breeds battered children. The children are left unattended. There is a mortality rate of three or four a week – all preventable.

(Federal Court of the Eastern District of
New York, 1972: *New York ARC v. Rockefeller*)

During this period, a medical experiment was carried out permitted by the authorities, but not by the parents or custodians of the clients. Children were deliberately infected with hepatitis virus, to try out a new vaccine.

The staffing of this institution was a big problem. An official report stated that:

the situation was critical. The care of the patients has been seriously deteriorating, resulting in high rate of absenteeism, lowering of morale, restlessness, irritation, increasing subordination, and what is potentially an explosive situation among the employees of the institution. It was indeed very difficult to find any personnel willing to work at Willowbrook. As a result, the turnover of the staff, which mostly had no training for the job, was very high.

(Rothman and Rothman, 1984)

The court took over the detailed supervision of Willowbrook; it lasted until 1986. During that time, some 2,600 of the 5,400 residents at Willowbrook were removed and entered into living arrangements in the community that were decent, safe and rehabilitative. Most of these alternative services consisted of small apartments for four to six persons, fully integrated in the community and with the presence of all necessary staff and the necessities for a good quality of life. Some other clients were transferred to residential care in other centres that were somewhat better than Willowbrook. By 1988, all clients of Willowbrook had left, and the institution was closed. The Federal Department of Health and Welfare and New York State have rules and legal standards.[8] The Joint Commission for the Accreditation of Hospitals supervises the care in residential institutions. These standards, however, had been seriously disregarded in Willowbrook. Annual inspections had been held as required, but no action was taken to correct the problems. Nobody was ever charged.

In 1999, state agencies in the United States reported 245,720 individuals with mental retardation and developmental disabilities living in nursing homes, psychiatric facilities, or congregate care (institutional) settings. In 2001, 542,000 children were in public care in the USA. It was estimated that of those, about 12,000 children under the age of 5 were in residential institutions (US Department of Health and Human Services, 2001). The conditions have certainly improved, but are still far from what should be attainable in the world's richest country.

Nameless children

I visited an Asian country in the 1990s at the official invitation of its government. On my arrival, the Director of Social Welfare gave an overview of the country's services for disabled persons. He invited me for an accompanied visit to a 'model' residential centre for 'custodial care' of severely disabled persons managed by his department. It was located in an isolated rural area, and surrounded by a high wall. Inside, there was a well-kept garden and the houses, built eight years before, were all in excellent condition. The cost for the centre was fully paid by the government.

The centre had 266 places, of which 229 were occupied. Some fifty staff were directly engaged in the care. The 'inmates' (the official term used) had severe disabilities. They had arrived as children from various other 'homes' in the country, at the request of the parents to whom the government had promised 'specialized care'. The pavilion I visited was their final destination in life. I was not shown the other residential buildings because 'the personnel were doing the annual cleaning', and so I could not enter. I heard screams and tumult from these pavilions; on hearing these, the Director was embarrassed and offered some improbable excuses.

The pavilion looked extremely orderly, which made me suspect that it had been specially prepared for my visit. It had a large dormitory with about fifty beds. Next to it were offices for the staff, bathrooms and other utility rooms: all impeccably clean. In the dormitory, the 'inmates' were lying in cage-like beds made of metal bars. It was difficult to establish any age or gender among these clients because their heads were shaved ('to avoid head lice'). Most of the beds were too short for their occupants, who were lying in crooked positions, with contractions in both arms and legs, their bodies permanently deformed. They were very emaciated; the muscles were mostly gone. I was informed that the clients were fed mashed food, using tubes or bottles. All were doubly incontinent; the personnel changed their nappies a few times a day. The windows were all open, but this did little to dispel the heavy odour of excrement and urine; most of the clients were wet in their beds. The children were all semi-comatose. I could not establish eye contact with any of them; they looked up to the ceiling or to the side of the bed, their eyes blank, unfocused, without expression. They did not seem to notice my presence. Nobody spoke or reacted to touch. Some of them were quietly engaged in sexual self-stimulation.

I interviewed the staff – none of whom had accompanied me during the two rounds through the dormitory. They were seated next door, and were reluctant to give any information at all. I asked for the medical records, and was informed that there were none, and that the staff did not know what the initial conditions had been. The Director told me that these children were the 'most severely un-trainable inmates'; the main disorder was mental retardation. The personnel had been informed that all possible remedies had already been tried and proven ineffective before their arrival. A few of the clients were on medication for epilepsy; no other medication such as sedatives was given (according to the Director – a statement that lacked credibility). The tasks of the staff were limited to feeding them, distributing medicines, washing them, changing the nappies, and keeping the premises clean.

Because I did not see any names on the beds, I asked for a list of their names. The nurse told me that on arrival the children did not have names with them, except for a few who had come from neighbourhood residential centres; the patients were now known only by their bed numbers. There were no records of addresses, parents or relatives, or of any birth dates.

With 40 hours of work per week per employee, there were 65 minutes of personnel time for each of the present 229 clients during each 24-hour period – totally insufficient, even for the 'basic care'. There were actually more personnel per animal in the zoo, which I had the opportunity to visit later on. No training programmes for the resident clients existed, just 'storage'. No parents or other family members came; and no children had ever been taken back home – quite naturally as they had no names. When I asked about the sexual self-stimulation, the personnel were very embarrassed and said that they had hoped that I 'would not notice it'. It appeared to me that this was the only remaining sign that here were still human beings, creating an ultimate moment of pleasure in a life that they had lost because of the unspeakable neglect so cruelly applied to them.

All naked

In an African country, I officially visited a large mental hospital built about 1870. Most of it was occupied by people with mental disorders, many of them lying on their beds the whole day, sleeping and heavily sedated – not moving and not speaking. In the more 'lively' parts of the hospital, there were 'tempest departments', where patients had their arms and legs strapped, some of them were chained to the walls in windowless cellars and screams filled the air.

There were two pavilions for the children and adults with mental retardation, one for males and one for females; each housed about seventy-five clients. Most of them had been admitted as small children. Whenever the door was opened, about five or six of them escaped into the courtyard, all of them naked and without shoes. They did not run far, and were quietly brought back in. Inside each pavilion, there were two large dormitories. All clients were undressed, and I was told that the hospital did not have enough budget for the laundry. Incontinence was common; the place was smeared with excrement and urine, reflecting the chaotic state of affairs. Disorder reigned everywhere. The beds had no sheets; many mattresses were broken and dirty, with traces of excrement. Some of the clients were extremely friendly and obviously glad to meet us, utter strangers. The ward for the mentally retarded girls and women was similar.

About 100 metres away, separated by a barbed-wire fence, was the occupational therapy unit. There two therapists were training five of the newly arrived children, who were wearing dresses and shoes. The therapists told me that the quality of the 'care' was deplorable; none of the mentally retarded clients should ever have been admitted to this asylum. The therapists were trying to convince the government to close it all down, to ask as many of the families as possible to take their children back home, and to offer families or foster families economic support and day-care, and move the adults to homes in their birth communities.

United Kingdom: abuse in children's homes

The Waterhouse Inquiry in 2000 published a report dealing with accusations of abuse and neglect in forty residential child care facilities in Wales. The residents were mainly children removed by the authorities from malfunctioning families, or because of the children's behaviour. Problems of paedophilia and sexual abuse in these institutions had first been exposed by a senior child care official working for the local council from 1976 to

1987. In 1987, she was dismissed after breaking ranks and informing the police of her observations. She was vilified and condemned at every turn, and despite her innumerable approaches to the Welsh Office, the Department of Health, the Home Office, various Home Secretaries and Ministers of Health, and to the Prime Minister, she only encountered apathy and insurmountable obstacles.

In 1991, the matter was exposed by a television channel and two newspapers. The Welsh police mounted a huge investigation and subsequently referred some 800 allegations to the Crown Prosecution Service. This damning report was, however, suppressed. Fewer than 3 per cent of these referrals proceeded to trial to the dismay and mystification of many of the victims and of the adults who knew the extent and nature of the abuse.

The Wales Child Abuse Tribunal of Inquiry was announced in 1996, after more than a decade of mounting public and political concern. It was chaired by Sir Ronald Waterhouse. The tribunal took evidence from 575 witnesses and from 259 complainants alleging abuse while they were in residence. Some 9,500 social services files were made available and 3,500 statements were made to police. There were 43,000 pages of evidence of complaints about some forty homes, as well as foster placements. Most attention was focused on sexual abuse of boys by staff and others outside the care system, but there was also sexual abuse of girls and boys by women staff. Physical and emotional abuse were also common, including hitting and throttling children, bullying and belittling them. Punishments included scrubbing floors with toothbrushes, or performing garden tasks using cutlery. The inquiry found that the quality of care, and standard of education, were below acceptable levels.

The majority of complaints were made against the deputy principal at Bryn Estyn home:

> He regularly invited resident boys – five to six at a time – to his flat for 'recreation'. These boys were given drinks (including some alcohol) and light food and were watching television, playing cards, board games etc. The boys were required to dress in pyjamas without underwear. If they were wearing underpants, they were ordered to remove them. The deputy principal had a number of favourites who were sexually assaulted at these parties.

> The lives of these already disturbed children were grossly poisoned by a leading authority figure in whom they should have been able to place their trust. They felt soiled, guilty and embarrassed. Most had trouble in their future sexual relationships.

There had been widespread physical and sexual abuse of boys and, more limited, of girls, in some 40 local authority homes – much of it by senior administrators and care workers. Some of the children had for a period of over ten years been continually abused by the principals of the homes. Life in such homes was a form of purgatory or worse from which children emerged more damaged than they had entered. The Tribunal criticized the staff of the homes, the social services, the Welsh Office, and the central Government for inaction.

(Waterhouse Inquiry, 2000)

The main offender was convicted in July 1994 and sentenced to ten years in prison.

Children in detention

I have visited closed prisons and halfway houses in several countries and seen examples of both good quality and of absolute hell. Those in Nigeria are 'life threatening' (US Department of State, 2000). To find children in prisons in developing countries is common. In some developing countries, the prison does not offer food, so unless the family comes with it all the time the prisoner will not survive. Inside, drug abuse, peer violence, sexual abuse and mental disorders are some of the overriding problems, including among juveniles. Shackling of prisoners is routine in many countries. The shackles are tight, heavy and painful, and reportedly have led to gangrene and amputation in several cases. In Pakistan minors were shackled routinely and sexual abuse of child detainees by police and guards is common (US Department of State, 2003). Some children develop drug habits while in these institutions and are supplied with drugs by their guards. A high proportion of them have been childhood victims of sexual, physical and/or emotional abuse, neglected educationally, live in inadequate housing and are malnourished.

Children in detention are frequently subjected to violence by staff, as a form of control or punishment, often for minor infractions. In at least seventy-seven countries corporal and other violent punishments are accepted as legal disciplinary measures in penal institutions (Global Initiative, 2006). Children may be beaten, caned, painfully restrained, and subjected to humiliating treatment such as being stripped naked and caned in front of other detainees. Girls in detention facilities are at particular risk of physical and sexual abuse, mainly when supervised by male staff (Report of the Special Rapporteur, 1999).

Over 9 million people in the world are kept in penal institutions (Walmsley, 2006). Half are in three countries: the USA, China and Russia. Among them are about 1 million juveniles (Sickmund, 2004). Most of these are charged with petty crimes, and are first-time offenders. Many are detained because of truancy, vagrancy or homelessness.

In most countries, a child less than 10 years old cannot be charged with a criminal offence. A common legal rule (*doli incapax*) is a presumption that a child aged 10–14 is 'incapable of crime' because of immaturity. This does not, however, imply that society takes no action: the child may be sent to a foster family or be referred to a detention institution for juveniles where in principle there will be access to appropriate rehabilitation programmes: counselling, education, survival skills training, group work, health care and gradual return to the community. Some countries treat juvenile offenders with a degree of leniency: suspended sentences, access to non-institutional rehabilitation and education programmes, community work and social control/supervision.

Some very young children live in prisons because their mothers are there; many become pregnant because they are raped by prison guards. Approximately 10 million children in the USA have had one or both parents incarcerated. These children and young people have little or no voice about who, in the absence of the parent, is the primary care-giver, who will take care of them, or if they will be allowed to visit or communicate with the incarcerated parent (Reed and Reed, 1997).

Juveniles under the age of 18 commit a relatively high proportion of all crimes, and those of them sentenced for violent crime have more than doubled during the last thirty years in the United States. In the USA, some 150,000 juveniles were estimated to be in custody in 2005 out of whom at least 10 per cent were in prisons for adults (Sickmund, 2004). At least 2,225 offenders in the USA serve life without parole (LWOP) sentences for crimes committed before they were 18; a few were as young as 13 at the time of the offence. An estimated 59 per cent were sentenced to LWOP for their first-ever criminal conviction. Thirteen other countries have laws that allow children to be sentenced to LWOP, but outside the USA there are only twelve such cases (Human Rights Watch and Amnesty International, 2005). A high proportion (some say all) of the youths in jails and prisons have mental disorders, but their access to treatment is limited. In the USA, 11,000 incarcerated youths in 1996 committed 17,500 acts of suicidal behaviour (US Justice Department, 2002). An estimated 12 per cent have mental retardation (Petersilia, 1997). Among infectious diseases tuberculosis, hepatitis and AIDS are the most common, and many prisoners are infected during their period of incarceration.

The UN Special Rapporteur in 2000 stated at the UN General Assembly:

> The conditions of detention for children in pre-trial centres and prisons continue to be of concern. Severe overcrowding, unsanitary conditions and inadequate and/or insufficient food and clothing are often exacerbated by a shortage or absence of adequately trained professionals. The resulting lack of appropriate attention to the medical, emotional, educational, rehabilitative and recreational needs of detained children can result in conditions that amount to cruel or inhuman treatment.
>
> The Rapporteur continues to receive information according to which children were allegedly at risk of deliberate acts of torture, including forms of sexual abuse. Children in detention are severely abused, humiliated, physically restrained, strip searches are carried out and some spend time in total isolation. Other prisoners and the staff are responsible for the very high degree of violence inside prisons; children should never be incarcerated.

A report from Brazil (a country that has adopted one of the most progressive juvenile justice laws) states:

> many facilities are decaying, filthy, smelly, dangerously overcrowded (some have occupancy rates of 130% above the legal levels), and failing to meet basic standards of health and hygiene. Beatings by prison staff using pieces of wood are common, and complaints of ill-treatment are never investigated by state detention authorities. At night some youths are obliged to defecate and urinate in plastic jugs, because the guards will not let them out to the toilets. Many sleep on rat-infested floors; cellblocks often have standing water on the floor.
> (Bochenek and Dalgadoi, 2006)

In 1985 the United Nations issued UN General Assembly Resolution 40/33, 'Minimum Rules for the Administration of Juvenile Justice' (the Beijing Rules), and in 1990 UN General Resolution 45/113, 'Rules for the Protection of Juveniles Deprived of their Liberty'. It appears that in many countries the extent of compliance is low or non-existent.

Research has been carried out on many programmes that describe efforts to facilitate the transfer of juvenile criminals back into community life (Reddington and Wallace, 2004). Early intervention programmes are important and cost-effective (Greenwood, 2005): by strengthening the family, supporting core institutions, promoting delinquency prevention, intervening immediately and effectively when delinquent behaviour occurs, and identifying and controlling the small group of serious, violent, and chronic juvenile offenders, juvenile crime rates can be lowered. Childhood violence increases criminality, thus its prevention should be cost-effective.

In spite of the abuse and neglect described above, it is not proposed to close all child 'homes'. In many situations, such as when children are removed from malfunctioning or abusive families, they must be received into a substitute home. The options for a substitute meso-system are discussed in Chapter 6.

5
Children On Their Own

A large number of children – other than those in residential institutions – live without a family. Six groups of uprooted children are described below: orphans, child soldiers, street children, refugee children, child labourers and child prostitutes.

Orphans

The word 'orphan' means different things in different cultures. In many, it is a child who has lost both parents (double orphans) by death, or by permanent separation. Half-orphans are those have one surviving parent. The term 'social orphan' is used for children who live on their own without parents. In 2005, UNICEF estimated the number of orphans in Africa at 38 million, 12 per cent of the population (11 million due to AIDS), in Asia 65 million, 6 per cent of the population (5 million due to AIDS), and in Latin America 9 million, 5 per cent of the population (2 million due to AIDS). There are a total of 112 million orphans (28 million due to AIDS). The proportion of half-orphans is not known. The number of AIDS orphans is increasing, especially in Africa. Adult AIDS victims – since 1981 25 million have died – often leave behind many dependent children. In many developing societies, the extended family takes care of orphaned children. In AIDS-epidemic areas not enough adults of the extended family may now be left to take care of this traditional function. Building orphanages is generally considered the most expensive and – because of the negative effects described in the previous chapter – the least desirable solution. In the view of most experts, the best solution for the developing nations is to set up an alternative model of institutions involving the transformation of children's homes into community-based resource centres that help families support children in the community.

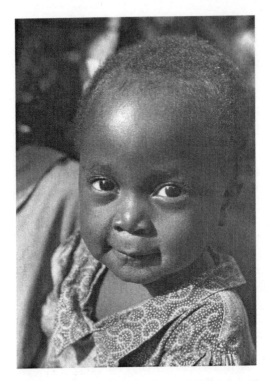

Photo 4.   **AIDS orphan.** *This girl from Tanzania is an AIDS orphan. She was taken care of by an international non-governmental organization. The international community does provide excellent help for some, but unfortunately not enough. For that reason, AIDS/HIV infections continue to spread. © World Health Organization.*

Such centres would provide day-care (thus partly relieving substitute parents), support groups, counselling, training in parenting skills, and skills training programmes for older orphans. Where circumstances prevent immediate care, institutionalized care is best used as a temporary measure until more appropriate placement can be arranged. Many governments and NGOs support programmes for the orphans in developing countries, and the funds are welcome, but insufficient. No organization has yet published estimates of the requirements for funds to implement such a programme. If just half of the 112 million orphans in the developing countries were to receive supporting programmes costing US$2 per day per child (corresponding to the World Bank poverty level), the total annual costs would amount to US$41 billion.

Child soldiers

The UN Convention on the Rights of the Child states, 'States Parties shall take all feasible measures to ensure that persons who have not attained the age of fifteen years do not take a direct part in hostilities. The Parties shall ensure protection and care of children affected by an armed conflict' (article 38). In 1998, the recruitment of children under the age of 15 and their use in hostilities was identified as a war crime by the statute of the International Criminal Court. The Court established in the Netherlands has jurisdiction to prosecute those responsible for the use of child soldiers.

In 1996, Mrs Graça Machel carried out a UN study[9] on the impact of armed conflict on children: some 300,000 children under the age of 15 were used as child soldiers and exposed daily to horrific violence. The report covered all parts of the world where armed conflicts had taken place during the last decade. Child warriors have been used in over thirty countries, among them: Angola, Colombia, Democratic Republic of Congo, Iraq, Lebanon, Liberia, Sierra Leone, Sudan and Uganda. According to UNICEF, in just one decade, 2 million children have been killed, up to 5 million have been disabled, 12 million made homeless, 300,000 forced to fight, 1 million orphaned or separated from families, and 10 million have been psychologically traumatized.

Thousands of Sierra Leonean boys and girls have been abducted to provide slave labour for troops. Thousands of children were not just quietly asked to join, but abducted by force by the 'rebels'. New recruits in Sierra Leone were often forced – as part of their initiation – to murder their parents. These children took part in all forms of warfare. They had their own AK-47s and M-16s and used them at the front lines of combat. They acted as spies, messengers and as advance human mine detectors and they were engaged in suicide missions. Many were drugged to overcome their reluctance to carry out the killings, beheadings, hangings, rapes and burnings of their victims alive. In Sierra Leone, Foday Sankoh, a rebel leader, expected his soldiers to subsist by eating the flesh and drinking the blood of freshly killed victims; some of them were their own family members. In Uganda, a rebel group that calls itself The Lord's Resistance Army, led by Joseph Kony, has abducted more than 20,000 children. Some are forced to fight, some carry bags, others have sex with the fighters. By way of initiation, many are obliged to club, stamp or bite to death their friends and relatives, and then lick their brains, drink their blood and even eat their boiled flesh. A 14-year-old girl soldier in Sierra Leone stated: 'I've seen people get their hands cut off, a ten-year-old girl raped and then die, and so many men and women burned alive. So many times, I just cried inside my heart because I didn't dare cry out loud' (Human Rights Watch, 2004).

The development of lighter weapons – such as the AK-47 – means that boys as young as 8 can be armed. The smallest boys are placed closest to the enemy. In war, they are said to be fearless. Children are often less demanding soldiers than adults are. They are cheaper to keep as they eat less and are easier to manipulate. 'The unpredictability of small children makes them better fighters' (Human Rights Watch, 2004). Some are sent into battle high on drugs to give them courage. In combat children are often captured and threatened. They fight for whoever controls them in order to stay alive. In continuous civil war, many children have fought for both sides. Thousands of Sierra Leonean boys and girls have been abducted to provide sex services and slave labour for troops; many acquire sexually transmitted diseases and HIV/AIDS. Now a second generation of child soldiers is being born of girl soldiers forced into sexual slavery. In Uganda, Human Rights Watch (2004) interviewed girls who had been impregnated by rebel commanders, and then forced to strap their babies on their backs and take up arms against Ugandan security forces.

According to Human Rights Watch (2004) in Colombia, tens of thousands of children have been used in the various military or rebel armed forces. Government-backed paramilitaries recruited them as young as 8. Guerrilla forces used children to collect intelligence, make and deploy mines, and serve as advance troops in ambush attacks. In southern Lebanon, boys as young as 12 were conscripted by force into the South Lebanon Army (SLA), a pro-Israeli auxiliary militia. When men and boys refused to serve, fled the region to avoid conscription, or deserted the SLA forces, their entire families were sometimes expelled from their homes. The issue is still unresolved, and will remain so until the vague threats of punishment from the warlords are replaced by action that ends the offenders' present impunity and sends them to prison.

Street children

One might distinguish between children on the street, who have homes to which they return almost every day; and children *of* the street who have chosen the street as their home: it is there they seek shelter, livelihood, and companionship; they may have occasional contacts with their families. There is no globally consistent way of calculating data on street children. Prevalence estimates by several organizations (Street children,

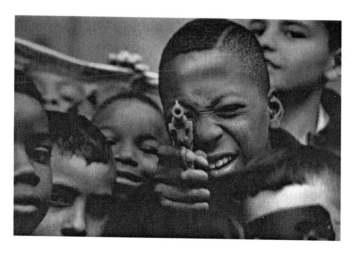

Photo 5. **Street boys in a Latin American country.** *Many of them join gangs and make the community unsafe.* © *World Health Organization.*

2006) are available for countries with 71 per cent of the world's population. In these, the total number of children of the street is reported as 5.8 million. Based on these data one might extrapolate that globally some 6.5 million are living homeless of the street. Some 20 million more children might be on the street. These are most likely underestimates. India might have 18 million street children: a proportion belong to families, where all members live of the street. A large-scale India study (Kacker, 2007) revealed that 67 per cent of all street boys and 68 per cent of all street girls had been physically abused and 55 per cent had been sexually abused. A study of drug-using street-involved youth in Vancouver, Canada, revealed high prevalence rates of 73 per cent for physical abuse; 32 per cent for sexual abuse; 87 per cent for emotional abuse; 85 per cent for physical neglect; and 93 per cent for emotional neglect (Stoltz et al., 2007).

Street children live from begging, doing small jobs such as selling trinkets or polishing shoes, some enter prostitution, and some join criminal gangs. Criminal child gangs may fight battles against each other for territory. Some children have run away from home or they have been thrown out by the parents; the reason is sometimes parental child abuse. Some have been abandoned, and some of them are in night shelters.

These children are targets of sexual and economic exploitation, trafficking for organs, general violence, and assassination and abuse by police and security forces. Many acquire sexually transmitted diseases, including HIV/AIDS. When apprehended by the police – innocent or not of crimes – they might be put in 'preventive custody' or in prisons with adults, where many are raped. Such custody may last for years. Their rights to competent legal assistance are mostly denied (Human Rights Watch, 1996b). In Colombia in the 1990s, thousands of children were murdered by 'death squads'. Indian street children are routinely detained illegally, beaten and tortured and sometimes killed by police. Several factors contribute to this phenomenon: police perceptions of street children, widespread corruption and a culture of police violence, the inadequacy and non-implementation of legal safeguards, and the level of impunity that law enforcement officials enjoy.

Most of Brazil's street children expect to be killed before they are 18. Between four and five adolescents are murdered daily in Rio alone. The murders are carried out by the police and by drug gangs. The death squads have met with little opposition from ordinary people, who feel threatened by gangs of children. Some members of the police force also fear the children, who are becoming knowledgeable witnesses to corrupt criminal activities by officials in the drug and prostitution business (Jubilee Action, 2000).

In many countries some parents abandon their children, some as young as 8 years old, sometimes by bussing them to a nearby big city and leaving them on the street. One example, describing my recent observations in a Caribbean island, follows.

Parents on this island bring their teenage children from the rural areas to the capital. When they arrive, the parent just leaves the child outside the bus station and disappears. The reasons for abandoning these children are poverty, poor school performance, disobedience or 'troublemaking' by the children at home. Some are mentally retarded and some are as young as 8 and do not know how (or do not want) to return back home; they stay on the street. Many go to sleep and share food in a big empty warehouse in the harbour.

Most of the young girls are soon picked up by men and taken home to serve as a combination of home-helpers and sexual partners. Therefore, the population at the warehouse is mainly boys. The boys live from begging on the streets or small jobs. Several are sexually exploited. Food is from the rubbish or stolen. Some of them catch infectious diseases and die. From time to time the police harass them and confiscate their earnings from begging. The killing of street children so widely practised by the police in Brazil and Guatemala did not seem to be common in this island. However, the boys I talked with were undernourished, looked unhealthy and were very frightened. The local psychiatric hospital was studying these children and through counselling managed to return some of them home after an intensive search for the parents. Others were given shelter by NGOs and referred to vocational apprenticeships. All services for children with mental retardation were at that time centralized to the capital. If decentralized day-centres had been available, the practice of abandoning these children would diminish.

Street children are often addicted to alcohol or drugs and need detoxification and rehabilitation. No global data are available, although all countries report that a high proportion of the children are exposed to drugs and/or alcohol, and that almost all children try them. Some do not come from poor families. Tyler et al. (2004) showed that 75 per cent of all homeless and runaway adolescents in Seattle had experienced sexual and physical abuse at home. Sullivan and Knutson (2000b) collected data in the USA about 39,352 children who had run away from hospitals and 40,211 who had run away from schools. The children in their study most likely to run away were those with behaviour disorders, mental retardation and some type of communication disorder. The most common factors associated with runaways were physical and sexual abuse, and high levels of domestic violence; they also had shown low academic performance, poor school attendance and more family stress factors.

Matchinda (1999) sampled 210 street children in Yaounde, Cameroon. The major reason for running away from home was combined severe physical and psychological abuse by the parents. A 2004 report about a group of similar children in Ethiopia confirms their high vulnerability: 55 per cent had been raped and a further 26 per cent had been sexually assaulted (Lalor, 2004a). Rajani and Kudrati (1996) carried out a study of street children in Mwanza (a large city in Tanzania) and noted that only 5 per cent of boys' and 15 per cent of girls' sexual behaviour is 'stereotypical prostitution'. The initiation rite of forced anal sex with new boys in the group was widespread – a 'rite of passage' in identity formation. Boys that were more docile were then frequently abused by the more dominant ones. This form of abuse of boys – as 'faggots' – was the worst form of humiliation among street boys. Street girls adopted a social role of adult sexual beings with the primary responsibility to satisfy one's male partner. Their relationships had little mutuality, and were frequently rough or even violent and characterized by power and intimidation. Because the continuum between love and abuse is so blurred, and because they have very low self-esteem, street girls often accept violence and humiliation in the pursuit of love and connection. This confusion undermines their ability to seek healthy options. A study by the International Labour Organization (2001) of juvenile prostitution revealed that common reasons for girls to leave home were 'problem with father', fights and maltreatment and poverty.

Huang et al. (2004) made a study of 115 abandoned street children (who agreed to be interviewed) in La Paz, Bolivia; 95 per cent were abused by the police, 84 per cent were absent from school, 26 per cent were engaged in robbery, 88 per cent inhaled paint thinner, 58 per cent used alcohol, and 53 per cent had a serious medical problem; the risks increased rapidly with age. These authors also made a comparison with thirty-five formerly abandoned street children in La Paz, Bolivia, who chose to enter a local orphanage; it was evident that operating homes for them had a positive effect. Such small, well-equipped homes with loving, competent personnel and good health and education programmes are mostly successful.

Child labourers

Article 32 of the UN Child Convention protects children from economic exploitation and work that is likely to be hazardous to the child's development, or to interfere with the child's education. It calls on states to take legislative and other measures, including sanctions and penalties, to guarantee this protection to children. The 174 member states of the International Labour Organization (ILO) in 1999 adopted the Convention on the 'Prohibition and Immediate Action for the Elimination of the Worst Forms of Child Labour'. The term 'child' refers to anyone under the age of 18, and 'the worst forms of child labour' include the sale and trafficking of children, debt bondage, forced or compulsory labour (including the forced recruitment of children for use in armed conflict), using children for prostitution or the production of pornography, using children for illegal activities, particularly drug trafficking, and other work which is likely to 'harm the health, safety or morals of children'.

The ILO (2006) estimated that 218 million children between the ages of 5 and 14 work in developing countries, about half of them full time; 73 million are aged 5–9 years. Sixty-one per cent of these are in Asia, 32 per cent in Africa, and 7 per cent in Latin America. Here are some national, officially reported examples of child labour: Albania 4,700; Bolivia 800,000; Colombia 2.5 million; Ethiopia 3.5 million; India 100 million; and Philippines 3.7 million. Of those, 126 million were in hazardous situations or conditions, such as in mines, with chemicals and pesticides in agriculture or with dangerous machinery. They are everywhere; some are invisible, working as domestic servants, in workshops or on plantations. The ILO has calculated that some 6.6 million children are working under the 'worst conditions of labour' as defined in article 3 of Convention 182 (not including those engaged in prostitution, see below). Of those, 5.7 million are in forced or bonded labour, 0.6 million in illicit activities and 0.3 million in armed conflicts. Slavery still exists; on a global scale it is estimated to involve between 15 and 30 million people.

There are many examples of underage work-related child violence. In India, I received an informal document describing the conditions during bonded labour of young boys. They were locked up day and night, worked 12–14 hours per day, and were given no salary and very little food. If they tried to run away, their 'owner' would shoot to kill them. The parents had sold them to pay debts to local loan sharks. In the India national study (Kacker, 2007), 65 per cent of working children were under pressure to work from their unemployed parents and 76 per cent handed over their earnings to the parents. Fifty-two per cent of the boys and 48 per cent of the girls reported physical abuse; 62 per cent of both reported sexual abuse. Other reports on child labour confirm the high risk for children of exposure to chemical and physical health hazards. In Bangladesh, the sexual abuse of child domestic workers is widely recognized (Rahman, 1995). Hadi (2000) studied a group of 4,643 children aged 10–15 years in villages in Bangladesh. Twenty-one per cent of the children were in the labour force, although this was forbidden by law. Of these children, 2.3 per cent were physically abused, 2 per cent were financially exploited, 1.7 per cent were forced to engage in inappropriate activities and 3 per cent were forced to work long hours. Out-of-school children and the children of illiterate, landless and unskilled labourers were most likely to be abused.

In a world where 130 million children receive no education at all and where most other children finish primary school – if they get that far – before the age of 12, there must be alternative occupation by that age. There are, states the ILO, degrees between exploitation of bonded children who are locked up day and night, undernourished and shot at if they try to run away, and practices that are more benign: for example, helping their families with daily chores, looking after younger children, assisting with cooking, doing light tasks in agriculture or animal husbandry or at the market and age-appropriate apprenticeships. Aggressive elimination of all jobs for children is seen as a 'negative approach' and might result in sending the children to the street to find alternative 'income' through begging, crimes or prostitution. Some organizations recommend the use of international economic sanctions to decrease child labour, or targeting certain employers or governments. However, such approaches have proven nearly impossible to monitor and the ILO estimates that only about 5 per cent of all working children are engaged in export industries.

One should seek better means for the prevention of 'the worst forms of child labour', and – since the 'extra' income is needed in poor families all over the world – try to arrange alternatives for unemployed adult family members. When secondary school education becomes the rule, child labour should decrease considerably.

Many development organizations provide assistance to remove children from hazardous environments, providing rehabilitation and social reintegration. They are given access to individualized gradual and nuanced programmes with free basic education and meals at school. If there are no family contacts, permanent lodging and food has to be found and, if possible, vocational training. Other organizations have helped to reduce child labour by providing jobs for their unemployed parents.

Refugee and displaced children

Article 22 of the Child Convention grants special protection to refugee children, especially if they are not accompanied by their parents or if they are fleeing war. Like all children, they have under the Child Convention the rights to life, physical integrity, adequate food and medical care, education, and to be free from discrimination, exploitation and abuse.

The UN High Commissioner for Refugees (2007) co-ordinates the activities related to refugees, but there are considerable political, financial and logistical challenges in protecting the human rights of refugee children. By the end of 2006 the number of refugees (9.9 million), displaced persons (12.9 million) and asylum seekers (740,000), stateless persons (15 million) and others under the protection of UNHCR has surpassed a record 33 million, of whom some 45 per cent are children under the age of 18 and 11 per cent under the age of 5. They were uprooted by increasing persecution, intolerance and violence around the world. Half are in Asia. In 2006 persons internally displaced included 4.3 million Palestinians, 4 million Iraqis, 3.5 million Afghans, 2 million Colombians and 2 million Sudanese. UNHCR, just like other international assistance organizations and NGOs, has severe budget problems; 'donor fatigue' has limited their resources. By the end of 2006, 45 per cent of all refugees were children under the age of 18, and 11 per cent under the age of 5. Refugee children are vulnerable. They suffer human rights abuses in countries of asylum: hazardous labour exploitation, aggression, neglect, denial of education, poor health care, sexual violence, cross-border attacks, kidnapping, militarization of refugee camps, and recruitment as child soldiers. They may be abducted, mutilated or murdered.

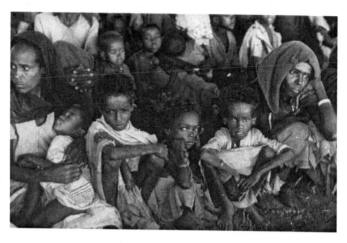

Photo 6.   **Refugees.** *Women and children waiting for food and shelter, while the men have stayed behind to continue the battle. Once uprooted, they may stay away from home for many years.* © *World Health Organization.*

Child prostitutes

Child prostitution is increasing rapidly; sex exploitation of children is spiralling out of control. This is explained by several factors: poverty, wars (with sex service demand by soldiers), increased tourism, and lack of viable opportunities for earning a living. The AIDS epidemics have increased the 'market' for underage sex workers, who are seen as uninfected, preferably virgins, and some aged 10–12 years. In some countries it is believed that sex with a virgin girl will cure an AIDS-infected man, and will also help a poor man to become rich (Lalor, 2004b).[10] Rekart (2005) estimates that at present globally there are 9 million girls and 1 million boys in prostitution. Not all have joined the sex trade voluntarily. Some have been sold by their parents to pay off debts to a local moneylender, and some have been lured away by promises of jobs. Some have been kidnapped on the street: in India it is estimated that 25 per cent of child prostitutes have been abducted and sold. In Lithuania 10–12-year-old children living in residential centres have been used as actors in pornographic movies (ECPAT, 2005). Child trafficking and outright 'exportation' of 'candidates' for sex work sometimes include children from neighbouring countries: this decreases the risk that they will run away. The brothel owner often forbids the young girls or boys to go out and confiscates their identification papers; in effect they are 'slaves'.

They are threatened with being killed or disfigured with acid if they try to get away. In many countries sex work is decriminalized for adult workers: if not, local bribes are paid to the police to close their eyes. Brothel owners are known for making 'arrangements' for underage prostitutes, as their presence is illegal.

Religious temple prostitution (Devadasi cults) has been practised for hundreds of years in Hindu religion areas (Sen and Nair, 2004; Varhade, 1998; Human Rights Watch, 2006). These cults originate from very ancient higher-caste temple traditions. Girls aged 5–9 from poor, low-caste homes are dedicated by an initiation rite to the deity in the local temple during full moon. After a girl is married to the deity by special rite, she is branded with a hot iron on both shoulders and her breast. She is then employed by the temple priest. Sometimes, even before menarche, she is auctioned off for her virginity; the deflowering ceremony is the privilege of the highest bidder. The market value of a girl falls after she attains puberty, when she is said to have no recourse other than prostitution. Yellama is represented as the principal goddess worshipped but the practice of Devadasi is prevalent in many other temple towns and with many other deities. By law, Devadasi prostitution has been forbidden in India since 1935 but efforts are still being made by the government and some NGOs to eradicate it. In spite of the illegal status of the Devadasi girls, 4,000–5,000 new girls are recruited each year. In Delhi they constitute 50 per cent and in Mumbai, Pune, Solapur and Sangli about 15 per cent of all prostitutes.

Global estimates on child prostitution were published by Rekart (2005). The estimates of the annual incidence of health complications appear in Table 5.1. Rekart estimates that the total global number of

Table 5.1 Health complications among 10 million child prostitutes, annual incidence (modified after Rekart, 2005)

Complications	Annual incidence (%)
Substance abuse	90
Post-traumatic stress disorder	67
Papilloma virus infection	45
Rape	25
Physical assault	25
Sexually transmitted diseases	23
Abortions	21
Hepatitis B infection	20
Attempted suicide	16

child prostitutes is 10 million, of whom 9 million are girls and 1 million are boys. Children born to prostitutes have a very high frequency of health problems, such as HIV infections; many die early. The annual occurrence of adverse health effects in infants born to child prostitutes are assessed at: 190,000 infant deaths, 237,000 with complications related to sexually transmitted (non-HIV) diseases, 250,000 HIV infected, 55,000 deaths from HIV infection, and 8,000 are infected with papilloma virus.

Sex work is extremely dangerous, and the harm that results includes violence (physical assaults, rape, murder), numerous infectious diseases, pregnancies often followed by abortions, alcohol and substance abuse, mental health complications and malnutrition. Most prostitutes have a history of adverse childhood experiences. A study by the US Justice Department (2003b) showed that in the USA 325,000 children are sexually exploited annually. Of that figure, 121,911 ran away from home and 51,602 were thrown out of their homes by a parent or guardian. They are not all poor: 75 per cent of children who are victims of commercial sexual exploitation are from middle-class backgrounds. Forty per cent of the girls who engaged in prostitution were sexually abused at home, as were 30 per cent of the boys. A Canadian study (Farley et al., 2005) of first nations sex workers in 2005 revealed that 82 per cent had a history of childhood sexual abuse, by an average of four perpetrators; 72 per cent reported childhood physical abuse. Ninety per cent had been physically assaulted and 78 per cent raped while working as prostitutes. Seventy-two per cent of them met the criteria for post-traumatic stress disorder. Ninety-five per cent wanted to leave prostitution; 86 per cent had experienced homelessness. A 2003 study (Pedersen and Hegna, 2003) of 10,828 children aged 14–17 (response rate 94.3 per cent) in Oslo, Norway, revealed that the adolescents who sold sex were 1.4 per cent of the sample. There were three times as many boys as girls; most of the clients were assumed to be homosexual or bisexual men. Most of the children were under the legal age of 16 when they started. There was no association with socio-demographic variables or residential area in Oslo; some children were from upper- or middle-class families. Adolescents who take part in these activities run a considerable risk of acquiring a sexually transmitted disease, drug use, or delinquent and criminal behaviour.

Many people with important positions are involved in child abuse, knowing that it is a crime; they may appear as socially well-functioning. Sex tourism to child prostitutes in countries such as Morocco, Sri Lanka, Philippines and Thailand involves well-to-do men, who only rarely receive prison sentences. Production of child pornography and human trafficking requires organizations with large economic resources. Many expatriates have been investigated for sexual exploitation of the people in developing countries they are there to help. These offenders seldom get caught; most escape unscathed because of high-level protection.

Many government and non-governmental programmes exist to prevent and punish child trafficking, child pornography and child prostitution. Unfortunately, they are totally insufficient. It is imperative to help children to escape from sex work, and to reduce the adverse health consequences.

Violence against children in cyberspace

Assisted by the internet new forms of child violence have appeared during the last decades. These include child pornography (see p. 29) and 'live' online sexual abuse for paying customers, online sexual solicitation, cyber stalking and bullying, and access to illegal and harmful materials. Child exploiters use cyberspace to network for child sex tourism and trafficking. ECPAT International (2005) reports that

> the effects of new technologies are pervasive, cause deep and lasting physical and psychological damage to the child victims, and are outstripping the resources of law enforcement agencies. Weak laws and fragmented industry action is exposing children around the world to increasingly serious violence. The child pornography industry is worth billions of dollars a year, although most child sex abuse images are traded for non-monetary gain. The main free-to-view sites have been traced to the Commonwealth of Independent States, the USA, Spain, Thailand, Japan and the Republic of Korea. More than half of the child sex abuse images sold for profit are generated from the United States and nearly a quarter from Russia. These countries are also the main hosts of commercial child pornography websites, followed by Spain and Sweden. Millions of child sex abuse images circulate online, and through mobile phones and peer networks. Interpol's shared child pornography database contains images of between 10,000 and 20,000 individual child victims, of whom fewer than 350 have ever been located. Urgent, wide-ranging actions are needed by governments, the industry and all sectors of the community to combat the rise in violence against children in cyberspace.

Trafficking

Trafficking in human beings is defined as the recruitment, transportation, transfer, harbouring or receipt of persons for the purpose of exploitation. Most trafficking is carried out using force, coercion, fraud or deception; for children often by persons who abuse a position of trust or power or employ outright abduction or theft. Some of it has been described above. The exploitation includes among others the following forced activities: prostitution, participation as solders in wars, labour (see above), participation in pornographic movies or internet sex, other practices that amount to slavery, servitude, or removal of organs; some children are known to have been killed to provide 'total organ harvest'. People smuggling is defined differently to 'trafficking', as is does not involve the use of force.

The extent of international child trafficking is not known precisely; the US State Department has estimated that between 600,000 and 820,000 men, women and children are trafficked across international borders each year – approximately 50 per cent are minors (Fleck, 2004; US State Department, 2005).

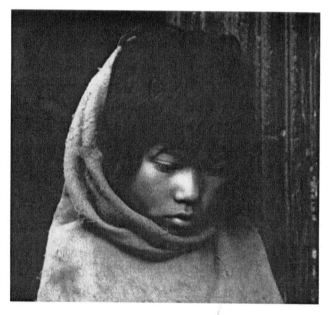

Photo 7.   **Nepalese girl in Kathmandu.** *She may not know it, but 5,000–10,000 girls like her are abducted each year from the streets or sold by the parents for prostitution.*[11] *Millions of children are trafficked each year. © World Health Organization.*

Trafficking is forbidden in international legislation by:

- The Convention concerning the Prohibition and Immediate Action for the Elimination of the Worst Forms of Child Labour or Worst Forms of Child Labour Convention (ILO, no. 182, 1999), ratified by 132 countries.
- The Protocol to Prevent, Suppress and Punish Trafficking in Persons, Especially Women and Children, supplementing the United Nations Convention against Transnational Organized Crime (UN General Assembly, 2000).
- The European Convention on Action Against Trafficking in Human Beings (2005), signed by 34 countries.

Human trafficking is one of the economically biggest international criminal industries. Many national judicial systems, the international police and the customs authorities are involved in the attempts to control it. Many children's charities are helping to take care of children who manage to escape and repatriation is common (Wolthuis and Blank, 2001; Brian et al., 2004). In spite of these efforts, there has been a 'dramatic' rise in this form of exploitation of children.

The children described in this chapter need to find homes, either with substitute parents, or if that is not possible, in a well-staffed, high quality child residential institution. The issues related to such transfers are discussed in the next chapter.

6
Parent Deprivation: Consequences and Alternatives

Children who are brought up away from their parents in an institution suffer many negative and destructive effects. The degrading effects are physical, psychological, social, and mostly long-lasting. The residential system is no substitute for the care, the attachment and the emotional development that develop in a family setting. However, it may sometimes be unavoidable to remove a child from its family home for social or for 'moral' reasons, or because of parental abuse; this must be seen as an ultimate and least desirable solution.

The research into childhood deprivation in institutions has been published in a large number of books and in scientific journals. At the end of an extensive review of all 92 such articles published between 1940 and 1989 Lie (1999) formulated these conclusions:

1. Institutional care, particularly in inadequate orphanages with few care-givers and poor stimulation, is disastrous for the child.
2. Different forms of deprivation – maternal, emotional, sensory, perceptual and opportunities for imitation – interact and cause the disorders observed.
3. All available studies agree that those who grow up in orphanages are handicapped, and also when compared to infants who grow up in inadequate families.
4. Observations made even in adequately equipped and staffed orphanages, supervised by the most distinguished experts, have nevertheless shown that many children in long-stay orphanages have a high prevalence of problems, with difficulties persisting into adulthood and into the next generation.

Frank et al. (1996), reviewing 'a large body of medical knowledge', state that:

> infants and young children are uniquely vulnerable to the medical and psychosocial hazards of institutional care, negative effects that cannot be reduced to a tolerable level even with massive expenditure. Scientific experience consistently shows that, in the short term, orphanage placement puts young children at increased risk of serious illness and delayed language development. In the long term, institutionalization in early childhood increases the likelihood that impoverished children will grow into psychiatrically impaired and economically unproductive adults.

Attachment

Normal attachment develops during the child's first two to three years of life. Problems with the care-giver–child relationship during that time, orphanage experience or breaks interfere with the normal development of a healthy and secure attachment. There are wide ranges of attachment difficulties. If an infant's needs are not met consistently, in a loving, nurturing way, attachment will not occur normally and may manifest itself in a variety of symptoms. When the first-year-of-life attachment cycle is undermined, mistrust begins to define the perspective of the child and attachment problems result. The developmental stages following the first three years continue to be distorted and/or retarded.

It should be noted that this description relates to Western 'modern' families, who live on their own. In other situations, there are multiple nurturing figures: grandparents, older siblings, aunts and uncles, long-time family employees and so on. Attachment also develops with them. This is often seen in developing countries. Another factor that contributes to early attachment in the developing countries is the mother's habit of strapping the infant to her back and carrying it along during the day, until the next baby arrives and takes its place. The attachment process may still be disturbed, however, by a variety of circumstances. This has serious consequences for the future of affected children. Details are given in Chapter 8.

Family support

In the developed countries, the alternative to residential care could be technical and economic support to the families: using community-based and home care services, day centres for training and for education in inclusive facilities. The World Health Organization has published a monograph by the well-known psychiatrist Bowlby (1951), who states:

> There are today governments prepared to spend up to 10 pounds a week on the residential care of infants who would tremble to give half this sum to a widow, an unmarried mother, or a grandmother to help her care for the baby at home. Indeed, nothing is more characteristic of both public and voluntary attitudes towards the problem than a willingness to spend large sums of money looking after children away from their homes, coupled with a haggling stinginess in giving aid to the home itself. These problems should be solved by methods other than retaining the children in an institution.

In the poor countries government economic child support is rare. Until now it has been common to see the extended family helping, but in urban areas such willingness is declining. When there is no help infants may be abandoned or neglected, and some will die.

Substitute families

When needed for children who are by legal decision removed from their biological parent(s), arrangements should be made for substitute family-based care.

Adoption

Many countries have national legal adoption procedures. There has existed since 1993 the Hague Convention on Protection of Children and Co-operation in Respect of Intercountry Adoption.[12] Its key principles include: ensuring that intercountry adoptions take place in the best interests of children; and preventing the abduction, exploitation, sale or trafficking of children. By February 2007, seventy countries had ratified and three had signed the Convention. There are rules for the process by which parents give up their child for adoption. After an application by the adopting parent(s), there follows a determination of eligibility, and assessment of suitability, to adopt. These are mostly carried out by national authorities with specialized personnel and may be time-consuming. If one were to handle the adoption with respect to available scientific knowledge, all such children should be transferred to the adoptive parents within a period not exceeding six months, preferably even less. Many infants awaiting adoption, however, are sent to child residential institutions, and some stay for years. During that time they acquire RAD, with lifelong consequences for many. A study by the US National Adoption Center found that 52 per cent of adoptable children had symptoms of RAD (Boris et al., 1998). Governments should lose no time in speeding up the heavily bureaucratized adoption system that causes a lot of damage to defenceless children (Brodzinsky et al., 1992).

Foster parents

Foster parents in developed countries are usually paid for taking over the care of children who are biological or social orphans, or who have been removed by judicial authorities. An example of such a transfer appears in Box 6.1 (Helander, 2007).[13]

Sylvestre et al. (2002), in a Canadian report, estimated the prevalence of communication problems among children under the age of 3 taken into care by the authorities as a result of parental negligence. In a representative sample of eighty-four such children, 46 per cent presented problems in at least one area of communication. The seriousness of the condition increased with age; boys were more affected than were girls.

Foster parents may face many difficulties and need training and supervision. Neglected children may show lack of skills in daily life activities, they may be malnourished, and not used to proper hygiene. After transfer to foster parents, many physical consequences, such as weight and height, are often normalized within one year. Change of foster parents should be avoided, as it is traumatic for the children and may lead to adult consequences. For example, Marilyn Monroe's father left before she was born, her mother had a mental disorder, so she become a 'ward of the state', first staying in a 'child home' and then experiencing twelve different foster families. She felt unwanted and unworthy of love, growing up with her emotional needs unmet (Asbury, 2003).

Children who have been transferred for severe behavioural problems or early significant delinquency may need foster parents who are professionals (e.g. psychologists, social workers), a system that has been tried with success in some developed countries.

Residential homes

Residential homes for children removed from their parents may be the last resort when no other solution can be found, for example if one cannot find any substitute families willing to take care of them. Such homes should be very small, aiming at creating a family atmosphere, and large inputs for training, social education and professional

Box 6.1:   Children transferred from a residential centre to foster families

Twenty-eight children in a small town in Romania during the last few years have been transferred from the local residential centre to foster families. The children were 4–17 years old at the time of the transfer; 17 were girls, 11 were boys. All except one had lived in residential centres since soon after birth. They had been healthy infants abandoned soon after birth and had no disability when they arrived. The reason for institutionalization was poverty. All had been raised in at least two such centres since they were born; several had been to three or more centres. To transfer the children to foster families was a challenge, for they all had severe induced disabilities caused by the years spent in institutions.

The foster parents were carefully selected and trained before the change took place, and social workers are still giving them continuous support and advice. Twelve of the foster parents had previously been employed by the residential centre. They were all paid a salary for the work; their homes were nice and well-equipped. I have interviewed all parents and seen all the children twice. The parents told me that they were happy with their 'new children', and the social workers confirmed that there were no major problems for the children to adjust to the new homes.

During the children's stay in the centres, their functions had become affected, to the degree of severe disability. Only four were fully continent, one was wetting and twenty-three were both soiling and wetting. Fourteen could not eat alone, and twenty-six could not wash themselves. Many were unable to dress alone and some had mobility problems.

Sixteen of the children had been transferred already in 2001 and 2002, thus at my examination they had been with the foster parents for two to three years. Within months after the transfer to the foster families, most of the 'functional' deficiencies described above had been overcome with training. All were fully continent. Only one child still had problems walking, all but one was eating alone, but nine still needed help with washing.

Twelve other children were transferred in 2004, and had only been with the foster parents for three months when I saw them for the last time; there was not yet much change, except that now only eight rather than eleven children were both soiling and wetting.

But there were also emotional and behavioural problems. All twenty-eight children had pronounced post-traumatic stress disorder, with nightmares, depression and anxiety, and crying. They were overly dependent on constant affection, and some had difficult behaviour. These symptoms have been slow to disappear; in some there have been minor improvements.

The most striking symptoms were their speech problems. Only one could speak (a child admitted at age 5 already speaking) when they left the centre. Even after daily training by the foster parents during three years, none of them is able to speak more than a few very simple short syllables (no child was originally autistic or had hearing problems). This will make it difficult for them to attend school and find jobs and incomes as adults. The speech problems are likely to remain unresolved for life; children who have not learnt to speak phonemes before the age of 6 will never speak: probably the brain cells involved in speech have been 'pruned off'.

Brain scans of children from Romanian orphanages show decrease of brain size and grave disturbances of brain function (Perry, 2002); see p. 147.

advice – if available – should be sought. Treatments with dyadic psychotherapy for RAD have proven effective and should be integrated.

Residential homes of this type are found in many developing countries. Quite a lot of them are managed by NGOs for the groups of children mentioned in Chapter 5. Many of those that I have visited have good qualities, and are different from the mostly huge government-managed institutions that were described in Chapter 4.

In Part III, the evidence will be presented about the violence against children who live in their birth homes, and of the short- and long-term consequences of child violence.

Part III

Damaging Effects of the Meso-system: Childhood Violence in Birth Families and its Consequences

7
Prevalence of Childhood Violence

In the previous chapters, we dealt with the children whose micro-system lacked the most important component of the meso-system: the parents. This chapter will examine how common violence is among 'ordinary' children, who live with their birth families.

Sexual abuse

Many studies originating in Western countries differentiate between three levels of child sexual abuse:

1. Non-contact (exhibitionism, verbal threats, harassing or inappropriate proposals, photographing sexual parts of children and adolescents, showing children how to masturbate, asking the child to masturbate);
2. Contact without penetration; and
3. Penetration/intercourse.

In the studies appearing below, different definitions of levels of reported sexual abuse have been used (see pp. 29–31). One specific issue is whether to include non-contact sexual abuse. WHO (Andrews et al., 2003), when applying a *narrow* CSA definition (criteria 2 and 3 above), had a prevalence of 19 per cent; those who applied a *broad* definition (criteria 1, 2 and 3 above) had a 23 per cent prevalence rate. When only one question was asked to assess CSA, the prevalence was 14 per cent; with more than one question it went up to 23 per cent. Other studies (Gorey and Leslie, 1997) use *narrow* CSA to include only criterion 3 above, *middle* includes 2 and 3 and *broad* 1, 2 and 3. Cultural factors have to be kept in mind while reading published studies. In some countries verbal sexual harassment, and forced kissing and hugging are taboos and are included in the statistics of sexual abuse (see Ethiopia, Table 7.1., India and Israeli Bedouin-Arabs in Table 7.4); in many countries, this is serious abuse.

Sexual abuse in developed countries

There are few prospective longitudinal studies of risk factors for sexual abuse. Fergusson et al. (1996) followed, from birth to age 16, a cohort of 1,265 children born in Christchurch, New Zealand, in 1977. At 18, retrospective reports of sexual abuse before the age of 16 were obtained and risk factors that had been prospectively assessed were examined. Of the 1,019 subjects interviewed at age 18, 10.4 per cent indicated that they had been sexually abused (17.3 per cent females and 3.4 per cent males). Major risk factors were: female gender of the victim, marital conflict between parents, poor parental attachment, paternal overprotection, parental alcoholism, and other social problems. The level of prediction was, however, weak. Collin-Vézina and Cyr (2003) studied trans-generational transmission of sexual violence and found that of parents who themselves were molested in childhood, one-third of the men and half of the women went on to molest their own children. Ertem et al. (2000) made a review of all articles concerning such transmission and found that only one of ten studies fulfilled all desirable scientific criteria; that study showed an increased relative risk of intergenerational physical abuse of 12.6.

Recidivism is common; Doren (1998) calculated that the lifetime rate for extra-familial sexual abusers is 52 per cent and for rapists 39 per cent; the percentage of new offences at the end of twenty-five years was 26 per cent for rapists and 32 per cent for child molesters. Arszman and Shapiro (2000) analysed the records of thirty-one offenders who confessed between 1994 and 1999. The perpetrators confessed 101 acts of sexual abuse of 47 victims, some of whom were victimized multiple times. Out of the 47 victims, 45 were old enough to provide a history describing 111 acts of abuse. Holmes and Sammel (2005) made a study of abuse rates among criminals. They found that 10–20 per cent of all non-criminal boys were sexually abused. In comparison, the rates among criminals are much higher: 33 per cent of male juvenile delinquents, 40 per cent of sexual perpetrators, and 76 per cent of serial rapists reported CSA. Thirty-one per cent of women in prisons in the USA in 1991 and 95 per cent of prostitutes had been sexually abused as children.

Holmes and Slap (1998) have undertaken a meta-analysis of 166 studies of boys, published in peer-reviewed journals, representing 149 samples.

The authors conclude that sexual abuse of boys is 'common, under-reported, under-recognized, and underrated'. The US Department of Health and Human Services (1997) stated that boys experience 48.5 per cent of all childhood abuse. In the past, abuse of boys may have been underestimated. Terry and Tallon (2005) have compiled a major review of the literature on sexual abuse. Sperry and Gilbert (2005) culled an archival data set containing retrospective reports of childhood sexual experiences for instances of sexual abuse by child peers. They found 8 per cent of females and 4 per cent of males reporting at least one experience of sexual abuse before the age of 12 (mean age 8.2) by a child peer. These experiences involved some degree of force, and were clearly unwanted, and were perceived as 'mostly negative'. Their findings suggest that child peer abuse may be associated with adverse mental outcomes. A Canadian study (Fischer and McDonald, 1998) was made of 1,037 cases of child sexual abuse obtained from police files. A comparison was made between intra- and extra-familial abuse. The results showed (1) earlier onset, longer duration, higher levels of intrusion, and greater physical and emotional injury for intra-familial victims; (2) less use of physical/verbal force, or enticements, and greater use of instructions 'not to tell' by intra-familial offenders; (3) more convictions and longer jail sentences for intra-familial offenders; and (4) no intra- or extra-familial differences in victim sex preference.

Other studies were made in the Czech Republic (Rarboch, 1996), Denmark (Fabricius et al., 1998; Riis et al., 1998), Finland (Sariola and Utella, 1994), Greece (Agathonos-Georgopoulou and Brown, 1997), Japan (Nakamura, 2002; Ikedar, 1995; Tarimura et al., 1995), Norway (Bendixen et al., 1994), Poland (Deres and Kulik-Rechberger, 2001), and the United Kingdom (Mackenzie et al., 1993; Morris et al., 1997). These generally confirm reported sexual abuse prevalence of 15–20 per cent. In some countries it is lower (Documentation Française, 2002) and in others it is higher.

Sexual abuse in developing countries

In developing countries, talking openly about sex is often a taboo, even among professionals. There is little or no knowledge about symptoms of abuse and neglect in general. The truth is slowly 'seeping in' from abroad, and initially becomes known to professionals in the health and social services. Crimes become apparent, such as infections of minors by sexually transmitted diseases, physical damage, and detection of pregnancies among underage girls (Haj-Yahia and Tamish, 2001), many caused by incest and rape, which are cultural taboos. When the evidence becomes

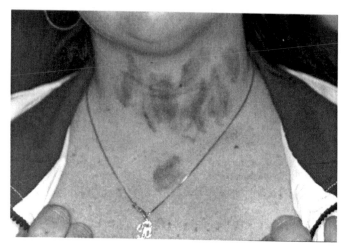

Photo 8.   **Abused teenage girl.** *This 13-year-old girl was drugged by her date and then raped. The offender left sucking marks on her neck. Credit: Dr James Williams, Volcano Press, USA.*

better known, the avalanche of knowledge emerges and the demands for action start. The level of abuse of all types in the developing countries will eventually be identified as being on the same or on a higher level than in the 'affluent' nations. Some developing country studies reveal that boys have the same or higher sexual abuse rate compared to girls (South Africa: Petersen et al., 2005; Israel: Zeira et al., 2002; India: Kacker, 2007). This may be typical in several other countries with a high rate of peer abuse of boys. Many articles from developing countries confirm a high incidence of CSA, although there are many cultural constraints hampering the account of sexual abuse. In Pakistan (US State Department, 2004) evidentiary requirements for sexual offences include that four adult male Muslims must witness the act. Half of all rape victims there were juveniles. However, very few rapes were reported to the police because the women risk being prosecuted for adultery; alleged 'adultery' is the reason for 80 per cent of the women who are in jail in that country. In Ecuador (US State Department, 2004) a woman can only file a complaint for rape if she can produce a witness. Of 3,083 rapes reported, 656 persons were charged but only 118 prosecuted.

A large proportion of sexual abuse is related to socialization into unequal gender relations, rape myths, peer pressure and sexual urge. A detailed example from South Africa follows (Box 7.1.).

Box 7.1: Sexual behaviour among the youth in South Africa

Petersen et al. (2005) report from South Africa one of the highest rates of sexual violence in the world: at least 44 per cent of females and 29 per cent of males had experienced childhood sexual abuse, girls aged 12–17 being at particularly high risk. There are multiple streams of influence for adolescent boys and girls becoming either victims or perpetrators of sexual violence. In several representative groups of high-school children/adolescents aged 13–16 years, in-depth individual interviews and 'focus group' discussions were carried out. The adolescents mentioned the following factors:

(1) *Cultural/environmental influence*: The boys are socialized from an early age into traditional patriarchal notions of masculinity, which promote and legitimize unequal gender power relations. Rape myths are held by many, for example that men are unable to control their sexual urges. Sexual violence is a strategy used by boys/men to put girls/women in their place if they become too independent and assertive. Sexual abuse of children was understood by the researcher as a mechanism that was sometimes used to punish the mother of the child, if she did not comply with her partner's demands. Sex was viewed as a commodity that could be exchanged for favours, normally food or money. Sexual abuse within and without the family was often condoned because of economic dependence on the abuser. Poverty plays a direct role in increasing a child's vulnerability to falling victim to sexual abuse; disparities in wealth interfacing with materialist values emerged as risk influences contributing to intra-personal anger and increasing the risk of boys becoming perpetrators of sexual violence. There is also the absurd and perverse notion that having intercourse with a virgin will cure HIV/AIDS.

(2) *Situation context/normative influences*: Social norms and social pressures prescribe that boys/men should have sexual relations as a marker of their masculinity. Boys/men who do not have a partner commit rape to show masculinity. Perceived norms are weakening the traditional protective role that brothers have played in protecting their sisters from rape and abuse by other boys; there is a 'sell-out' as part of boys' friendship with other boys. Lack of an adequate role model from fathers emerged as a risk: they were often absent from home, or were poor models leaving the mothers with the burden of raising their sons on their own. Modelling

of violence against girls/women is contributory when such violence is regarded as normative behaviour. When boys reach puberty, there is poor parental monitoring or outright neglect; this increases the possibility of affiliation with negative peer groups. Traditional parental support is eroding, and that includes the girls. The formal justice system is inadequate, and community social controls have been eroded.

(3) *Intra-personal level influences*: There is evidence that a child who is abused and neglected is likely to become a sexual abuser later in life. Abused girls in particular, but also some boys, later lack assertiveness and refusal skills as a consequence.

In South Africa, as in many other countries, the low status of women contributes to their victimization. Female genital mutilation, for example, affects some 135 million women (see p. 34). Education should include learning to change the present aggressive attitudes and behaviour of the males and the submissive behaviour of the females.

During the last thirty years of civil wars and unrest, rapes of thousands of women and underage girls have been committed as part of a 'strategy of intimidation' in Algeria, Angola, Bosnia, Colombia, Democratic Republic of Congo, Liberia, Rwanda, Sierra Leone and Uganda.

Small-scale studies of childhood sexual abuse have been published from Bahrain (Al-Mahroos et al., 2005), Bangladesh (Rahman, 1995), Botswana (Mathoma et al., 2006), Cameroon (Rwenge, 2000; Menick and Ngoh, 2003), El Salvador (Barthauer and Leventhal, 1999), Ethiopia (Lakew, 2001; Mulugeta et al., 1998), Hong Kong (Tang, 2002), Hungary (Csorba et al., 2006), Indonesia (Hakimi et al., 2001), Lesotho (Brown et al., 2006), Malawi (Lema, 1997), Malaysia (Sing et al., 1996), Papua New Guinea (Johnson and Ambihaipahar, 1999), Pitcairn Island,[14] Republic of Korea (Hong et al., 2004), Singapore (Yiming and Fung, 2003), South Africa (Adedoyin and Adegoke, 1995; Howard et al., 1991), Sri Lanka (Miles, 2000), Swaziland (Mathoma et al., 2006), Tanzania (Rajani, 1998) and Zimbabwe (Watts et al., 1998). The selection below reflects the presently available results from a variety of countries; the quality and methods used differ. Some studies were presented in Box 2.1 (p. 31) and more are appear in Table 7.3 (Combined abuse), (pp. 111–15). The specific problems affecting most of these studies are the high attrition rates and under-reporting among the responders, described in Chapter 2.

Table 7.1 Prevalence of sexual abuse, selected studies

Country Authors	Type of study, comments	Results
Antigua and Barbados University of California, 2006	Sample of women	30% reported undesired sexual contact with a relative or with someone more than 5 years older than them before age 16.
Australia Goldman and Padayachi 1997	Group of undergraduate students	18.6% male, 44.6% female forced into unwanted sexual acts; incest had a prevalence of 10% of males, 19% of females.
Congo Courtois et al. 2001	Survey of 292 high-school students: 39% of girls and 61% of boys, 14–25 years old	88% of the boys have sexual intercourse at the age of 15, vs 72% of the girls at 16; sexual intercourse under duress 29%
Costa Rica University of California, 2006	Costa Rica college students	32% of women and 13% of men reported unwanted sexual activity during childhood.
Costa Rica Heise et al. 2002	Study of pregnant girls aged 12–16, in hospitals	95% of pregnant girls aged 12–16 subjected to incest or rape.
Ethiopia Worku et al. 2006	323 female students from grade 9 (age about 14–15 years)	Prevalence of CSA 69%, 7% unwanted pregnancy, 6% sexually transmitted disease.
Germany Wetzels et al. 1995	Sample of 2,104 women aged 20–59	15% reported that they had been victims of (attempted) violent intercourse.
Great Britain Cawson et al. 2000	Young adults (aged 18–24) in retrospective self-reports	16% had experienced contact sexual abuse 11% unwanted sexual assault before age 13.
Ireland McGee et al. 2003	Random selection of adults (n = 3118) Telephone interviews Response rate 71%	20% of women reported contact and 10% non-contact childhood sexual abuse. 16% of men reported contact and 7% non-contact childhood sexual abuse. 67% of abused girls and 62% of abused boys were abused before the age of 12. For 58% of girls and 42% of boys, the abuse lasted more than one year.

(Continued)

94

Table 7.1   (Continued)

Country Authors	Type of study, comments	Results
		Women reported 42% life-time sexual abuse or assault (penetration/attempted penetration 31%), men 28% life-time sexual abuse or assault (penetration/attempted penetration 21%). 28% of the women and 20% of the men were re-victimized by a different perpetrator.
Israel Schein et al. 2000	1005 randomly selected patients attending family practitioners, aged 18–55, response rate 81%	31% of females and 16% of males reported childhood sexual abuse. Victims knew 55% of the perpetrators. 26% of female and 7% of the male victims reported intra-family abuse.
Jordan Jumaian 2001	Male college students	27% sexually abused before age 14.
Korea, Rep. of Shim 1992	Population study	17% of women reported attempted or completed rape.
Morocco Alami and Kadri 2004	Interviews with a representative sample of 728 women, aged 20 and above	9.2% reported childhood sexual abuse. All those abused during their childhood suffered sexual disturbances as adults.
Nicaragua Olsson et al. 2000	Representative urban sample of literate men and women aged 25–44. 289 men and 322 women were invited to take part in the survey, and 53% of the men and 66% of the women participated	20% male, 26% female reported sexual abuse, occurring before age 19. Women were victims of attempted or complete rape twice as often as men. 1/3 of the men and 2/3 of the women were abused by family members. Median age at first abuse 10 years for both boys and girls.
Peru Heise et al. 1992	Study of pregnant girls aged 12–16, admitted for childbirth at hospitals	90% of the girls were pregnant because of incest or rape.
Romania Artemis, 2000	851 girls and 416 boys, aged 14 to 19 attending school, interviews	19% of the girls and 4% of the boys had experienced sexual acts against their will, in half of the cases by somebody they knew.

(Continued)

Table 7.1   (Continued)

Country Authors	Type of study, comments	Results
Sierra Leone Coker and Richter 1998	Population sample	50% of all women respondents had been coerced to have sex by a male partner. Many of them were underage. Sexually mutilated women were at a significantly higher risk.
South Africa Collings, 1991	Female university students Male university students	44% of 94 female students had experienced CSA or harassment; for half of them contact sex abuse. 29% of the male students had been victims of child sexual abuse.
South Africa Madu and Pelzer, 2001	414 high school students aged about 15–16	CSA rates were 60% for the boys and 53% for the girls. Among them, 87% were kissed sexually, 61% were touched sexually, 29% were victims of oral/anal/vaginal intercourse. 'Friend' was the highest indicated perpetrator in all patterns of sexual abuse. Many victims (87%) perceived themselves as not sexually abused as a child.
Spain Lopez et al. 1995	Representative sample of 1,821 persons	15% of males and 22% of females sexually abused before age 17
Sweden Krantz and Östergren 2000	Rural sample, women 40–50 years old	32% had experienced CSA; 16% sexual abuse as adults.
Switzerland Bouvier et al. 1999	Random sample of 1193 14–19 year-olds	11% of males and 34% of females had experienced CSA
Switzerland Torella et al. 1994 Niederberger, 2002	Initially representative sample of Swiss- German women, dropout rate 58%	Sexual abuse prevalence 40% overall and 15% for severe abuse. Average age of first abuse 11 years, 25% experienced first sexual abuse before age 9.
Taiwan Luo, 1996	Estimates based on official reports.	Annually over 10,000 sex crimes, 42% relating to children and adolescents. In a brutal child sexual abuse incident, 'the abuser dragged, with a bamboo stick, the intestines out of a dying 5-year old girl.'

(Continued)

Table 7.1 (Continued)

Country Authors	Type of study, comments	Results
Taiwan Luo 1996	Conclusion based on local culture	In 'Marrying my rapist?' Luo states 'patriarchal control over women's sexuality has been transformed into a cultural fetish for female chastity'
Tanzania Matasha et al. 1998	Random sample of 892 school children aged 12–19, in which 85% of the boys and 58% of the girls were sexually active. 14% of girls (mean age 14) had been pregnant; half had an illegal abortion	Nearly half of the sexually active girls and 7% of the boys reported their first sexual experience as forced. Half of the primary school girls had already had sex with adults, including teachers and relatives.
Tanzania McCrann et al. 2006	Sample of 487 university students, mean age 29 (20–53). No attrition	Prevalence rate for CSA 31% for females and 25% for males, at age 13.
Turkey Elal et al. 2000	Study of 1,597 college students by self report	CSA (broad definition) experienced by 16.0% of males and 28.0% of females.
Turkey Eskin et al. 2005	1,262 university students	28% reported at least one instance of sexual abuse during childhood, those with a homosexual or bisexual orientation had increased risk for suicidal ideation.
USA Felitti et al. 1998	Survey by Kaiser Permanente, (HMO) in California. It included 17,000 adults; 71% response rate; mean age 56 years	22% experienced contact sexual abuse during childhood or adolescence. 8% responders excluded because they did not reply to the questions about childhood sexual abuse, thus the prevalence might be higher.
USA American Indians Robin et al. 1997	Sample of 582 American Indians	49% of females and 14% of males had been sexually abused, 78% by family members. The victims showed a high frequency of subsequent psychiatric disorders.

(Continued)

Table 7.1 (Continued)

Country Authors	Type of study, comments	Results
USA Gorey and Leslie 1997	Review of 16 studies of child sexual abuse	Average prevalence of female CSA 22.3%; male 8.5%. Response rates 25% to 98%. In studies between 1969 and 1985 the response rate averaged 68%; after 1985 the response rate dropped to 49%. Those responding in surveys after 1984 reported systematically higher prevalence rates of abuse than those before 1984. Child abuse definitions influenced prevalence rates: female CSA, narrow definition 8.3%, middle 17.8%, broad 36.3%, male CSA narrow 6.6%, middle 7.2% and broad 11.5%.
USA Wyatt et al. 1999	Los Angeles County sample of 10,204 women aged 18–36 years	34% had experienced at least one incident of sexual body contact, 75% of those very severe before age 18. The refusal rate for the interviews was 29%. No changes in prevalence rate over the last 10 years. Most incidents were not reported.
Zimbabwe Nhundu et al. 2001	Teacher-perpetrated sexual abuse	All perpetrators were male teachers. 98 out of 110 victims were girls. The mean age of victims was 12 years; in 70% the abuse was penetration. 83% of teacher perpetrators were dismissed from their jobs.
21 countries Finkelhor 1994	Retrospective study of 21 countries	3%–29% of males, 7% to 29% of females, reported sexual abuse. Many studies showed females were abused 1.5 to 3 times more than were men. One third of the above was intrafamiliar.

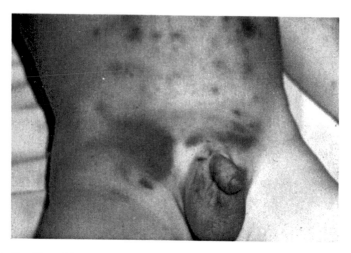

Photo 9. **Abused boy.** *Bruises on the lower abdomen, pubis or perineum should raise suspicion of sexual abuse. Credit: Dr James Williams, Volcano Press, USA.*

Physical abuse

There is less published information on physical than on sexual abuse. In many countries it is legal to physically punish children. It is forbidden by law in some seventeen countries. In twenty-four additional countries, corporal punishment in school is forbidden (Global Initiative, 2006). Most people everywhere sincerely believe that corporal, psychological and emotional punishment is beneficial for all children; parents and teachers argue that deliberately inflicted pain is 'character building' and vital to the 'development of strength and endurance' (Hesketh et al., 2000; National Clearinghouse, 2000). It is common to see that children also accept these beliefs.

Physical abuse in developed countries

Children suffer physical abuse from four major groups: parents, teachers, other children and outsiders. Working children have a high probability of being abused by their employer or supervisor.

The reported incidence and severity of physical abuse by parents tends to vary considerably in the world. This is partly objective reality and partly the result of inadequate or dishonest record keeping. Many experts share the opinion that physical abuse is more common than sexual abuse. Data registered by authorities are much lower than those based on

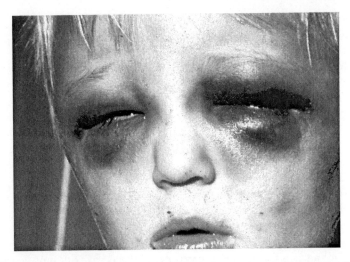

Photo 10. **Abused boy.** *Eye trauma resulting from direct blows to the face. Credit: Dr Barton Schmitt, Volcano Press, USA.*

sample surveys. In the OECD countries the number of reported cases of child abuse and neglect has risen, reflecting increasing awareness of the issue (Innocenti, 2003): in the USA, reporting increased five-fold over a period of twenty years. A 1997 federal law in the United States establishes the rights of parents physically to punish their children (Dietz, 2000). The US Prosecutor's Research Office has, however, in 2004 produced some guidelines for the courts (Vieth, 2004).

They state:

- Parental license to discipline is not a license to maim a child.
- Spanking preceded by an explanation of the infraction and followed by an affirmation of parental love looks like discipline. Take away an explanation of the infraction, take away the affirmation of love, and the conduct looks less like discipline. Add a litany of derogatory insults hurled at the child and a pattern and location of injuries unexpected from a spanking, and the picture of child abuse develops.

Teachers play a large role in physical punishment. According to the National Coalition to Abolish Corporal Punishment in Schools, 342,038 US schoolchildren were hit by teachers in 2000. In Canada, the Criminal Code allows 'reasonable' force on the part of a teacher or a parent as a disciplinary measure. A Mexican code reads: 'Persons exerting legal tutoring have the faculty to moderately correct and punish their children.'

McCormick showed in 1992 that 67 per cent of primary health care physicians and paediatricians sampled in the USA approve the use of physical punishment. Countries with poverty and lower general-education levels practise abuse of children more than the richer ones. In the USA, children living below the poverty level experience twice as much reported abuse than those above that level. Half of those investigated by the US Child Protection Services live in welfare-supported families. To beat children is seen by many parents as 'part of the normal upbringing'. In OECD countries 20–75 per cent of women report that their husbands beat them regulalry (Innocenti, 2003). Some of these countries are outside the Western sphere, and have higher rates. Severe physical abuse of intimate partners is noticeable not just among poor people and it often has severe traumatic effects on children: in many developing countries, 'wives' are as young as 12 years. When there is physical abuse of women, there is most often physical abuse of children. Small-scale studies of child physical abuse have been published for Bosnia-Herzegovina (Nikšić and Kurspahić-Mujcić, 2007) and Poland (Witanowska et al., 2002). More data appear in Tables 7.2 and 7.3.

Physical abuse in developing countries

Very high incidence numbers of 'childbeating' were found in Nicaragua: 69 per cent (Ellsberg, 2000); Papua New Guinea: 67 per cent (Johnson and Ambihaipahar, 1999); Turkey: 58 per cent (Dietz, 2000); and Kuwait: 86 per cent (Qasem, 1998). Most abuse, even when the health consequences are very serious, is never reported to the police and the perpetrator is virtually assured of impunity. Immigrants might 'travel with or inherit' their ethnic attitudes and behaviours, originating in their 'root' countries. Ferrari (2002) compared 150 parents in the USA of Hispanic, African and European descent. A history of childhood abuse was found to be predictive of the use of both physical and verbal punishment by mothers, but not for fathers. Cultural factors/beliefs were predictive of fathers' parenting behaviours, but not mothers'. Ethnicity, as a demographic variable, continued to be a significant predictor of parenting behaviours and attitudes for all parents, controlling for cultural factors. Hesketh et al. (2000) published a questionnaire-based study about the views and experiences of 331 paediatricians and nurses, made in eight hospitals in two provinces in Eastern China, one rather wealthy and one very poor. The response rate was 98 per cent. None of them had any training in the recognition and management of child abuse. When asked about their professional experiences of clinically observed child abuse, almost none was mentioned. Eighty-six per cent would not consider it to be child abuse when faced with an injured child. Almost all believed that physical punishment is widely used by Chinese parents and half of the respondents stated that beating as punishment was acceptable at any age.

Community violence is common in developing countries: fist fights and use of guns, knives, machetes and other hand weapons are very common. In some parts of the world – such as the border between Chad and Sudan – not only men, but also women, carry knives with them all the time 'for their own defence' (Helander, 2003). A UNICEF study in Somalia (Helander, 1988) (before the civil war) covered four district hospitals, each of them serving about 100,000 people. The author states that 'it was surprising to find that in the hospital records dating two years back, the only patients admitted for treatment in the hospital consisted of hundreds of cases listed as "wounds" (dhawac). The hospital staff described these "wounds" as resulting from domestic violence and other forms of community fighting. Other patients coming to the hospital had not been admitted as in-patients.' Witnessing such family and community violence is traumatic to children's health.

Awareness of violence is increasing in the developing countries. The level of abuse of all types in the developing countries will eventually be identified as being on the same or on a higher level compared to the 'affluent' nations. Small-scale studies of childhood physical abuse have been published from Bahrain (Al-Mahroos et al., 2005), Cambodia (Nelson and Zimmermann, 1996), Ghana (Forjuoh, 1995), Kenya (Sukjumbe and Bwibo, 1993), Kuwait (Al-Moosa et al., 2003), Mexico (Baker et al., 2005), Nigeria (Chianu, 2000) and Palau (Collier, 1999). Some studies were presented in Box 2.1 (p. 31) and more appear in Table 7.3 (Combined abuse, pp. 111–15).

Emotional/psychological abuse

Emotional/psychological abuse of children is difficult to research because it is not easy to detect, assess and substantiate; a great deal of it goes unreported. It is, however, probably the most prevalent of all forms of abuse. Several authors state that emotional abuse is often more destructive than other abuse.

The Canada Department of Health (1995) survey of women found that 36 per cent had experienced emotional abuse while growing up. In the Kaiser study (Felitti et al., 1998), 11 per cent of the responders had been

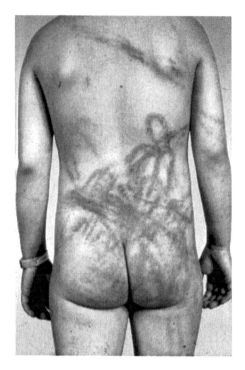

Photo 11.   **Whip injury.** *This 10-year-old child was beaten with a braided rope. Credit: Dr James Williams, Volcano Press, USA.*

psychologically abused as children at home. Scher et al. (2004) report from a US representative community adult sample (98 per cent response) a prevalence of 34 per cent of childhood emotional abuse and emotional neglect. In the national India study (Kacker, 2007) the emotional abuse rates for children aged 5–18 was 50 per cent for both boys and girls. The WorldSAFE study (WHO, 2002) reveals the following examples of psychological punishment by the mother during the last six months: (a) yelled or screamed at her child: Chile 84 per cent, Egypt 72 per cent, India 70 per cent, Philippines 62 per cent, and USA 85 per cent; (b) cursed at the child: Egypt 51 per cent, USA 24 per cent; (c) threatened to kick the child out of the household: Philippines 26 per cent; (d) threatened abandonment: Egypt 10 per cent, India 20 per cent, Philippines 48 per cent; (e) threatened with evil spirits: Egypt 12 per cent, India 20 per cent, Philippines 24 per cent; (f) locked the child out of the household: Philippines 12 per cent.

Table 7.2 Prevalence of physical abuse, selected studies

Country Authors	Type of study	Results
Canada Macmillan et al. 1997	Community sample of 9.953	31% (severe 11%) of males and 21% (severe 9%) of females physically abused.
Chile Vargas et al. 1995	Sample of children and parents in (1) state and (2) private schools	80% of parents in group (1) and 57% in group (2) admitted child battering; mothers were leading abusers. Children reported parental physical abuse: 86% in state and 54% in private schools.
Egypt Youssef et al. 1998a, 1998b	2,401 high school pupils, aged 11–20, parents' and teachers' behaviour studied	38% severely punished by parents; of those, 26% reported fractures, loss of consciousness, concussion, and permanent disability. In 25% the victims required medical consultation. The risk of corporal punishment increased with low parental education, unskilled father, father's use of alcohol, living in cramped quarters, and constant fights and quarrels among family members. 80% of the boys and 62% of the girls incurred physical punishment from their teachers. 26% of the boys and 18% of the girls suffered injuries (contusions, fractures, and loss of consciousness).
Ethiopia Ketsela and Kebede 1997	Sample of 649 school- children: parental punishment	78% of all schoolchildren physically punished; 21% urban and 64% rural children reported bruises and swelling, only 6% visited a health centre.
Germany Pfeifer et al. 1999	Sample 14,000 pupils age 15–16	During the last 12 months, 15% had been subjected to physical abuse.
Great Britain Leach 1999	London Maternity service, clinical sample	97% of all 4-year-olds were physically punished, half of them more than once a week. 25% of these children were regularly hit with straps or canes.

(Continued)

Table 7.2 (Continued)

Country Authors	Type of study	Results
Hong Kong Tang 1998	1019 children under 16, selected randomly	Minor physical violence 53%, severe battering to 46%. Highest rate of severe violence among boys aged 3–6, mainly by mothers. These findings 'can be understood in light of the cultural values concerning parent-child relation and child-rearing practices in contemporary Chinese societies; filial piety obliges parents to assert authority and inflict punishment.'
India Segal 1995	Selected sample of 319 adult professionals Interviews and test instruments	57% had been engaged in 'normal physical violence,' 42% in abusive behaviours, and 3% in extremely violent behaviours with their children.
Israel Benbenitshty et al. 2002	Representative sample of 5,472 students aged 9–12 years. Scale for physical and psychological maltreatment	Physical and psychological maltreatment by school staff recorded. 33% reported emotional maltreatment, 22% at least one instance of physical maltreatment. Most vulnerable: males, students in Arab schools and in schools with low-income and low-education families.
Jamaica Gardner et al. 2003	1,710 randomly selected secondary school children	33% had been victims of violence and 60% had family members who had been victims of violence. 82% thought that violent television could increase aggressive behaviour.
Republic of Korea Hahm et al. 2001	Population study	67% of the parents had whipped their children, and 45% had kicked, hit or beaten them.
Spain Paúl et al. 1995	Under-graduate students sample	29% physically abused before age 13; 7.5% had injuries.
Thailand Isaranurug et al. 2002	Sample of 212 sixth grade students	95% violently treated by parents, 77% beaten by cane or belt. 95% emotional (scolded using rude language) violence.

(*Continued*)

Table 7.2   (Continued)

Country Authors	Type of study	Results
Turkey Bilir et al. 1998	16,000 children	36% physically abused before age 5.
USA Flisher et al. 1997	Community sample of 660 9–17-year-olds and caretakers in New York and Puerto Rico	26% of the sample physically abused.
USA Trocme and Lindsey, 1996	Population sample	94% of 3–4 year old children smacked, spanked, or beaten. 40% of children aged 13 were regularly hit; at 15, 25% were still hit or beaten by their parents.
USA Straus and Stewart, 1999	Nationally representative sample	Parents hit 35% of infants, 94% of 3–4-year-olds, 50% of 12–year-olds, 33% of 14 year-olds an average of six times a year. Severe hitting (with a belt or a paddle) was 28% between ages 5–12.
USA Holmes and Sammel, 2005	Random sample of 298 men	51% had a history of childhood physical abuse, 73% were abused by parent.
Database study, Europe Lampe, 2002	MEDLINE, PubMed, Psyndex, Psycinfo	Physical abuse ranged from 5% to 50%. There were large differrences in definitions and data gathering techniques.
Study of 19 countries Douglas and Straus, 2006	Study of 9549 students in 36 universities	56% (range 13–73%) corporally punished by parents. Rate of partner assault 30%; partner injury 7%. Students who had experienced high rates of corporal punishment showed higher rates of assaulting and injuring a dating partner.

While frequently applying psychological and emotional abuse, schoolteachers in many developing countries cause great harm. Community abuse is often directed towards immigrants, and members of minority ethnic and religious groups.

Nhundu and Shumba (2001) studied teacher behaviour in Zimbabwe. They revealed a high incidence of 'belittling, absence of a positive

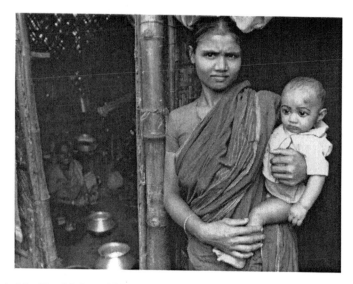

Photo 12.   **Head injury.** *This poor family lives in a peri-urban slum area. The child has been hit on the head by the father © World Health Organization.*

emotional atmosphere, verbal abuse, shouting, scolding, use of vulgar language, humiliation and negative labeling of pupils, and terrorizing of pupils by teachers'. The female teachers were the main perpetrators. In a representative sample of 202 residents aged 16–25 in Bangkok, 32 per cent reported emotional abuse (Jirapramukpitak et al., 2005).

Combined physical and psychological abuse by peers and siblings includes name-calling, hitting, pushing, social exclusion, threats, bullying and theft. An often cited estimate of bullying is that 50 per cent of children aged 6–10, and 25 per cent of children aged 11–16 get bullied regularly. Other estimates suggest that one child in seven is bullied, and that 85 per cent of that bullying is by peers. WHO's Global School-based Health Survey (2003), based on data from fifteen developing countries in 2003, assessed that 20–65 per cent of all children were bullied during the last thirty days. In this study, reporting from thirty-five countries in Europe and North America, WHO found that on average 34 per cent of all 11–15-year-olds were bullied during the previous few months. Many children have at some time experienced such abuse; in some countries, this abuse may be daily and less vulnerable persons may perhaps think that it is 'normal'. However, others may suffer and show withdrawal and depression or may commit suicide.

Care neglect

Care-giver neglect is the most common reason for registration by social child-protection agencies in the developed countries. In the USA (US Department of Health and Human Services, 2007) in 2005, 63 per cent of all registered cases (which are just 1 per cent of the population) concerned neglect. The parents or care-takers failed to provide the daily needs for food, clothing, accommodation, schooling, appropriate education at home, health care, security, and/or a 'moral' and healthy environment. Neglectful parents are not a homogeneous group. Among them are, for example, teenage mothers who may have been thrown out of their parents' homes, parents with substance dependence, indifferent parents with unwanted children, mentally ill parents, families living in unsafe conditions, care-giver in prison, parents exposed to domestic violence, and families living in poverty or with low economic status often in combination with unemployment. Some neglect is intentional, but most is circumstantial.

Parents of neglected children may have their parental rights suspended or terminated. In several developed countries, some 2–10 per 1,000 children are annually taken into care for these reasons. Such public action is rare in the developing countries.

In the USA approximately 1.3 to 1.5 million, or 2 per cent of the national population under 18, run away or are thrown out of home by their parents each year; many of them are neglected and/or abused, and some are killed. Some population data about neglect are available: Romania 11 per cent (Roturo, 1996); in the UK (Cawson et al., 2000) 18 per cent of respondents had experienced some absence of care in their childhood and 20 per cent had experienced less than adequate supervision.

The prevalence of care-giver neglect is high in many poor countries. Such neglect was studied in a random sample of 1,164 children in China (Pan et al., 2005): 28 per cent of children aged 3–6 years were neglected, boys more than girls, and the highest prevalence was in single parent families (43 per cent). In other studies the figures are: Brazil: 26 per cent (Gonçales et al., 1999); Iran (Sheikhattari et al., 2006): neglect at home 83 per cent, at school 66 per cent; Kenya (African Network, 2000): 22 per cent of all children reported intentional parental neglect.

Straus and Savage (2005) reported on the prevalence of neglectful behaviour by parents of university students in seventeen countries (six in Europe, USA and Canada, two in Latin America, five in Asia, Australia and New Zealand). Between 3.2 per cent and 36 per cent (median

12 per cent) of the sample reported neglect. It should be noted that university students rarely come from poor families.

Structural neglect (see p. 21) is not caused by the care-givers. It is closely related to poverty; in the developing countries there are about 1,000 million severely neglected, poor children. Most experience bad housing, many are without clean, safe water and sanitation. Some 130 million do not attend school at all, and for most of those who do, the quality of education is low. About 350 million are malnourished because of lack of food. One-quarter of all children do not have access to primary health care. In many such countries 20 per cent of all children die before the age of 5. Structural poverty with neglect also exists in the more developed countries; there its combined prevalence may be estimated at 100–200 million. The overwhelming majority of child neglect is structural, and is massive. A detailed review appears in Chapters 12 and 13.

Economic abuse and exploitation

Economic abuse or exploitation of an underage child includes work, services or other activities benefiting a person who is in a position of responsibility, trust or power, or has authority over the person abused. Descriptions and prevalence data appear in Chapter 5.

Combined abuse and neglect

Combined abuse and neglect is common; it appears that sexual and physical abuse are sometimes combined and accompanied by verbal psychological abuse and neglect.

There are few numerical studies showing the combinations of sexual, physical and psychological abuse. One such study of partner abuse was published by Ellsberg et al. (2000) from Nicaragua. Among 360 women, 263 had been abused. The most common form was psychological, reported by 257; 77 of the women had experienced a combination with sexual abuse and 109 with physically abuse, and 74 with both. There was an overlap between physical and sexual abuse: of 188 physically abused women, 74 had also been sexually abused. Abuse of pregnant women may cause damage to the foetus with serious consequences (Chapter 9). In the USA, American Indians, Alaskan natives and African Americans have a higher combined abuse and neglect rate than the white population (National Clearinghouse, 2000). A description of combined physical and emotional abuse in Palestine appears in Box 7.2.

Box 7.2: Combined abuse in occupied Palestine

Haj-Yahia and Abdo-Kaloti (2003) published results of research on combined psychological and physical abuse in Palestine using a convenience sample of 1,185 students from thirteen private Palestinian secondary schools in the West Bank and Jerusalem. The main findings were that 37 per cent of children had witnessed their fathers cursing the mother, using abusive language, or calling the mother names and threatening to hit her. Thirty-one per cent had witnessed their fathers slapping, pushing or kicking the mother, or attacking her continuously with a stick, club or other harmful objects. During their adolescence, 37 per cent of the participants had witnessed their fathers ridiculing and attacking the ideas of their mothers, and cursing them for being a failure. Twenty-five per cent had witnessed their fathers throwing, smashing, hitting and kicking something while attacking their mothers, or saw their fathers strangle or trying to strangle their mothers. The lower the father's education, the greater was the likelihood that the mother had been psychologically and physically abused. Participants living in rural areas, or in refugee camps, reported more father-to-mother abuse than those living in urban areas. The more the families were exposed to political stressors, the more the fathers abused the mothers.

In an analysis of mother-to-father violence during childhood, 11 per cent of the participants had witnessed their mothers threatening to hit, or throwing something at, the father, and 27 per cent witnessed the mother ridiculing the father and accusing him of being a failure. Eight per cent of the participants had witnessed the mothers slapping, pushing, kicking, attacking or shoving the father. During their adolescence, 38 per cent of participants had witnessed the mothers arguing heatedly with the fathers, and yelling or doing something to insult him; 5 per cent indicated that they had witnessed their mothers throwing, smashing or kicking something on/at their fathers; and 3 per cent had witnessed their mothers strangling or trying to strangle their fathers.

The student participants and their siblings in over 50 per cent of cases reported that their parents had argued heatedly with them and their siblings, cursing them, using abusive language, calling them names and yelling at them, or doing something to insult them. Forty per cent had been threatened with direct physical attacks; 19 per cent reported that the parents had threatened them and their siblings with a knife, a gun, a stick, a chair, or with some other kind of injurious or lethal weapon. Thirty-five per cent had witnessed the parents attacking their children continuously with a stick, club or other harmful object. The lower the income of the family, the poorer the housing conditions, and the lower the level of education of the parents, the more elevated and frequent became the psychological and physical abuse.

In Palestine, the combined effects of occupation, military and civil violence, poverty and unemployment have led to widespread frustrations, and to the breakdown of many intra-familial relations (see Khamis, 2000: Table 7.3). Physical and verbal aggression are at extremely high levels. Haj-Yahia and Tamish (2001) have researched sexual abuse in another article, and shown that such abuse among Palestinian children living in Israel was very high, especially among boys, and exceeded the prevalence among Jewish Israeli teenagers. Similar situations exist in other countries with high population stress.

Child death caused by violence and neglect

In 2000, throughout the world there were an estimated 57,000 homicides of children under the age of 15 (WHO, 2002). Infanticide still goes on in the industrialized countries, as evidenced by Innocenti (2003), Glass (1999), and Southall et al. (1997). Fatal violence against children aged under 5 in high-income countries is estimated at 2.2/100,000 boys and 1.8/100,000 girls. In low- to middle-income countries, the rates are two to three times higher. The highest homicide rates for children under the age of 5 are in Africa: 17.9/100,000 boys and 12.7/100,000 girls. All child murders are under-reported (Innocenti, 2003).

In a report of 459 forensic autopsies of battered children (aged 0–4) by the Japan Society of Legal Medicine (1995) it was found that the cause of death was head injures in 35 per cent, suffocation 8 per cent, strangulation 7 per cent and drowning 7 per cent. Among the assailants were the biological mother in 49 per cent of the cases, the biological father in 16 per cent and a stepfather in 10 per cent. The battered children were emaciated and had stunted growth in 31 per cent; there were abrasions and bruises in 32 per cent, numerous internal injuries (bowels, liver and lungs), subdural haematoma in 32 per cent, oedema in 17 per cent, and thymus atrophy in 13 per cent. Some of the murdered children

Table 7.3 Combined abuse and neglect, selected studies

Country Authors	Type of study and comments	Results
Arab peninsula Al-Mahroos 2007	Reports from professional contacts about observed physical and sexual abuse and severe neglect, some of it combined	27 cases from Kuwait, 11 from Saudi Arabia, 5 from Oman, 150 from Bahrain. Yemeni population-based surveys revealed widespread use of corporal punishment and cruelty to children, ranging from 51%–81%. Child abuse is ignored or may even be tolerated; abused children continue to suffer, most abusers go free, and unpunished. Very difficult to break silence, respond to and prevent child abuse and neglect.
Brazil Gonçales et al. 1999	976 children from Rio exposed to domestic violence	39% exposed to physical abuse, 26% to neglect, 26% to psychological abuse, and 7% to sexual abuse; 44% referred to Court.
Canada Trocme et al. 2002	Representative sample of 7,672 officially reported child maltreatment investigations (total 135,573, = 2.2% of all children)	Maltreatment was substantiated in 45% of the investigations and in an additional 22% remainned suspected. Causes for investigation: physical abuse (31%), sexual abuse (11%), neglect (46%), emotional maltreatment (37%), extreme veral abuse (13%). Many children suffered from combinations.
Haiti Martsolf 2004	Study of 258 outpatients, study included five types of child maltreatment	60% of the women and 86% of the men reported at least one type of childhood maltreatment at the moderate to severe level. Of the total sample, 54% had scores indicative of major depression and 44% reported an average score of 'somewhat bothered' by 37 physical symptoms.
India Kacker, Ministry of Women and Child Development 2007	Multistage purposive sampling design. Questionnaire used. Total sample 18,200, response rate 96% Included (i) children aged 5–18 in five groups: (a) living	Children: physical abuse 73% of boys, 65% of girls; by mothers 51%, by fathers 38% by others 11%. In 15% the abuse resulted in swelling or bleeding or causing serious physical injury to the child; sexual abuse 48% of boys, 39% of

(Continued)

Table 7.3 (Continued)

Country Authors	Type of study and comments	Results
	with family not in school; (b) living with family in school; (c) in institutional care; (d) working; (e) on the street;	girls; emotional abuse 50% of boys, 50% of girls. Only minor differences between the five child groups. 65% of children going to school were physically abused there. In institutions the caregivers are often the abusers. The prevalence of sexual abuse was higher in upper and middle classes compared to the lower classes. The majority of the abusers were known to the child. 21% suffered severe sexual abuse, more boys than girls.
	(ii) Adults aged 18–24; rate of abuse before age 18	Adults: physical abuse 53% of men, 47% of women; sexual abuse 61% of men, 41% of women; emotional abuse 51% of men, 49% of women.
	(iii) Stakeholders: older persons, working, mostly parents	45% of stakeholders felt that physical punishment was necessary. The most suitable forms of punishments suggested by them were: scolding and shouting 35%, slapping, beating with a stick 11%, locking up the child and denying food 11%. 32% said that children should work.
Iran Sheikhattari et al. 2006	Sample of 1,370 school students aged 11–18	Physical maltreatment at home 40%, at school 44%; mental maltreatment at home 78%, at school 66%; neglect at home 83%, at school 66%. Rural children more maltreated than urban, females less than males.
Israel Khuory-Kassbri 2006	Nationally representative sample of 17,465 Students in grades 4–11, 9% attrition. Report of school staff abuse	Primary schools: 31% emotionnal and 24% physical abuse; Junior high schools: 35% emotional, 25% physical, 8% sexual abuse. High schools 35% emotional, 18% physical and 8% sexual abuse. Sexual abuse of boys (9.7%) higher than of girls (6.4%). Arab students much more abused than Jewish.

(Continued)

Table 7.3 (Continued)

Country Authors	Type of study and comments	Results
Israel Elbedour et al. 2006	217 Bedouin-Arab female high school students, aged 14–18 years	During last month at least once had been physically abused by father 37%, by mother, (44%) by siblings 44% at least once during the previous month. Psychological abuse by family members 50%. Sexual abuse 31%; in addition 16% requests for sex, which are considered abusive in this culture.
Palestine Khamis 2000	1000 Palestinian school children aged 12–16. Of these, 6% had a physical or sensory disability, 12% were working.	14% had been physically abused by a family member. 24% affected by the political violence, (a family member killed, injured, imprisoned, or their homes demolished by the occupying forces). 9 children reported sexual abuse. Children living with a single parent less abused than those with two parents at home. Disabled children more abused than non-disabled. Economic hardship was a significant cause. Psychological maltreatment was less common where families followed traditional values: dominance by the men and submission by the women, children more obedient and submissive to authority. The overwhelming effects of the political situation were clear.
Portugal Machado et al. 2007	Representative sample of 2,391 parents Portugal in two-parent families with children under-18.	26% reported at least one act of emotional or physical abuse towards a child during the previous year; 12% was physical and 22% emotional. The self-reported support for physical punishment was higher in parents who reported using abusive behaviour.
Romania Rotoru 1996	488 parents and 796 school pupils in Romania were studied.	14% reported verbal aggression; 16% of the parents admitted such abuse. 28% of the pupils said they

(Continued)

114

Table 7.3   (Continued)

Country Authors	Type of study and comments	Results
		had been physically punished and 23% reported severe punishment. Parents admitted to administering physical punishment in 26% and severe in 22%. 11% of the children said they had been neglected, 9% of the parents admitted such neglect. In rural areas, abuse and neglect more common than in urban.
Russia Berrien et al. 1995	Sample of 412 children aged 11–16 in a school for 'intellectually talented children' in Siberia, drop-out rate 9%	29% severely physically abused by parents, 4% required medical attention. 46% had witnessed abuse of other children. For 98% punishment included psychological distress, restrictions, strict verbal reprimand, and enforced labour; 2.4% refused to stay in parents' home.
South Africa Madu 2001	559 high school children aged about 13–16	Self reported prevalence rates of abuse: 71% were psychologically abused (14% extreme), 27% physically abused, 35% emotionally abused and 10% ritually abused. It appeared that these various forms of abuse are widespread, suggesting that a much more serious problem may exist than has been recognised.
Turkey Vahíp and Doğanavşargil 2006	Combined community studies	Physical violence in 36% of families, verbal violence in 53%, 46% of all children physically abused. 72% of women subjected to psychological, physical or sexual violence during past and present pregnancies.
USA US Department of Health and Human Services 2007	National data, based on reports from 2005 (3.6 million children: 1.2% of the population reported)	62.8% of victims experienced neglect, 16.6% physical abuse, 9.3% sexual abuse, 7.1% psychological maltreatment, and 2% medical neglect. In addition, 14.3% of victims experienced other types of maltreatment such as abandonment, threats of harm to the child, or congenital drug addiction.

(Continued)

Table 7.3 (Continued)

Country Authors	Type of study and comments	Results
USA Scher et al. 2004	Representative community sample of 9000 adult men and women, aged 18–65. Telephone interviews using a Childhood Trauma Questionnaire, 98% response rate	35.1% (men 41%, women 30%) of the sample met criteria for at least one form of childhood maltreatment; 13.5% (men 13%, women 14%) met criteria for more than one form. Most common: physical abuse and physical neglect (42%), and emotional abuse and emotional neglect (34%), sexual abuse 15%; many co-occurring. Persons with no schooling or elementary education compared to college educated have significantly higher odds ratios for emotional neglect (3.63) and for physical neglect (2.47).
USA American armed forces Rosen and Martin 1996	Sample of 1,060 male and 305 female soldiers (mean age 26 years)	49% of women and 15% of men reported a childhood history of sexual abuse. 48% of the women and 50% of the men had a history of physical abuse. 34% of females and 11% of males had experienced both.
USA Finkelhor et al. 2005, 2007	Nationally representative sample of 2,030 children and youth aged 2 to 17 years	53% were victims of physical assault in the study year; 27% of a property offence; 14% of child maltreatment; 8% of sexual victimization; 36% had witnessed violence or experienced another form of indirect victimization. Only 29% had no direct or indirect victimization. The mean number of victimizations for a child or youth was 3. A child or youth with one victimization had a 69% chance of another during a single year. Children experiencing four or more different kinds of victimization in a single year (poly-victims) comprised 22% of the sample. Results suggest that cumulative exposure to multiple forms of victimization over a child's life-course represents a substantial source of mental health risk.

were mentally retarded, in others the disability was induced by long-term cruelty, abuse and neglect.

In several African countries, I was informed about the practice of putting newborn babies to death by starvation on the advice of the traditional midwife (Amoako, 1976). Most of these babies were visibly deformed or were a younger twin (twins are in some countries seen as a bad omen). Killing, by neglect or abuse, a yet-to-be-named infant appears to be socially acceptable among very poor families, who already have 'too many mouths to feed'. Laime (1997), in a Peruvian rural study, followed twenty-three local children under the age of 7 over one year. Young children are thought to have 'loose body–soul connections', making them vulnerable to diseases. Traditional health concepts such as 'uraña' (fright) explain the deaths among children – caused by neglect – in a 'culturally acceptable' way.

From Senegal, Menick (2000) reviewed 164 cases of infanticide diagnosed over twenty-seven years. Infanticide was caused by mothers with mental disorders in only 3 per cent of cases. The main reason for the killing by Muslim mothers was that they were unmarried, and in their families a pregnancy before the wedding was dishonourable. Attitudes of rejection are similar in Christian and Hindu families in many other developing countries. Another reason for child murder by married mothers was that the husband was away abroad working, sometimes for several years, and children whom he had not fathered were unwelcome.

Kassim et al. (1995) report on childhood deaths caused by physical abuse in Malaysia: 766 cases were registered by the authorities, the average age of children being 2 years and 5 months. Most frequent causes of death were intra-cranial haemorrhage and intra-abdominal trauma. The traumas were all very severe: perforated intestines, liver rupture, aorta rupture, strangulation, cervical and skull fractures, poisoning; two newborns died after having been thrown into the river.

In most poor countries, little official attention is paid to the causes of children's deaths. Most are buried next day. Few pathologists are available to examine suspicious deaths. The data in Table 7.4 reflect the negative attitudes among parents towards girls in some Asian countries and the lack of any community programme to help them (Fikree and Pasha, 2004). The table compares the male to female infant population from censuses in five Asian countries. The extremely high male to female ratios for Harayana and Punjab are the highest recorded in the world (Premi, 2001; Ravamudan, 2003).

An estimated 40 million females are 'missing' in China's population statistics (Coale and Banister, 1994). Gendercide and fatal child

Table 7.4   Male/female ratio in Asian countries recorded as live births

Country/age group	Males to females %, total
Bangladesh 1988 (0–1)	107.0
China 1930–1940 (0–1)	118.0
1982 (0–1)	107.6
1999 (0–1)	119.5
India 1970 (0–1)	106.6
2001 (0–6)	107.9
Harayana & Punjab 2000	126.1
Pakistan 1988 (0–1)	109.0
World total 2000 (0–4)	104.6

Source: UN population data 2002.

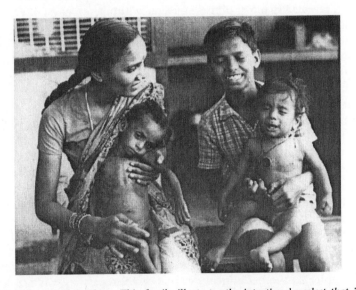

Photo 13. **Child neglect.** *This family illustrates the intentional neglect that is a common experience for girls and the reason why so many of them die before the age of 5. This Indian mother and her older son are holding 2-year-old twins, the well-fed twin brother to the right and the seriously malnourished twin sister to the left of the photo.* © World Health Organization.

neglect are common in many countries; girls and children with a disability are common victims. Among those responsible for these losses are 'orphanages' and other 'child protection institutions'. A preference for boys can be seen, for instance, in China where 85 per cent of children sent to 'orphanages' are girls (Chan, 1995; Croll, 2001; Lavely, 2001). In Japan during 1980–90, 191 newborn infants were abandoned in coin-operated lockers in the railway stations (Kouno and Johnson, 1995); when found most were dead.

The same preference for sons is very visible in India; this is accompanied by an excessive mortality among girl infants, and selective abortion as soon as the gender of the unborn child is known (Allahbadia, 2002; Arnold et al., 1998). Thousands of newborns – especially girls – in South and South-East Asia are abandoned behind bushes, with the rubbish, in suitcases, in trains, in the forest, on the steps of orphanages or drowned. In India there are many reports that indicate filicide through neglect. The highest number comes from the Kallar community, Tamil Nadu. An average 1,200 children are born annually in this area, and of those, some 600 are girls. The government hospital made a study which revealed that 570 of these girls die within a few days; physicians attributed this to maternal filicide (Sabu, 1997).

The under-5 mortality rate in 2005 was 89/1000 in the developing countries, more than twenty times higher than in the most developed countries (Sweden 3.4/1000 – in 1930 it was 59/1000 – equivalent to the average of what is now reported by the developing countries 75 years later). Of the 110 million children born annually at present in developing countries, at least 9 per cent die before the age of 5, which equals 10 million a year. Many deaths (estimated at 40 per cent, which includes gendercide, neglected and disabled children) are caused by abuse and avoidable neglect.

Violence experienced by disabled children

A review follows of the violence against a very vulnerable group: children with disabilities most of whom live with their family. The methodological difficulties in analysing the prevalence of disability were described in Chapter 2. Another difficulty is that disabled persons may not have fully understood that they have been victims of abuse or neglect during their childhood. Some of them, such as those who have severe mental retardation, speech impairments, deafness or autism, may not be able to communicate their experience of violence. Prevalence assessments are constrained by the fact that many, especially girls in the developing countries, die very young. The assessments below are based on available scientific surveys, official data (reports to the police or authorities), and my own observations and examinations of children. Most underestimate the problems. Some studies are made on non-representative samples, are convenience studies or are 'anecdotal'. Some of those interviewed have been asked to complete questionnaires under the supervision of persons who were the offenders and they may not have dared to tell the truth. More comprehensive data gathering is needed.

Prevalence of violence against disabled children

There are a number of scientific studies of the prevalence of violence against children with disabilities. Govindshenoy and Spencer (2007) reviewed all population-based studies published from 1996–2006 and concluded that the evidence base for an association of disability with abuse and neglect is weak. Children with disabilities are seen by most researchers as exposed to an increased risk compared to normal children. Table 7.5 shows the results from ten studies, almost all from the USA. I have been unable to find any published population study of childhood abuse and neglect of children with disabilities from developing countries.

Sobsey and co-workers (Sobsey and Varnhagen, 1990; Sobsey and Doe, 1991; Sobsey et al., 1995; Sobsey, 2000) published detailed studies about violence and abuse in the lives of people with disabilities. Maltreatment occurs during the victims' childhood. Sobsey (2000), in a convenience sample of 152 people with disabilities, found that 60 per cent had experienced penetrative sex, 62 per cent had been abused ten times or more, 42 per cent had physical injuries after the abuse, 95 per cent of the victims reported emotional problems, and 58 per cent were infected with sexually transmitted disease. Half of them were under 21 when the abuse started: 36 per cent 7–17 years old, and 7 per cent 1–6 years old. Eighty-three per cent were females and 17 per cent males. Sobsey et al. (1995) found that the following factors contributed to vulnerability: 32 per cent inadequate knowledge or impaired judgement, 24 per cent lack of assertiveness or too much compliance, and 13 per cent too much trust in others. For 67 per cent the abuse occurred at home and for 11 per cent it occurred in the vehicles used for their transportation to programmed activities; 20 per cent took place in institutions that the victims visited because of their participation in rehabilitation programmes. The offenders had an average age of 34 years; some were as young as 10 and some over 80; 89 per cent were male. The victims knew 90 per cent of the offenders. Only 20 per cent were family members, 49 per cent paid caregivers. Some offenders had abused up to 70 people before arrest. Only 25 per cent of sexual abuse cases involving people with DD were ever reported, Non-disclosure promotes an environment ready for continued victimization. Only 8 per cent of the offenders were convicted.

Table 7.5   Violence against children with disabilities, selected studies

Country Author	Groups researched for childhood violence	Prevalence
USA Ammerman et al. 1989	Multi-handicapped children in two US psychiatric institutions	39% sexually abused
USA Zigler 1979	Mentally retarded (MR) children	45% extensive physical abuse or neglect
USA Sullivan et al. 1991	Deaf boys and deaf girls	54% childhood sexual abuse of boys and 50% of girls
USA Chamberlain et al. 1984	Adolescent girls with MR	25% sexually abused
USA Tharinger et al. 1990	Sexual abuse and exploitation of children and adults with MR and other handicaps	88% exploited, most during childhood, 35% girls had physical evidence of sexual abuse, 6% were sexually assaulted, 6% got sexually transmitted disease
USA Welbourne et al. 1983	Blind females	50% sexually abused, mostly during childhood
Sweden Lundqvist et al. 2004	Mentally ill women in therapy	25% to 77% experienced childhood sexual abuse
USA American Academy of Pediatrics 2001	Review of maltreatment of children with disabilities	Children with disabilities are 1.8 times more likely to be neglected, 1.6 times more likely to be physically abused and 2.2 times more likely to be sexually abused
USA Valenti-Hein and Schwartz 1995	Persons with developmental disabilities (DD)	90% will experience sexual abuse, mostly before age 18. 49% will experience 10 or more abusive incidents
Sullivan and Knutson 2000a	Population study (merger of school and official social and police records) of 46,900 children, 8% (3,262) had a disability	Rate of maltreatment among disabled children 31%; among the non-disabled 11%. 84% neglect, 49% physical abuse and 9% sexual abuse (many combined). Victims: behaviour disorder (53%), speech/language problems (37%), mental

(Continued)

Table 7.5 (Continued)

Country Author	Groups researched for childhood violence	Prevalence
		retardation (28%). Neglect, physical abuse, emotional abuse and sexual abuse were about four times higher than among non-disabled. Maltreatment started in preschool (29%), elementary school (35%), middle school (23%), and high school (13%). Most perpetrators were family members. The study is likely under-reporting, as some disabled children are not in school and official records are incomplete.

The New York State Office of Mental Health (1989) reported on child abuse at a children's psychiatric centre. Over several years many young children (aged 5–12) were engaged in sexual activity with other children; these incidents occurred and persisted because of deficient management, clinical and supervisory practices at the facility. Many disabled children are regularly teased or bullied at school by other children, especially if they are small and weak.

Violence against children with disabilities in developing countries

In the developing nations, there are few children as maltreated as those with disabilities. Exact information from these countries is seldom available; one has to rely on informal information. I have interviewed responsible administrators and professionals in some fifty developing countries and they have all confirmed that such abuse is very common, especially in boarding institutions and special schools. The Secretary (top civil servant) of the Union Ministry of Social Welfare in India told me that in his country this was the most abused group. Sexual abuse is often combined with other physical and psychological abuse, intimidation, threats, bullying and, when possible, with economic exploitation. Some articles have been published from developing countries: Bode et al.

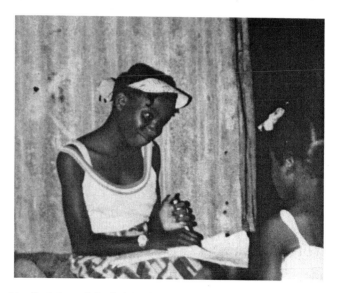

Photo 14. **Training of deaf girl.** *This teenage girl from the Caribbean was almost totally deaf. Deaf girls are among the most abused, but she was taken care of by the local community-based rehabilitation programme. She was protected and taught lip-reading and sign language, and was able to finish high school. © World Health Organization.*

(2001) report from Nigeria on widespread parental abuse and neglect of children with congenital deformities; the abuse was detected when these children were hospitalized for surgery.

Some disabled children end up as beggars or prostitutes; many die because of gross neglect or from sexually transmitted diseases. Poverty has many hidden corners and bitter disillusionment follows these human beings. There are few people – or nobody – to protect them. In the absence of published evidence, a few author-observed instances of abuse follow.

Abuse in a home for disabled adolescents

A physically disabled (wheelchair user) European expatriate went to an African country to set up a 'home', for which he had obtained the necessary funds at home. He rented a villa in the capital and built dormitories. He then 'collected' a dozen or so disabled adolescent boys, whom he lodged and fed. There was no rehabilitation or job-training. By court order, he was also custodian of five non-disabled young male criminals just out of prison. One day the expatriate had a fatal accident.

The local church took over and employed a couple to look after the boys. When they went through the belongings of the expatriate, they found his diary. In it, he had recounted in graphic detail his sexual 'experiences' with all those who were in his custody. Interviews with the boys confirmed the story; they had never dared to complain, for the expatriate threatened them with being thrown out on to the street or sent back to prison. Besides, they thought that nobody would believe them – the expatriate had good connections with high-ranking officials and the church.

Special schools in developing countries

In a boarding high school for blind students in a West African country, the principal informed me that he had taken over the school only three months earlier. The reason was that the previous principal and about half of the specialized teachers had been fired. They had had extensive sexual contacts with the blind girls some of whom had become pregnant. When a pregnancy was detected, the girl was asked to return to her family and was not allowed back.

In another African country, a group of deaf people from Sweden visited several boarding high schools for deaf and hard-of-hearing adolescent boys and girls. They communicated with the students using sign language. The visitors found out that the teachers had sexually abused almost all girls and boys. Several girls had left the school when they became pregnant; that was the end of their 'special education'.

In a Middle East country, a male employee was sexually abusing several mentally retarded boys in a residential centre. He was discreetly moved away – to another school for mentally retarded boys! The responsible doctor at the Ministry informed me about many similar cases.

A paediatrician in an Asian country described the conditions of the children in the local blind school. Almost all children were already sexually abused by the age of 7. No parent dared to report the abuse to the police because they feared, firstly, that the police would take no action and, secondly, that the children would be dismissed from the school, the only special education establishment available.

Early death of disabled children

In countries with a very high under-5 mortality rate (sub-Saharan Africa and South Asia) the observed prevalence of disability among children aged 0–9 is only about one-third of that in developed countries (such as the UK). These deaths are explained by parental neglect and

Table 7.6   Results of disability survey in Gujarat, India, 1997

Type of disability	% of all disability, both genders	% of all disability, males	% of all disability, females	Difference male as % of female
Blind	8.4	5.0	3.4	+47
Vision impairment	9.2	5.8	3.5	+66
Deaf	19.4	13.1	6.3	+108
Orthopaedic impairment	56.7	38.4	18.3	+110
Mental retardation	6.3	4.1	2.2	+86
Total	100.0	66.4	33.6	+99

extreme poverty resulting in malnutrition accompanied with untreated respiratory infections and diarrhoea.

The results from a prevalence study in the state of Gujarat in India (BMA, Ahmedabad,1997; see Table 7.6) shows that the prevalence of disability is twice as high in the male group as in the female one. Although small gender differences may be expected, the numbers reveal a larger degree of fatal neglect of disabled girls than of disabled boys. It is highest in the groups with polio and with deafness.

Yacoub et al. (1995) have published a study of a cohort of newborn children in Pakistan followed up until the age of 24 months. They found a rate of severe mental retardation of 11/1000. The mortality due to neglect of these children, aged 2–24 months, was 36 per cent, all caused by respiratory infection.

In the developed countries, a decrease in the mortality of disabled children has taken place. Annerén (2002) researched Down's syndrome children in Sweden. In 1920–30 the life expectancy was 2.3 years, in 1950–60 15 years, in 1970–80 45 years and in 1990–2000 57 years. Instead of letting these children die untreated (in accordance with the cost-utility concept) from congenital heart defects and leukaemia, they are now treated and survive. By contrast, in 1982, the Indiana Supreme Court in USA ruled that doctors and parents could allow the starvation death of a retarded infant (Encyclopaedia Britannica, 2003). Based on studies of 1,164 known homicides and 63 attempted homicides of persons with developmental disabilities, Sobsey et al. (1995) concluded that 'mercy-killing' of disabled children is frequent and that the murderer usually receives a lenient or no punishment.

The conclusion is that at least 50 per cent of all children with disabilities experience sexual, physical and emotional abuse and neglect, often in combination.

Other violence and trauma

In addition to interpersonal violence, there are millions of child victims of wars, civil wars, ethnic cleansing, and similar events. Several hundred have occurred during the last thirty years. In these cases, not only are people killed but millions of civilians (one-third is under-18) are wounded, raped and tortured or exposed to army, police and prison staff brutality. They are robbed of their houses, their properties are destroyed, family members are killed or disappear. Violence occurs increasingly in schools, in transportation vehicles, and as random shootings in public places – especially in countries with an abundance of private guns.

Other events that traumatize the surviving victims are natural disasters such as earthquakes, flooding, hurricanes, land slides, tsunamis, droughts and fires. Another group consists of manmade disasters: toxic, chemical and nuclear accidents, mine explosions, dam collapses and transport accidents. During the period 1994–2003, a total of 2.7 billion people were affected by such events; on average one disaster took place every day (Louvain University, Belgium, 2004). Many of them, including children, become disabled because of these events; physical and mental health problems will follow them for the rest of their lives.

Estimates of the global prevalence of childhood violence

The 2008 world population is estimated at 6,750 million (UNCTAD, 2007). There are some 2,300 million children (under the age of 18) in the world, 200 million in the developed regions and about 2,100 million in the developing regions (UN Population Division, 2007). When estimating the global prevalence of childhood violence, greater weights will be given to the data from developing countries. For example, in South Asia there are 440 million children in India, 55 million in Bangladesh, 79 million in Pakistan, 20 million in Myanmar, and 16 million in Nepal; the total comes to 610 million. From these five countries there are only 'usable' data from India; these will be extrapolated to its neighbours: their combined weight is considerable for the global estimate. In China, there are 360 million, in Taiwan 6 million, in Hong Kong 1 million, in Democratic People's Republic of Korea 9 million and in the Republic of Korea 11 million; thus in this region, there are 388 million children; the few data from these countries are quantitatively important for the global esti-mates. These two geographical regions together have half of the children in the developing regions. Africa has about a quarter, 450 million, and Latin America 185 million children. Examples below are from Box 2.1 and Tables 7.1, 7.4 and 7.6. The studies below demonstrate high preva-lence rates. Many have low attrition rates, and it is unlikely that respon-ders to anonymous interviews would invent abusive events (Chapter 2).

Abuse

Childhood sexual abuse (information from 64 countries)

Developed countries: Australia (Goldman and Padayachi, 1997), male 19 per cent, female 45 per cent; Ireland (McGee et al., 2003), male 24 per cent; female 30 per cent; Israel, Jewish population (Schein et al., 2000), male 16 per cent, female 31 per cent; Sweden (Krantz and Östergren, 2000), female 32 per cent; Switzerland (Niederberger, 2002), female 40 per cent; USA (Finkelhor et al., 1990), male 16 per cent, female 27 per cent; USA (Gorey and Leslie, 1997), broad definition male 12 per cent, female 36 per cent.

Developing countries: China (Chen et al., 2004), female 26 per cent; Costa Rica (University of California, 2006), male 13 per cent, female 32 per cent; India (Kacker, 2007), male 48 per cent, female 39 per cent; Israel, Arab population (Elbedour et al., 2006), female 31 per cent; Jordan (Jumaian, 2001), male 27 per cent; for Peru, Cáceres et al. (2000) determined lifetime coercion rates among adolescents. Of those with het-erosexual experience, males reported 20 per cent, females 46 per cent; of those with homosexual experiences, males reported 48 per cent, females 41 per cent; Tanzania (McCrann et al., 2006), male 25 per cent, female 31 per cent; Turkey (Eskin et al., 2005), male and female 28 per cent; USA (American Indians) (Robin et al., 1997), male 14 per cent, female 49 per cent.

A conservative global estimate based on the above studies is that *about one-third of all now living persons was sexually abused before the age of 18.* The impression is that sexual abuse of males is in many studies under-reported. With a global population of 6.5 billion, the survivors (adults and children) of sexual abuse are assessed at about 2,100 million people.

Childhood physical abuse (information from 48 countries)

Many country studies show that very large proportions of children receive corporal punishment. This includes 80 per cent in Chile, 78 per cent in Ethiopia, 97 per cent in Great Britain, 69 per cent in India, 95 per cent in Thailand, and 94 per cent in the USA (parents hit 35 per cent of infants, 94 per cent of 3–4-year-olds, 50 per cent of 12-year-olds and 33 per cent of 14-year-olds, an average of six times a year). Below is a list of studies with data about severe punishment using straps or canes or whipping, causing bruises, lacerations, burns, bite marks, swelling, haematomas to the face or other parts if the body, bleedings, fractures, loss of consciousness, concussion and permanent disability.

Developed countries: Canada (Macmillan et al., 1997), male 11 per cent, female 9 per cent; Great Britain (Leach, 1999), 25 per cent of all 4-year-olds regularly hit with straps or canes; Romania (Roturo, 1996), 23 per cent; Russia (Berrien et al., 1995), 29 per cent; USA (Straus and Stewart, 1999), severe hitting (with a belt or a paddle) 28 per cent.

Developing countries: Brazil (Gonçales et al., 1999), 39 per cent; Egypt (Youssef et al., 1998a, 1998b), 38 per cent severely punished by parents, 26 per cent reported fractures, loss of consciousness, concussion or a permanent disability. Teacher abuse: 26 per cent boys and 18 per cent girls suffered injuries (contusions, fractures and loss of consciousness); Ethiopia (Ketsela and Kebede, 1997), 21 per cent urban and 64 per cent rural children reported bruises and swelling from parental punishment; Hong Kong (Tang, 1998), 46 per cent; highest rate of severe violence among boys aged 3–6, mainly by mothers; India (Kacker, 2007), of the 73 per cent boys and 65 per cent girls who were physically abused, in 15 per cent they had swelling, bleeding or serious physical injury; Republic of Korea (Hahm and Guterman, 2001), 67 per cent of the parents whipped their children, and 45 per cent had kicked, hit or beaten them; Thailand (Isaranurug et al., 2002), 77 per cent beaten by cane or belt.

Physical abuse or violence towards children is extremely common. A conservative estimate of severe physical abuse provides *a global prevalence of 20 per cent*. Applying the estimate to the total global population of 6.5 billion, the survivors of such abuse are assessed at 1,300 million people.

Childhood psychological and emotional abuse (information from 58 countries)

Developed countries: Portugal (Machado et al., 2007), 22 per cent; Romania (Roturo, 1996), 14 per cent reported verbal aggression; USA (Scher et al.,

2004), emotional abuse and emotional neglect 34 per cent; Israel, Jewish population (Elbedour et al., 2006), emotional abuse 35 per cent.

Developing countries: Brazil (Gonçales et al., 1999), 26 per cent psychological abuse; China (Qin et al., 2008), 47 per cent emotional abuse; India (Kacker, 2007), emotional abuse 50 per cent boys, 50 per cent girls; Iran (Sheikhattari et al., 2006), mental maltreatment at home 78 per cent, at school 66 per cent; Israel, Arab population (Elbedour et al., 2006), psychological abuse by family members 50 per cent; Palestine (Haj-Yahia and Abdo-Kaloti, 2003), 37 per cent; South Africa (Madu, 2001), 35 per cent emotionally abused; Thailand (Jirapramukpitak et al., 2005), 32 per cent emotional abuse; Turkey (Vahíp and Doğanavşargil, 2006), verbal violence 53 per cent.

Over 75 per cent of all children experience parents yelling and screaming or cursing at them (World Health Organization, 2002); in some countries they are threatened with evil spirits or told that they will be sent away.

Psychological and emotional abuse are very common. It is concluded that at least 50 per cent of all people have been emotionally or psychologically abused in a major way during their lives. This would include long-term, very upsetting or repeated verbal, psychological and emotional aggression at home, at school, at work, or during leisure activities. Some of these abusive acts occurred in combination with physical and/or sexual abuse, or with physical neglect. *Severe psychological abuse during childhood is conservatively estimated at 30 per cent*; this implies that the surviving victims are 1,900 million individuals.

Table 7.7 sums up the prevalence estimates of childhood abuse made below.

Table 7.7 Global estimates of the prevalence of childhood abuse

Type of abuse	Basis of estimates	Estimated global prevalence victims (of adults and children)
Sexual	33% abused during their childhood. Female sexual mutilation: 135 million	2,220 million
Physical	20% severely abused during their childhood	1,350 million
Emotional/ psychological	30% severely abused during their childhood	2,020 million

Neglect

Child care-giver neglect

In the developed countries, it appears that 1–4 per cent of all children are annually investigated by child protection authorities for child maltreatment. While child neglect is the type of maltreatment most frequently reported to and acted on by official agencies, its proportion of all maltreatment in the general population is comparatively smaller. In studies using such reports, the proportion of neglected children is: Canada (Trocmé et al., 2002), 46 per cent, and USA (US Department of Health and Human Services, 2007), 63 per cent. Some general population data are available: Brazil (Gonçales et al., 1999), 26 per cent; China (Pan et al., 2005), 28 per cent; Iran (Sheikhattari et al., 2006), neglect at home 83 per cent, at school 66 per cent; Kenya (African Network, 2000), 22 per cent; Romania (Roturo, 1996), 11 per cent; UK (Cawson et al., 2000), 18 per cent of respondents had experienced some absence of care in their childhood and 20 per cent had experienced less than adequate supervision. Straus and Savage (2005) summarized data from seventeen countries (six in Europe, USA, Canada, two in Latin America, five in Asia, Australia and New Zealand): the median was 12 per cent.

The published evidence based on representative populations in developing countries is scant. In the absence of enough such data the global prevalence of child care-giver neglect is estimated at 12 per cent.

Child structural neglect

Calculations of structural neglect are presented in Chapter 13. The victims are children for whom the society has not provided adequate health care, nutrition, education, permanent shelter, safe living and other

Table 7.8 Global estimates of the prevalence of childhood neglect

Type of neglect of children	Basis of estimates	Estimated global prevalence of victims, children only
Care-giver intentional neglect	Child authorities' reports and population surveys, a balanced estimate of the 1,200 million children not included below is 12%	140–150 million
Structural care neglect of children	Children living in poverty both in the developed and developing countries	1,100 million

conditions necessary for their development. Most is related to poverty. Globally the prevalence is estimated at over one billion children, in the developing countries; in the developed ones there are about 100 million children under the poverty level.

When calculating the combined global prevalence we need to take into account the frequency of *exposure to multiple forms of childhood violence*. Kessler et al. (1995), in a US sample, calculated the lifetime prevalence of trauma (rape, molestation, physical attacks, combat, shock, threat with a weapon, accident, natural disaster with fire, witness gross violence, neglect, physical abuse and other qualifying trauma) to be 61 per cent for men and 51 per cent for women. For about half of them, there had been more than one such trauma. Elklit (2002) studied 390 Danish schoolchildren aged 12–15 and found that 78 per cent of males and 87 per cent of females had been exposed to at least one potentially traumatic event. The most distressing subjective events were rape, suicide attempts, death in the family, serious illness, and childhood abuse. Seventy-four per cent of male Icelandic schoolchildren aged 12–15 years reported at least one traumatic event, as did 79 per cent of females (Bödvarsdóttir and Elklit, 2007).

Scher et al. (2004) found that one-third (35.1 per cent) of their sample met criteria for at least one form of childhood maltreatment and 13.5 per cent met criteria for more than one form. Finkelhor et al. (2005, 2007), in a US nationally representative sample of 2,030 children and youth aged 2–17 years, found that during the study year only 29 per cent had no direct or indirect victimization. The mean number of victimizations for a child or youth was three. A child or youth with one victimization had a 69 per cent chance of another during a single year. Felitti (2002) registered adverse childhood experiences (ACEs) in a very large middle-class US sample and found that only 36 per cent did not report any such experiences. Finkelhor et al. (2007) found that children previously victimized during Year 1 are at higher risk of continued victimization during Year 2, and that the poly-victims are at particular risk. Onset of poly-victimization in Year 2, in contrast to persistence from Year 1, was associated with violent or maltreating families, family problems such as alcohol abuse, imprisonment, unemployment and family disruption. Other studies are by Bifulco et al. (2002), Clemmons et al. (2003), Edwards (2003), and Rosen and Martin (1996) for American soldiers (see p. 115). Bifulco et al.'s study is from the UK; all others are from the USA. We do not have much accurate data from the developing countries to assist in this estimate, although Ellsberg (2000) has produced one study for Nicaragua (see p. 108).

Table 7.9 Social and biological orphans

Group	Estimated global prevalence, children
Children in residential institutions, including prisons	10 million
Biological orphans	112 million
Child soldiers	300,000
Street children	25 million
Child labourers	218 million
Refugee and displaced children	15 million
Child prostitutes	10 million
Trafficked children	400,000
Total	**390 million**

One more factor to consider is the influence on the prevalence rates of the groups mentioned in Chapters 4 and 5 (see Table 7.9). These groups, totalling 390 million (17 per cent of all children), are seldom included in 'ordinary' prevalence research studies, which often describe their participants as non-institutionalized persons, with a home address or a telephone or appearing in the voters' register. Social and biological orphans are under-represented in such surveys, and these groups suffer very high rates of all types of abuse and neglect (Table 7.9).

It would seem reasonable to conclude that *50 per cent of all people in the world have been victims of childhood abuse before the age of 18.* When child neglect is added, this global estimate is likely to be higher. Maltreatment of children takes place across all cultures and societies, and all economic, social and religious strata. *It appears to be higher in the developing countries than in the developed ones.*

The group of sexual perpetrators might be as large as the victims' group – some abuse several children, but one child may be abused by more than one person. Although parents dominate as abusers, adolescents may in some cultures may be responsible for a considerable proportion of such abuse (see p. 195). Among the perpetrators of emotional and physical abuse, parents, parent substitutes and teachers may be involved. Some abusers are previous victims now abusing others. We should note that for structural neglect the major part of the responsibility rests with government authorities.

These very high prevalence estimates are painful and disturbing and call for an examination of human nature. Even more troubling is the fact that the main group of perpetrators is the parents. Man's destructive behaviour seems to have few limits. The injurious consequences for the individual are reviewed in Chapter 8. These effects remain chronic for a very large proportion. Time does not heal; time conceals.

Although it is clear that childhood violence is extremely common, as well as frightening, this does not imply that it is too late or hopeless to turn the tide. Few perpetrators are 'monsters': most are frustrated, unhappy, traumatized by having been abused and humiliated during their own childhood, and misguided by an environment that does little to discourage violence and to prevent harmful and irrational child rearing habits.

8
Micro-system Consequences and Upstream Effects of Childhood Violence

'Childhood is not the shortest period of our lives but the longest as it stays with us until our death'

(Lombardo, 2001)

This chapter presents assessments of the health and social consequences for the victims of childhood violence. It includes a short estimate of the global judicial and economic burdens to society.

Health and social consequences

An important method used to measure the effects of childhood violence is used in the Adverse Childhood Experiences (ACE) studies by Felitti et al. (1991, 1998, 2002). It is based on observations of ten categories of adverse childhood experiences, taking place before the age of 18, among 17,337 adult Kaiser Health Plan Members, mean age 56:

1. recurrent and severe physical abuse;
2. recurrent and severe emotional abuse;
3. contact sexual abuse;
4. growing up in a household with an alcoholic or drug abuser;
5. a household member being imprisoned;
6. a mentally ill, chronically depressed, or institutionalized household member;
7. the mother being treated violently;
8. both biological parents not being present;
9. emotional neglect;
10. physical neglect.

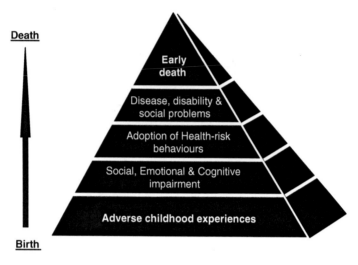

Figure 8.1   Consequences of adverse childhood experiences
Source: Felitti, 2003.

The experience of any of these categories was scored one point. Felitti and his co-workers have studied a large number of consequences related to ACE scores and published some fifty articles. Some of these studies include only the first eight categories listed above.

Somatic consequences of childhood violence

Persons subjected to physical abuse may have fractures, head trauma with brain damage, whiplash injuries, spinal cord injuries (caused by falls, gunshots and assaults with a knife), blindness, burns, wounds, cuts and other skin lesions, traumatic damage to interior organs, poisoning and other complications. It is common to see abused children with haematomas, burns from cigarettes or scalding, bruises from beatings and whipping, traumas to the head and eyes, periorbital haematomas and damage to abdominal organs; very often these traumas are repeated.

An estimated 135 million women have been sexually mutilated during childhood (for details see Chapter 2). Common immediate side-effects are: severe bleeding, tetanus and other infections, exquisite pain, and death. A majority of the survivors will have long-term problems with incontinence and urinary tract infections; sexual intercourse can be very painful. For some women, the sexual mutilation is repeated after the birth of the first child.

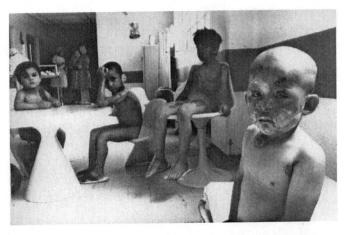

Photo 15. **Children with burns.** *Children in a hospital in a developing country. All of them have burns, many caused by the parents' neglect and some by physical abuse.* © *World Health Organization.*

Acute effects of sexual abuse are common: some studies report 20 per cent with severe somatic injuries – in many cases of the genital organs – requiring treatment (Sobsey, 2000). Sexually abused children may have vaginal infections and difficulties in sitting and walking. Kawsar et al. (2004), in a UK clinical study of 98 girls who had been raped or sexually assaulted (aged 0–16 years), found that sexually transmitted diseases had a prevalence of 26 per cent. Eighty-one per cent also reported current psychological difficulties and 15 per cent had attempted self-harm; 29 per cent were unknown to the social services. The high prevalence of AIDS and gonorrhoea among children is indicated by reports from Somalia (Ahmand, 1992), Cameroon (Menick and Ngoh, 2003), Botswana and Zimbabwe (Lalor, 2004a), South Africa (Collings, 1991) and by WHO (2002). In Zimbabwe 1.25 per cent of all children will have experienced abusive penetrative sex with an AIDS/HIV infected person before the age of 18. In Botswana, the figure is almost 2 per cent (Lalor, 2004a).

There are also many long-term secondary physical health effects, which appear when the maltreated children reach adulthood; these lead to increased mortality. The ACE study (Felitti et al., 1998) has shown that adults with scores of four or more categories of ACE have a prevalence of ischaemic heart disease of 5.6 per cent vs. 3.7 per cent for those with a zero ACE score, stroke 4.1 per cent vs. 2.6 per cent, chronic obstructive pulmonary disease 8.7 per cent vs. 2.8 per cent, hepatitis 10.7 per cent vs. 5.3 per cent, severe obesity 12.0 per cent vs. 5.4 per cent, and chronic headache 45 per cent vs. 25 per cent.

Physical and sexual abuse increases the risk of subsequent eating disorders with self-induced vomiting or use of laxatives and diuretics to reduce weight (Neumark-Sztainer et al., 1997). Chronic fatigue and headache, menstrual problems and gastro-intestinal disorders are more prevalent among persons with childhood sexual abuse (Taylor and Jason, 2001). Berkowitz (1998) found that gastrointestinal disorders increased from 10 per cent in non-abused populations to 33 per cent after CSA; 44 per cent of all women visiting gastroenterology practice had been abused; and 64 per cent of women with chronic pelvic pain had experienced CSA compared to 23 per cent of non-abused women (Leserman and Drossman, 2007).

The cautious global estimate is that *childhood violence has led to life-long somatic disability for at least 300–400 million people*. Some of this is associated with premature death.

Mental, behavioural and social consequences of childhood violence

The information below is based mainly on studies in developed countries (all, except those otherwise specified, were carried out in the USA).

Swanston et al. (2003) published a prospective study of 103 sexually abused children in Australia. These children were compared with a matched group of non-abused children studied during the same period. After nine years, 49 of the abused and 68 of the non-abused children were available for interviews. The abused children had significantly higher scores for depression, lack of self-esteem, anxiety, fearful behaviour and despair. They had histories of bingeing, self-induced vomiting, smoking, and using amphetamines, ecstasy and cocaine. All their families were classified as malfunctioning. Fergusson and Lynskey (1997) made a prospective study of a birth cohort of 1,265 New Zealand children followed to the age of 18. The group was assessed on exposure to physical punishment/maltreatment, with several measures of psychosocial adjustment. Much of the elevated risk that was identified among those physically abused had arisen from the social context within which harsh and abusive treatment occurs; exposure to such treatment during childhood leads to elevated rates of violent offending, substance and alcohol abuse, suicide attempts, being a victim of violence and mental health problems. Yanowitz et al. (2003) state that physical and emotional abuse by teachers leads to lower self-esteem, heightened aggression, academic difficulties and poor social interaction skills among the pupils.

Flisher et al. (1997) found that physical abuse was significantly associated with global impairment, poor social competence, major depression, conduct disorder, oppositional defiant disorder, agraphobia, over-anxious disorder, and generalized anxiety disorder. Knutson et al. (2005) established that when children are exposed to care neglect, supervision neglect and punitive care, the level of aggression increases significantly. Empathy-inducing, positive parenting practices give rise to less antisocial behaviour than punishment-based, negative parenting practice. Keily et al. (2001) studied a group of 578 children from their start in kindergarten until the eighth grade. Comparisons were made between maltreated and non-maltreated children; these showed that the children that were harmed early (before 5 years of age) showed significantly higher rates of behaviour problems than those who were maltreated after the age of 5 and those from the non-maltreated children.

Cognitive impairment

Child physical neglect has the most profound effects on cognitive functioning and academic achievement. Sameroff et al. (1987) showed that the average IQ scores of 4-year-old children are related to their exposure to a number of psychological and social risk factors. These include parental influences, such as rigid and punitive childrearing style, parental substance abuse, low parental educational attainment, father absence, poverty, and so on. In the ACE study (Felitti, 2003) the average IQ for children with zero, one or two of the factors is above 113. When a third and fourth risk factor are added, the average IQ score drops to 93; with the further addition of the fifth through eighth risk factors the average IQ score becomes 85.

Friedrich (1998) reviewed some additional factors, such as pre-abuse difficulties, stressful life events, level of IQ, and developmental differences; family variables, such as quality of mother–daughter relationship, problem-solving capacity of the family, pre-existing, long-standing and adverse psychosocial circumstances, substance abuse, single-parent families, and so on. Friedrich points out that CSA is often combined with physical and psychological abuse, domestic violence and neglect. Richards and Wadsworth (2004) analysed 1,339 representative males and females from the British National Survey of Health and Development. They found that early adverse circumstances were strongly associated with lower cognitive ability in childhood and adolescence, and were detectable on measures of verbal ability, memory and speed and concentration even as far as in midlife. Many abused children have delayed developmental milestones; after a traumatic event they may regress in cognitive development and in daily life abilities and communications skills. The authors state that in view of the persistence of child poverty in the industrialized world these findings give cause for concern.

Addiction

The ACE study (Felitti, 2003) relates self-reported alcoholism and use of injected illegal drugs to adverse childhood experiences. Figure 8.2 shows that there is more than a 500 per cent increase in adult alcoholism among subjects having an ACE score of four or more.

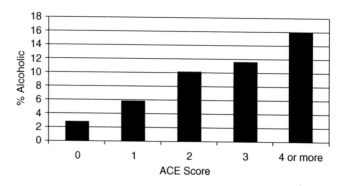

Figure 8.2   Relationship between alcoholism and adverse childhood experiences
Source: Felitti (2003).

The likelihood of injection of street drugs increases strongly and in a graded fashion as the ACE score increases (Felitti, 2002) (Figure 8.3). For instance, a male child with an ACE score of six, when compared to a male child with an ACE score of zero, has a forty-six-fold increase in the likelihood of becoming an injection drug user some time later in life.

Suicide attempts

The likelihood that an individual with an ACE score of four or higher will attempt suicide later in life is increased by ten times compared with an ACE score zero individual (Dube et al., 2001). Ystgaard et al. (2004) made a study in Norway of seventy-four hospitalized patients who had attempted suicide; among them they found a prevalence of severe sexual abuse of 35 per cent, severe physical abuse 18 per cent, neglect 27 per cent, antipathy 34 per cent, loss of care-giver 37 per cent, and exposure to family violence 31 per cent.

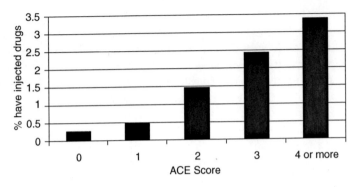

Figure 8.3 Relationship between injected drug use and adverse childhood experiences
Source: Felitti (2003).

Criminality

Child physical abuse has serious effects on aggression and subsequent violent behaviour. Physically abused or neglected children are more likely than others to commit violent crimes later in life. Several US studies have been made. Widom (2000) examined criminal records of children who had been abused and/or neglected and followed them over twenty-five years. At their approximate age of 33, she found that early childhood abuse and neglect increased the risk of arrest as a juvenile by 55 per cent and the risk of being arrested for a violent crime as a juvenile by 96 per cent. Abused and neglected children became chronic offenders 1.6 times more often than the controls. Zingraff et al. (1993) showed that abused and neglected children who had been removed from their homes were 4.8 times more likely to be arrested as juveniles and eleven times more likely to be arrested for a violent crime than the matched controls. English et al. (2002) reported that 19.6 per cent of abused and neglected children versus 4.1 per cent of the controls had a juvenile arrest record; 41.7 per cent of the abused and neglected group vs. 21.1 per cent of controls had an adult arrest. Rebellon and Van Gundy (2005) showed that parental physical abuse is associated with a doubling (97 per cent) in violent offence counts and an increase of 240 per cent in property offence compared with matched controls. Swanston et al. (2003) report that sexual abuse increases the odds ratio of juvenile (2.4) and adult (2.0) arrests. Douglas and Straus (2006) (see p. 105), in a large study of 9,594 students in thirty-six universities in nineteen countries, concluded that childhood experience of corporal punishment leads to higher levels of partner abuse.

Post-traumatic stress disorder (PTSD)

PTSD is highly frequent among victims of childhood violence. Specifically, sexual abuse, physical abuse, domestic violence and community violence are positively correlated with PTSD. In persons with PTSD the level of symptoms increases with the number and with the severity of traumas (Scott, 2007). For these patients the overwhelming traumatic event is re-experienced, causing intense fear, helplessness, horror and avoidance of stimuli associated with the trauma (WHO, 2002; Collings, 1995; Neumann et al., 1996). Briggs and Joyce (1997) showed that the severity of PTSD was proportionate to the extent of CSA and whether it involved sexual intercourse and the repetition of the abuse. There was a high level of co-morbidity with other mental disorders. Schneider et al. (2007) studied a sample of 3,936 women and reported that exposure to all types of child abuse (sexual, physical and emotional) was linked to a 23-fold increase in risk for probable PTSD.

The presence of memory defects among abuse victims is disputed. The common theory was that the victims were seeking unconsciously to forget the abusive event or repeated events. If pronounced, this mechanism was seen as symptom of a mental disorder: dissociation, which is characterized by a disruption in the usually integrated functions of consciousness, memory, identity and perception of the environment. According to this theory dissociation was seen to be employed by children who could not escape from the threat or abuse; it would be a means of mentally withdrawing from a horrific situation by separating it from conscious awareness. Studies by Mulder et al. (1998) have shown that among individuals exposed to physical childhood abuse, the rate of frequent dissociation is five times higher than in non-abused persons. As regards persons exposed to CSA, the rate is two and a half times higher; this increase, however, is not directly related to the CSA but to the degree of concurrent physical abuse and psychiatric illness. In contrast, Melchert (1998), studying 553 college students (of whom 27 per cent had been abused), failed to find any significant association between childhood abuse and any lack of memory of it. Widom et al. (2004) have disputed the general accuracy of retrospective reports of childhood violence. Alexander et al. (2005), however, have examined predictors of memory accuracy and errors twelve to twenty-one years after the abuse ended for individuals with legal experiences resulting from documented CSA. They showed that 'severity of PTSD symptoms was positively associated with memory accuracy'. Victims' memories are more distinct than are those of bystanders.

Other mental consequences

The mental consequences of CSA are multifaceted. Finkelhor and Browne (1986) proposed four mechanisms that would explain the outcomes:

- Traumatic sexualization, inappropriate conditioning of the child's sexual responsiveness and the socialization of the child into faulty beliefs and assumptions about sexual behaviour;
- Betrayal: the child's confidence and trust in persons who should protect him/her from harm have become shattered;
- Stigmatization: the child's positive self-image is disturbed by the shame that is instilled; and
- Powerlessness: intense fear of death and injury, and repeated frustration at not being able to stop or escape from the harmful experience or to get help from others; this is part of the post-traumatic stress disorder.

Among the psychological health effects Finkelhor and Browne list are fear, anxiety, depression, anger, hostility, inappropriate sexual behaviour, poor self-esteem, tendency towards substance abuse and difficulty with close relationships.

Childhood violence has negative effects on the biological capacity for attachment (Neumann et al., 1996). Without predictable, responsive, nurturing and sensory-enriched care-giving, the infant's potential for normal attachments will be unrealized. Problems with attachment lead to a fragile biological and emotional foundation for the forming of future relationships (Boney-McCoy and Finkelhor, 1996). The psychological impact for children witnessing violence, especially at home, is alarming; it may lead to PTSD, disrupted sleeping and feeding routines, poor weight gain, anxiety and rage, dropping out of school, drug use and running away from home (Knapp, 1998); the bonding process is also severely disturbed.

Manmade disasters (such as release of toxic substances, collapses of dams or bridges, traffic accidents, occupational accidents, wars and state-organized violence) expose people to traumas; the resulting mental health effects are similar to those caused by interpersonal violence. Natural disasters are common, and after disasters health symptoms are common (WHO, 1992). Some 80–90 per cent of all disasters occur in developing countries, where the population is unprotected and unprepared even when some disaster, such as flooding, is known to recur every year. In these countries the mortality and morbidity caused by disasters are high, and doubtless includes a large proportion of the 2 billion children who live there.

The prevalence of mental disability caused by childhood violence

Very large numbers of people underachieve because of a health condition. For example, in a US study with a response rate of 73 per cent, Kessler et al. (2003) estimated that the lifetime prevalence of an episode of major depression was 16 per cent; of these about 6 per cent had taken place during the most recent twelve months. Of persons with depression, many had experienced very severe, severe or moderate role impairment: 69 per cent at home, 54 per cent at work, 63 per cent in relationships, 71 per cent socially; overall 87 per cent had at least one of these role impairments; these indicate current disability. Most likely Kessler et al.'s assessments are too low; among the 27 per cent non-responders in his study there could be many additional persons with depression. WHO estimated that the global incidence of unipolar major depression was 109 million persons, and 59 million of them were disabled. These numbers are, however, probably underestimates as they are built on samples that had 13–55 per cent non-responders (WHO, 2001a). Mental disorders among care-givers are prevalent (see p. 177) and affect the mental health and behaviour of their children.

The disabling effects of abuse, neglect and violence are both somatic and mental. Persons with role impairments may appear, superficially, to function normally at work, in their families and in social contacts; however, by using deeper analysis, many are found to have significant disabilities (such as tiredness, decreased quality, quantity and creativity at work) due to mental and somatic disorders; or due to their daily frustrations, poverty and hunger. Parent role malfunctioning often leads to child violence.

Many health effects are lifelong and severely hinder normal functioning and lead to physical and economic dependence and restricted social participation. The prevalence of PTSD and other mental disorders have been studied in several surveys; the high frequency of co-morbidity is notable: it implies that the condition is severe, often long-lasting and difficult to treat. Many of the first studies of PTSD related to war victims, including camp victims from Nazi Germany.[15] Table 8.1 confirms the high prevalence of co-morbid mental disorders, and the many linkages between such disorders and childhood abuse.

The chronicity of PTSD was analysed by Kessler et al. in a 1995 study; it was part of the US National Co-morbidity Survey. Initially 8,098 participants aged 15–54 were included; the response rate was 82 per cent.

Table 8.1 Mental symptoms related to childhood violence

Authors Country	Groups of victims	Findings of mental symptoms
Ackerman et al. 1998 USA	204 children aged 7–13, referred to hospital after sexual or physical abuse or both	34% PTSD, 36% phobia, 29% ADHD, 36% oppositional defiance, 39% separation anxiety, 21% conduct disorder, 20% overanxious, 19% dysthymia; abused girls are more internalizing; boys externalizing.
Bödvarsdóttir and Elklit 2007 Iceland	Icelandic national representative sample of 206 students (mean age 14). Prevalence and impact of 20 potentially traumatic and negative life events	74% of the girls and 79% of the boys were exposed to east one event. Most common were the death of a family member, threat of violence, and traffic accidents. Lifetime PTSD 16%, subclinical PTSD (missing full diagnosis with one symptom) another 12%.
Chen 2004 China	Women students from medical school in China	26% abused before age 16, meian age 12. Victims reported higher levels of depression, less healthy; some had suicide thoughts, anxious of about attacks in the street, and had a higher proportion smoking and drinking alcohol than non-victimized students.
Elklit 2002 Denmark	Representative study of 390 Danish school children age 12–15	78% of males and 87% of females had been exposed to at least one traumatic event. Most distressing were rape, suicide attempts, death in the family, serious illness, and childhood abuse. Lifetime prevalence of PTSD 9.0%, subclinical PTSD another 14.1% .
Famuralo et al. 1996 USA	117 abused children removed from parental care	35% PTSD, high rates of ADHD, anxiety disorders, brief psychotic disorders, PTSD group had more mood disorders and increased suicide ideation.
Felitti and Anda 2003	ACE Study 17,337 adults (see above)	Population risks attributed to ACE: chronic depression 41%, suicide attempts 58%, alcohollism 65%, illicit drug use 50%, injected drug use 68%, as adults being sexually assaulted 62%, exposed to domestic violence 52%.

(Continued)

Table 8.1   (Continued)

Authors Country	Groups of victims	Findings of mental symptoms
Flisher et al. 1997 USA	Interviewed a community sample of 660 9–17-year-olds and their care-takers in New York and Puerto Rico	26% physically abused, this was associated with global impairment, poor social competence, major depression, conduct disorder, ODD, agoraphobia, overanxious disorder, and generalized anxiety disorder.
Kendall-Tackett, Williams and Finkelhor 1993 USA	A synthesis of 45 studies including comparisons with non-abused children	Victims of CSA had general PTSD (53%), promiscuity (38%), general behaviour problems (37%), poor self-esteem (35%), fear (33%), nightmares (31%), neurotic mental illness (30%), aggression including delinquency (29%), depression (28%), anxiety (28%), and inappropriate sexual behaviour (28%). Compared with non-abused children, the abused showed more PTSD and sexuallized behaviour. CSA strongly related to depression, aggression, and withdrawal. Separate comparisons for age groups 0–6, 7–12 and 13–18, yielded more focused and consistent findings than with mixed age groups. About 2/3 of the children had symptoms and 1/3 had not. About 2/3 showed recovery during the first 12–18 months after the event.
Nader et al. 1993 Kuwait	Kuwaiti children exposed to occupation and war	2 years afterwards, 70% had moderate to severe PTSD.
Shaw and Krause 2002 USA	US national survey of persons aged 25–74, 2,788 persons had complete data (response rate 61%)	24% experienced childhood physical violence with early onset of psychological disorder, setting in motion a vicious cycle of recurring disorder during the life course. Many somatic disorders are also related to such abuse.
Silverman et al. 1996 USA	Working class community. Sample of 777 kindergarten children screened	At age 21, 11% reported physical or sexual abuse before age 18. 80% of the abused met criteria for at least one psychiatric disorder. Compared with

Table 8.1 (Continued)

Authors Country	Groups of victims	Findings of mental symptoms
	for health development, behavioural, and academic factors. Follow-ups until children were 21. Because of school transfers, the attrition rate after 10 years was 22%, but after that time until age 21 95% could be interviewed	non-abused schoolmates, they had significant impairments both at age 15 and 21: more depression (23%), anxiety, emotional-behavioural problems (45%), suicidal ideation (18%), and suicide attempts (17%). At 21, physically abused males had 40% drug-abuse dependence (vs. 4% of non-abused) and 10% PTSD (vs. 0.6% of non-abused); for females PTSD it was 41.7% (vs. 3.4%). Sexually abused females had PTSD in 34.8% (vs.1.8%).
Stein et al. 1996 USA	Compared a group of 125 patients with anxiety disorders with a matched group drawn from a community sample	Childhood physical abuse: 16% of the male and 33% of female patients, in comparison sample 8%. CSA among 45% of women patients vs. 15% in the comparison group.
Straus et al. 1997 USA	National sample of 807 mothers of children aged 6 to 9 years. Follow-up after two years	44% of the mothers spanked their children during the week prior to the study, at an average of 2.1 times that week. The more spanking at the start of the period, the higher the level of antisocial behaviour (ASB) 2 years later. The change is unlikely to be owing to the child's tendency toward ASB or to confounding with demographic characteristics or with parental deficiency in other key aspects of socialization; those variables were statistically controlled. If parents replace corporal punishment by nonviolent modes of discipline, it could reduce the risk of ASB among children and reduce the level of violence in American society.
Walsh et al. 2007 Canada	Community sample of 3,381 women	Chronic pain was significantly associated with physical abuse, education, and age of the respondents and was unrelated to child sexual abuse alone or in combination with physical abuse, mental disorder (anxiety, depression, or substance abuse), or low income.

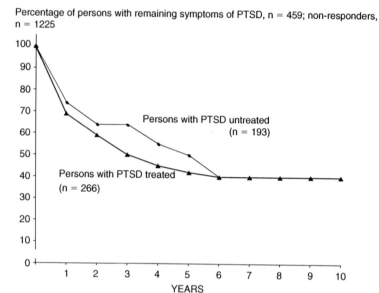

Figure 8.4   Survival curves based on duration of symptoms for respondents who did and did not receive treatment for PTSD, sample size 8098 (modified from Kessler, 1995)

Lifetime prevalence of PTSD was 5 per cent in men and 10.4 per cent in women. Survival curves during the first six years show recovery among 60 per cent (Figure 8.4). Of those with PTSD symptoms 266 respondents did and 193 did not receive treatment. Kessler et al.'s conclusion is that patients who received treatment had somewhat less (statistically significant $p < 0.05$) symptoms during the first five to six years; after that period – until the end of the ten-year observation period – there was no benefit from treatment. Their conclusions may be challenged: they were built on just 405 subjects, with 1,255 non-responders.

Based on the above study the proportion of victims who will remain chronically affected appears to be some 40 per cent, irrespective of psychiatric treatment; it may be higher, as many studies have significant attrition rates. Most exposed persons with these kinds of mental problems live in the developing countries, and there the availability of any Western-type treatment is very restricted: there is no money to pay for the medicines, and cognitive group therapy for violence victims may be culturally incompatible. All victims have a high frequency of significant role impairments. *It is estimated that one third of the victims of childhood violence remain with long-term mental disability (including significant role impairment). This would imply a global prevalence of persons with mental disability of about 1,000 million persons.*

Neurobiological correlates to childhood violence

It may be useful to give a brief account of the brain processes related to the mental consequences of childhood violence. The environment in which a child grows up, whether favourable or unfavourable, interacts with all the processes of neurodevelopment: neurogenesis, migration, differentiation, apoptosis, arborisation, synaptogenesis, synaptic sculpting and myelination (Perry, 2002).

The influence by child neglect on childhood brain development and function

At birth the brain has some 100 billion neurons. These have threadlike axons, but anatomically do not form a connected network; each cell is an independent unit. For a nervous signal to travel across the system, the axon releases a chemical product (neurotransmitter) to bridge the gap between its signalling axon and the signal-receiving dendrite of the adjacent nerve cell. A synapse is formed; during the first three years of life, in response to environmental stimulation, each nerve cell of a normal child forms some 15,000 synapses; totally some 1,000 trillion synapses (Eliot, 2001). If such a specific pathway is used often, there emerges a memory effect. If a certain pathway is not used, the nerve cell may disappear. This is seen among infants and very young children; they have at birth many more nerve cells than adults, but many of those unused will be 'pruned off'. The brain develops its functioning and ability to change because of its past and ongoing usage; the transmitting action leaves biochemical 'memory traces'. The memory systems of children who have not yet gone through the phase of 'pruning' are especially sensitive to the neurobiological processes triggered by abuse and neglect. If the environmental stimulation is severely reduced, such as among the abandoned children in the 'orphanages' described in Chapter 4, the development of synapses will be severely reduced (see Figure 8.5). Neglect in young children affects the early brain development resulting in excessive pruning off of neurons, much smaller brains, and loss of essential brain functions (see Box 6.1, p. 82).

The influence by violence-related stress reactions on childhood brain development and function

High levels of psychological or physical arousal, such as those caused by childhood violence, trigger stress reactions. These were first studied

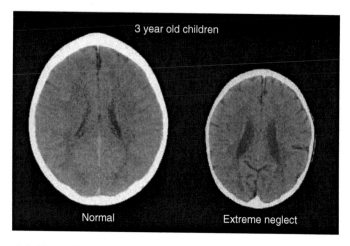

Figure 8.5   Brain CT scan with comparison between an extremely neglected and a normal child. The neglected child's brain is significantly smaller than average (3rd percentile) and has enlarged ventricles, cortical atrophy and a reduction of the head circumference. © B. Perry.

by Selye in the 1930s, who described the general adaptation syndrome to stress. It begins with an alarm reaction in the hypothalamus. This is followed by a stage of resistance, and, if the stressor is not removed, leads to a final stage of exhaustion: the general adaptation syndrome. The hypothalamus stimulates the sympathetic nervous system, activating the pituitary to produce adrenocorticotropic hormone (ACTH) which stimulates the adrenals to produce cortisol. The sympathetic nervous system increases the production of epinephrine and norepinephrine. These hormones mobilize the body to deal with the stressor. In the second stage of resistance, local reactions seek to normalize the hormone levels. If these responses are insufficient, exhaustion will follow and the hormonal levels become excessive. If this occurs, the person may become mentally disturbed, withdrawn or maladjusted.

Hormonal, biochemical, metabolic and anatomical correlates

High levels of cortisol caused by abuse depress brain cell function. Hippocampal damage identified by the anatomical decrease of its volume or depletion of its glucocorticoid receptors in PTSD leads to an increase in adrenal secretion. Impaired adrenocortical secretion leads to loss of granula cells in the hippocampus, which could explain the deficits in cognition. Because of stress, the hypothalamus increases or reduces the release of other hormones as well. The growth hormone is lowered in physically and sexually abused boys (Jensen et al., 1991). Women who have been sexually abused and developed PTSD have elevated levels of thyroid hormones (Friedman et al., 2005). PTSD patients (Bremner et al., 2003, 2005) have increased left amygdala activation with fear acquisition, and decreased anterior cingulate function during extinction, in comparison with controls. Anxiety disorders are related to an induced abnormal functioning of the amygdala. These overreact as stressful, abusive events and then hormones and other biochemical substances start 'flooding' the body. Emotional memory is centralized to the amygdala and the medial frontal cortex, which together with the hypothalamus control a wide variety of hormones. Fear and anxiety during traumatic events influence the biochemical agents used for neurotransmission. Because of their effects on the amygdala-hypothalamus brain regions, such emotions increase or reduce the release of hormones: cortisol, epinephrine and norepinephrine, gonadotropin-releasing hormone and growth hormone, to name just a few. The biochemical changes serve to encode emotionally charged memories so that the abuse victim may not be able to forget them.

Anxiety disorders, such as PTSD, are accompanied by important changes in the endocrine functions and in serotonin metabolism (Cicchetti and Rogosh, 2001; Gonzales-Heydrich et al., 2001; Newport et al., 2004; Rinne et al., 2002). With stress, not only is ACTH released but also endorphins that reduce pain. The noradrenergic system (related to the causation of anxiety, fear, sleeping problems and intrusive thoughts) malfunctions; in PTSD an elevated level of nocturnal noradrenergic metabolites has been found, which might cause the sleep problems. Nutt and Malizia (2004) suggest that the hallmark symptoms of PTSD may be related to a failure of higher brain regions (hippocampus and the medial frontal cortex) to dampen the exaggerated symptoms of arousal and distress that are mediated through the amygdala in response to reminders of the traumatic event. Taylor et al. (2006) conclude that neural responses to emotional stimuli are associated with childhood stress.

In PTSD, there are anatomical changes in the brain caused by traumatic events; they are 'upstream', secondary consequences. The hippocampus volume is reduced; its neuronal integrity and functional integrity are disturbed in PTSD (Shin et al., 2006; Driessen et al., 2000; Pederson et al., 2004; Schmal et al., 2004). Compared to normal subjects, subjects with PTSD have smaller intracranial, cerebral, and prefrontal cortex, reduced prefrontal cortex white matter, smaller right temporal-lobe volumes, and smaller volumes of the corpus callosum and its sub-regions.

Brain volume changes are positively correlated with the age at the onset of trauma and negatively correlated with the duration of the abuse (De Bellis et al., 2002). Early abuse has a deleterious effect on the brain cortical development (Knapp, 1998). PTSD causes a reduced neuronal viability in the prefrontal cortex (Mathew et al., 2004), and in the cerebellum (Anderson et al., 2002). In children with generalized anxiety disorder there is an association with pathological fear activation in the amygdala, ventral prefrontal cortex and anterior cingular cortex (McClure et al., 2007). Brain-scanning has shown that the blood flow to certain memory-related parts of the brain is redirected when the formerly abused person is exposed to retrieval of his or her memories of the childhood event (Shin et al., 1999). Sexually abused women with PTSD show increased amygdala activation with fear acquisition compared with controls (Bremner et al., 2005). A group of young women who had been exposed to severe childhood physical/sexual abuse were studied using positron emission tomography. Compared to a matched control group, they had reduced glucose intake in brain cortex areas involved in memory consolidation and retrieval that are part of a network of active brain regions that continuously gather information about the world around and within us and transfer this information to the cortex. Lange et al. (2005) have shown that early life stress is associated with smaller anterior cingulate cortex and caudate volumes. Close to 1,000 publications studying anatomical and functional alterations of the central nervous system using neuroimaging are now available. Etkin and Wager (2007) have recently published a meta-analysis of emotional processing in PTSD, social anxiety disorder and specific phobia. They suggest that the mechanisms for emotional dysregulation symptoms in PTSD extend beyond an exaggerated fear response.

The conclusion is that childhood violence has been shown to be associated with smaller volumes of parts of the brain, implying that cells have been damaged or have disappeared; evidently, this damage is widespread and combined with a 'cascade' of biochemical, hormonal and metabolic alterations.

Repair or replacement of damaged brain functions

It is currently debated whether damaged neocortical cells can be repaired or replaced. The conventional view was that nerve cells lacked this ability, and this appeared to be confirmed by clinical observations in several neurological diseases. However, in 1992 Reynolds and Weiss were the first to isolate neural progenitor and stem cells from mouse brain tissue.

Numerous experiments indicate that brain cells can re-form in mammals, including humans (Colucci-D'Amato et al., 2006). Complex factors are involved in cell renewal (Pluchino et al., 2007); how to foster repair is still insufficiently understood. Studies by Bhardwaj et al. (2006) using C14 techniques indicate that no cell division or replacement takes place in the necrotic nerve cells during the person's life from infancy to adulthood. The more specific question of whether the nerve cells which have been damaged or disappeared as a reaction to PTSD caused by childhood abuse can be repaired or replaced is influenced by the findings of Gould and Gross (2002). They showed that the presence of long-term stress reactions prevents the repair functions of adult stem cells in the brain. At present, there is no evidence that the widespread alterations of the function of the brain cells comprising changes in the brain biochemistry, metabolism, hormonal regulation and anatomy resulting from childhood abuse can be restored.

Resilience

People with a type of personality called hardiness have the ability to withstand even severe and prolonged stress. They are highly committed to what they do, have a strong need to control the events around them, and a willingness to accept challenges. These characteristics are likely to make them resilient also to the effects of childhood abuse. Other factors that contribute to resilience are social support from others, optimism, humour in the face of difficulty, and positive illusions. About one-quarter to one-third of all victims of childhood abuse and neglect appear to be resilient and do not develop the mental symptoms associated with the majority. McGloin and Widom (2001)have shown that resilient victims meet the criteria for success in eight domains: employment, homelessness, education, social activity, psychiatric disorder, substance abuse, official arrest and reports of violence. Twenty-two per cent of 676 substantially abused and neglected individuals met these criteria and were therefore considered resilient.

In Kendall-Tackett et al.'s (1993) review, about one-third of the abused college students were resilient. Barnes and Bell (2003) suggest that the factors included in resilience include: (1) intellectual and physical ability, toughness; (2) adaptive psychological factors (ego resilience, motivation, humour, hardiness, and perceptions of self), emotional well-being, hope, life situation, optimism, happiness and trust; (3) spiritual attributes; (4) attributes of post-traumatic growth; (5) interpersonal skills and relations, connectedness and social support; (6) positive life events and socio-economic status.

Himelein and McElrath (1996) described a group of 180 female college students (responders 97 per cent), of whom forty-five (26 per cent) reported contact CSA before the age of 15. They then made an in-depth study on a sub-sample of twenty CSA survivors. They showed that the resilient group revealed a greater tendency to engage in four cognitive strategies: disclosing and discussing CSA, minimization, positive reframing, and refusal to dwell on the experience. Positive illusion is strongly associated with psychological well-being. It appears that there are no studies of resilience published from the developing countries; in these, cultural and socio-economic factors leading to resilience may be very different. Outcomes of childhood violence generally worsen as risk factors pile up in children's lives, and then, resilience is less common (Masten, 1997; Egeland et al., 1993; Garmezy and Masten, 1994). At very high levels of trauma, no child is expected to be resilient until a safe and more normative environment for development is restored. Thus, in cases of massive trauma due to war or chronic child abuse, resilience refers to good recovery after trauma has ended. It is possible for a child to be resilient and still suffer from residual effects of trauma. Resilience does not mean invulnerable or unscathed (Masten, 1997).

Disturbance of attachment

The attachment process is very important. A person's capacity for attachment is defined as the lifelong ability to maintain emotional relations. Such relations are a necessary part of human life: to learn, to love, survive and procreate. Without emotional relationships the person will remain distant, isolated, self-absorbed, and without close friends. Loving and caring relations make life a pleasure. The attachment process involves the human brain. The attachment process is set up right after birth by neurobiological networks (Schore, 1994), as described above; if not maintained by constant stimulation, the network will be disturbed and with it the attachment process. The neurobiological processes that take place have a lasting effect during adult life. Most signs of attachment can be seen early and will lead to the capacity in childhood to recognize close family members and friends, develop love, sharing and empathy and to reduce aggression. Childhood abuse and neglect can destroy this security. Four infant attachment styles have been identified: (1) secure, (2) avoidant, (3) resistant-ambivalent, and (4) disorganized-disorientated:

> Infants with a secure pattern of attachment typically protest when they are separated from their caregiver, and they attempt to regain closeness to the caregiver upon reunion. The avoidant attachment

style involves behaviours that resemble rejection. Infants with this pattern tend to ignore the caregiver's departure and return and actively avoid the caregiver's attempts to regain contact. The resistant-ambivalent pattern is characterized by a preoccupation or fixation on the caregiver in which the caregiver is alternately sought for comfort and rejected. The disorganized style of attachment is typically seen in infants who have been maltreated by their attachment figure. They exhibit conflicted behaviours such as simultaneously reaching for and turning away from the caregiver. This is most likely related to the inherent conflict between the attachment object being both the cause of distress and the infant's only potential source of comfort from distress. The disorganized attachment style is thought to be most correlated with psychopathology.

(Hardy, 2007)

Maunder and Hunter (2001) made a meta-analysis of studies published from 1966 to 2000. Although more research is needed, they concluded that existing data can be organized into a model that describes attachment insecurity leading to disease risk through three mechanisms: increased susceptibility to stress, increased use of external regulators of affect, and altered help-seeking behaviour. They concluded that there is an association between attachment insecurity and physical illness. Sleep disorders may be caused by insecure attachment (Sloan et al., 2007). There is a relationship between borderline personality disorder (BDP) and insecure attachment. BDP has a high prevalence, and is often chronic and disabling; patients show a pattern of chaotic and self-defeating interpersonal relationships, emotional lability, poor impulse control, angry outbursts, frequent suicidality, and self-mutilation (Levy, 2005). Agrawal et al. (2004) reviewed thirteen empirical studies that examined the types of attachment found in individuals with BPD. All these studies concluded that there is a strong association between insecure attachment and borderline personality disorder. The types of attachment found to be most characteristic of BPD subjects are unresolved, preoccupied and fearful. In each of these attachment types, individuals demonstrate a longing for intimacy and at the same time concern about dependency and rejection. The high prevalence and severity of insecure attachments found in these adult samples support the central role of disturbed interpersonal relationships in clinical theories of BPD. The authors' review concludes that these types of insecure attachment may represent phenotypic markers of vulnerability to BPD. Brennan and Shaver (1998) also found attachment style to be correlated with personality disorder.

Other studies were made by Boris et al. (1998), Cicchetti et al. (1990) and Carlson (1998).

Yoo et al. (2006) have made a study of 494 Korean children. Parental insecure attachment was associated with the development of the psycho-pathologies and psychiatric illness of their children.

Crandell and Hobson (1999) compared children to twenty mothers with secure attachment style with those to sixteen mothers with insecure style. The quality of mother–child interactions was assessed by video-taping and by rating with the Belsky Parent–Child Interaction System. Using the Stanford-Binet test, children of secure mothers scored nineteen points higher compared to children of insecure mothers. The adjusted mean difference was twelve points when maternal IQ, education, and family socio-economic status were taken into account.

A study in Ireland (Marsa et al., 2004) serves to illustrate the importance of attachment during early childhood. The authors compared four groups: twenty-nine child offenders, thirty violent offenders, thirty non-violent offenders and thirty community controls. A secure adult attachment style was four times less common in the child offender group than in any of the other three groups. Ninety-three per cent of the sex offenders had an insecure adult attachment style. The sex offenders group, when compared to the community group, reported significantly higher levels of maternal and pubertal overprotection during their child-hood. Compared with all three comparison groups the sexual offenders reported significantly more emotional loneliness.

Based on evidence of the disturbances seen in children with attach-ment difficulties, the WHO in ICD-X and the APA in DSM-IV included 'Reactive Attachment Disorder' (RAD) among the list of mental disorders of infancy or early childhood. RAD is defined as a psycho-physiological condition with markedly disturbed and developmentally inappropriate social relatedness in most contexts; it begins before 5 years of age and is associated with grossly pathological care. This pathological care-giving behaviour may consist of any form of neglect, abuse, mistreatment or abandonment. Due to violence by care-givers, RAD sufferers have dif-ficulty forming healthy relationships with them, with peers and with families. RAD can reportedly be diagnosed as early as the first month of life. There are several articles describing dyadic treatments for RAD (Becker-Weidman, 2006; Hughes, 2003; Speltz, 2002).

Neurobiological mechanisms underlie the formation of bonding in infants and children. Based on research it is known that oxytocin (OT) and vasopressin (VP), which are part of the neurohypophyseal peptide (AVP) system, are critical for the establishment of social recognition and bonding, and for the regulation of emotional behaviours. Fries et al. (2005) have recently published a study of a group of eighteen children who had been abandoned at birth to 'orphanages'. They had then resided there for an average of seventeen months. After that period, they had transferred to adoptive homes where they had been for an average of thirty-five months at the time of the study. The results of the measurements of the OT and AVP peptides were compared with twenty-one children of the same age who had been reared by their biological parents. Early neglect leads to decreased levels of OT and AVP. The study showed that even after three years of rearing in relatively stable, enriched and nurturing family environments following the 'orphanage' experience, the normal levels of OT and AVP had not been restored. Social deprivation inhibits the AVP system, which is critical for recognizing familiar individuals, a key component in social bonding. The data provide a potential explanation for how the nature and quality of children's environments shape the brain-behavioural systems underlying complex human emotions. More about oxytocin and vasopressin in the regulation of human behaviour follows in Chapter 9.

A programme which results in the strengthening of early attachment should contribute to improving the parents' attitudes to the child: it will create a home atmosphere of love and empathy; it will inhibit aggression and reduce the risks for future child abuse, intentional neglect and adult mental disorder. It is recommended as a part of the Child Defence and Support Programme (Chapter 14).

Judicial upstream consequences

Child abuse and neglect may lead to interventions by social protection agencies and to judicial action against the perpetrator. A meta-analysis of twenty-one US studies of criminal justice decisions related to child sexual abuse was published in 2003 by Cross et al. The rates of referral to prosecution, filing charges and incarceration varied. The rate of carrying the case forward without dismissal was high: 72 per cent or greater. For cases carried forward, plea rates averaged 83 per cent and conviction rates 94 per cent. Diversion, guilty plea, and trial and conviction rates were the same for child abuse and all violent crimes.

The US Justice Department Bureau of Statistics (2002) concluded that for the period 1994–8 only 32 per cent of sexual assaults against persons aged 12 or older were reported to law enforcement. A three-year longitudinal study by the Bureau of 4,008 adult women found that 84 per cent of the respondents who identified themselves as rape victims did not report the crime to the authorities. No current studies indicate the rate of reporting for child sexual assault, although it is generally assumed that these assaults are similarly under-reported.

Finkelhor and Jones (2004) report that that between 1991 and 1997 the number of individuals incarcerated in US state correctional facilities for sex crimes against children rose 39 per cent, from 43,500 to 60,700, having already more than doubled from 19,900 in 1986. These totals do not include the large numbers of sexual abusers who receive sanctions which do not involve incarceration for a year or more. About 60 per cent of all known child sex offenders are under conditional supervision in the community. Incarceration may have diminished the incidence of sexual abuse.

The situation in South Africa (population 45 million) may serve as comparison. The South African Human Rights Commission stated that in 2002 there were about 173,000 cases of child abuse on the rolls of South African courts (Conradie, 2003). (There are 747 courts and 273 prisons in South Africa.) The conviction rate was 7 per cent. The daily average of incarcerated persons was 181,000, representing 80 per cent overpopulation; one-third of them were awaiting trial. Three and a half thousand incarcerated persons have been sentenced to life imprisonment.

The judicial system has no capacity anywhere close to dealing with the enormous numbers of crimes against children – nor will it ever have, should the present crime level persist. The global number of persons known to be in prisons for all crimes is just about 9 million. The costs to the society of the judicial consequences are very high.

Economic upstream consequences

Calculations have been made both for small groups of affected children and for countries. A detailed review was published in 2004 by WHO. WHO quotes the US estimate of losses due to violence as being 3.3 per cent of GDP. A main part relates to lost earnings and opportunity cost of lost time. The costs of violence in percentage of GDP are: for Brazil 10.5 per cent, Colombia 24.5 per cent, El Salvador 24.9 per cent, Peru 5.1 per cent and Venezuela 11.8 per cent. Daro (1988) cautiously calculated the cost in lost earnings of a group of 24,000 maltreated children living in the USA as US$658–1,300 million per year. Irazuzta et al. (1997) made cost estimates for thirteen abused children out of a total of 937 who were admitted to paediatric intensive care units in the USA. While the abused children represented only 1.4 per cent of all admissions, they had the highest severity of illness, seven of them died (of head trauma), and an additional four left the hospital with severe residual symptoms. These results were worse than those of any other group of children in emergency care. The medical bills for the acute care averaged US$35,641 per abused child (daily charges US$5,294). In this report, no calculations of the post-hospital costs were made.

The studies of costs related to childhood violence show large differences – it is not easy to make these calculations. Still, even the highest are very conservative and mostly built on official incidence reports, which underestimate the reality. Estimates of costs for treatment of the victims most often only cover short-term expenditure, but not care for the long-term consequences described above (addiction, risk behaviour, chronic mental disorders, and increased disease and disability rates). Most childhood abuse is hidden; although these victims may indeed seek health care, a very large proportion of the doctors are not in the habit of routinely asking about childhood violence, and the victims seldom volunteer such information. These costs are insufficiently recognized:

- decrease of educational achievements (reflecting decreases in cognitive functions);
- the victims' rehabilitation, including reintegration to society;
- loss of quality and creativity at work (not just unemployment, underemployment and absenteeism);
- the community effects of the doubling of violent and non-violent criminality;
- family problems, such as with the next generation of children of abused parents;
- and finally, economists are never seen to include the costs of lost dignity and human suffering in their calculations.

Heckman et al. (2006a) have pointed out that neglect-related damage to children's neurobiological development will lead to reductions of the future quality of a country's workforce. Such changes carry a high economic cost (Heckman et al., 2006b). The productive work time lost by employees with a major depressive disorder was estimated in a US study (Stewart et al., 2003) at 5.6 hours/week vs. the normal 1.5 hours/week. The two-week prevalence of any depressive disorder was 9.4 per cent; the production losses – for this disorder alone – in the USA amounted to US$31 billion/year. Anda et al. (2004), in a cohort of 9,633 employed persons, found that worker performance impairment among persons with ACE score four was twice that of those with score zero.

We may cautiously convert the direct and indirect costs cited for the USA to an approximate estimate of the global costs of violence. The GNP of the USA in 2001 was 29 per cent of the global GNP. To assess global costs one may use extrapolation based on the assumption that the direct and indirect costs are proportional to the combined GNPs (71 per cent of the global GNP) of the group of 221 countries and territories outside the USA. The result of this calculation is US$1.4 trillion. The size of this global, annual estimate emphasizes the urgency of finding preventive alternatives.

Part IV
Roots of Violence

9

Causes of and Contributors to Childhood Violence and the Potential for Primary Prevention

To initiate and provide resources for preventive and curative child violence services for populations is a role for communities and governments: the exo- and macro-systems. The information in this chapter will clarify some of the basic issues. It seeks to do the following:

(a) Identify the major causes and contributors to child violence. Why are people abusing children; do they have diseases or genetic factors that explain their aggression; or is it caused by adverse environmental factors in their lives? How much is related to alcohol use? What are the roles of social, cultural and economic factors? Is the problem the lack of family life preparation: they never got a chance to acquire the knowledge and skills for their most important task in life: educating their children? Do we live in a violent, uncaring and indifferent society that does little to meet families' needs and prevent the damage to our children? Is child protection failing? Do people learn how to become violent? Are there cultural factors, such as those related to gender?

(b) Estimate their relative prevalence. This not easy because we lack information about the exact occurrence of violence, especially in the developing countries. Childhood violence may also be the result of combinations of causes.

(c) Analyse the present knowledge about the effectiveness of preventing each of the causes and contributors; again our knowledge is mainly based in the developed countries and may not be transplanted to other cultures.

(d) Suggest priorities for preventive action. Should prevention be targeted just at families which have been reported to protection authorities, or should it be a programme for all?

The factors discussed imply interaction between all levels of the human ecology system. The information below comes mostly from North American and European sources; if existing, data from the developing countries are included.

Health-related causes appearing in childhood

Pregnancy and delivery complications

Mednick (1971) studied the records of violent criminals in the Danish penal system. Fifteen of the sixteen most violent criminals were found to have had an extraordinarily difficult birth and the sixteenth had an epileptic mother. In a second study, Kandel and Mednick (1991) compared pregnancy and delivery events between three groups: (a) 15 violent criminals, (b) 24 property criminals and (c) 177 non-offenders. Delivery complications such as ruptured uterus, umbilical cord prolapse, difficult labour, etc., were correlated to violent offending. Kandel and Mednick's conclusion was that 80 per cent of violent offenders rated high in delivery complications, compared with 30 per cent of property offenders and 47 per cent of non-offenders (the significance level is low as their numbers are small). Raine et al. (1990) reported a significant association between birth complications and early maternal rejection, and violent crime at age 18. While only 4.5 per cent of the subjects had both risk factors, this small group accounted for 18 per cent of all violent crimes. The effect was specific to violence and was not observed for non-violent criminal acts. Beck and Shaw (2005) studied birth records in addition to longitudinal data that were collected on 310 low-income boys followed from birth until 10 years of age. Perinatal complications emerged as a predictor of antisocial behaviour but only in the context of other family risk factors. According to maternal reports, boys experiencing high levels of perinatal complications, parental rejection and family adversity showed significantly higher levels of antisocial behaviour than did boys with lower levels of these risk factors. This finding was partially corroborated by young people's self-reports: boys experiencing high levels of perinatal complications and family adversity reported more antisocial activity than boys experiencing no risk or risk in only one domain. Nathanielsz (1999) has extensively reviewed the role of pregnancy and birth complications for the health of children.

A team at the University of Groningen in the Netherlands studied two consecutive cohorts totalling 3,162 singleton infants born in 1975 and 1978 and then followed them for twenty-five years (Tuin-Bastra, 2004). Obstetric data were collected and quantitatively scored using a list of seventy-four items describing the pre- and perinatal condition of the mother and of the foetus. Data included social and economic variables, past pregnancies, non-obstetric condition of the mother, obstetric aspects of the pregnancy, parturition and the child's immediate postnatal condition. For sub-samples, follow-up data on childhood detailed neurological status (Touwen et al., 1980) to diagnose clusters of dysfunctions were collected; and school performance tests and standardized questionnaires of behavioural and emotional problems were applied, including interviews with the teachers and the parents. The latest part of the study includes a follow-up of a sample aged 20–25 years. The social and economic status was noted as well as the present habits of smoking, alcohol consumption and substance use. Psychiatric interviews were made using a General Health Questionnaire (Goldberg, 1972). This was followed by the administration of the sub-scales of Symptom Checklist 90 (Derogates, 1977) for depression and anxiety and an interview, using the Composite International Diagnostic Interview (CIDI) form (Robins et al., 1988), which covered twelve sections of DSM-IV disorders. Complications during pregnancy and at delivery lead to a higher frequency of serious emotional problems, especially externalizing behaviour among boys, and to underperformance in school. The consequences are in line with conduct disorder. In young adulthood, it is associated with a significantly higher prevalence of anxiety and depression, and a high prevalence of co-morbid psychiatric disorders, alcohol and substance use, and smoking.

Some recent articles about biochemical factors related to pregnancy and birth complications have been published. De Weerth et al. (2003) report that children to mothers with high prenatal cortisol level display more crying, fussing and negative facial expressions. Huizink (2003) found that (1) high amounts of daily problems in early pregnancy were associated with a lower mental development score at 8 months; (2) high levels of pregnancy-specific anxiety in mid-pregnancy predicted lower mental and motor development scores at 8 months; and (3) early morning values of cortisol in late pregnancy were negatively related to both mental and motor development at 3 months. Niederhofer and Reiter (2004) showed a significant correlation between prenatal maternal stresses, prenatal temperament of the child and his/her school marks at the age of 6 years. Davis et al. (2007) examined 247 full-term infants. Elevated levels of mothers' prenatal cortisol at 30–32 weeks' gestation, but not earlier in pregnancy, were significantly associated with greater maternal report of infant negative reactivity. Prenatal anxiety and depression predicted infant temperament. There were clear associations between maternal cortisol and depression. Glynn et al. (2007) report that among breastfed infants, higher maternal cortisol levels were associated with increased infant fear behaviour; this reaction did not exist among the formula-fed infants.

During their pregnancies high proportions of women – especially in developing countries – are subjected to psychological, physical or sexual violence by their partners; this causes biochemical and hormonal stress reactions, among them increased cortisol levels (Pico-Alfonso et al., 2004). If a pregnant woman is exposed to such abuse her elevated cortisol will transfer via the placenta to the foetus and may influence its developing brain and neural system. Such stress may be more pronounced if these mothers are malnourished, anaemic, and have episodes of recurrent communicable diseases. Disturbances to the supply of energy or of other chemical components that serve to build the foetus' brain or to regulate its functions before the delivery may result in damage to the neural cells. After birth, the infant's metabolism is regulated by hormones such as catecholamines. These perinatal disturbances of the oxygen supply or other complications might harm the parts of the neural system that are involved in emotional regulation and may explain the Groningen findings of clusters of neurological dysfunction combined with emotional and behaviour problems among children, lasting into adulthood.

Conduct disorder

(i) Diagnosis and prevalence

Conduct disorder refers to a group of behavioural and emotional problems in youngsters. These children and adolescents have great difficulty following rules and behaving in a socially acceptable way. They may exhibit (DSM-IV, 1994):

(a) aggression towards people and animals;
(b) deliberate destruction of property;
(c) deceitfulness, lying or stealing;
(d) serious violations of rules: staying out at night, running away from home, truanting from school, precocious sexual activity, early involvement in prostitution;
(e) poor school performance; poor relations with peers, some expelled from school because of their behaviour or problems with the law.

Such children may have a combination of mood disorders, anxiety, PTSD, substance abuse, ADHD, learning problems, or thought disorders.

Rates of depression, suicidal thoughts, suicide attempts and suicide itself are all higher in children with conduct disorder (Shaffer et al., 1994). Between a quarter and a half of highly antisocial children become antisocial adults (American Academy of Child and Adolescent Psychiatry, 2004).

Conduct disorder is more common among boys than girls; the rate among boys in the general population ranges from 6–16 per cent, for girls 2–9 per cent. It can start early, before the age of 10. Oppositional defiant disorder is sometimes a precursor. The first sign of an emerging conduct disorder with aggressive behaviour may occur by the ages of 4 or 5 and may then be stable. Parents often react negatively to these children, withdrawing love and punishing them.

(ii) Aetiology

The aetiology of conduct disorder is not fully known. Twin studies have indicated a role for psychosocial components, but also for genetic ones. The gene GABRA2 is significantly associated with childhood conduct disorder (Dick et al., 2006). This gene produces parts of the receptor for the brain's primary inhibitory neurotransmitter, γ-aminobutyric acid (GABA). When GABA binds to the GABA-receptors on a nerve cell, it inhibits the firing of that cell. GABA is also involved with the body's responses to alcohol, such as loss of physical co-ordination, effect on mood, and alcohol withdrawal symptoms.

Frequent risk factors are diseases causing brain damage, child abuse and traumatic life experiences. Lack of bonding to the parents is common due to maternal rejection, separation from parents, institutionalization, parents' mental disorders, parental marital discord, large family size, crowding, and poverty.

(iii) Treatment

Children with conduct disorder without treatment may become unable to adapt to the demands of adulthood and continue to have problems with relationships and holding a job. They may become delinquent and antisocial (Stouthammer-Loeber et al., 2001).

Their treatment is complex because of the child's uncooperative attitude, fear and distrust of adults. Parents need assistance in devising and carrying out special, long-term behaviour therapy programmes and medication in the home (American Academy of Child and Adolescent Psychiatry, 2004). Loeber (1991) has challenged the notion that many children outgrow early conduct problems. The stability of antisocial behaviours is often underestimated. Data suggest that the malleability of child behaviours decreases as children grow older, leading to a higher continuity of antisocial behaviour possibly from early adolescence onward.

A recent meta-review of psychosocial treatments for children and adolescents identified eighty-two studies conducted between 1966 and 1995 involving 5,272 young people (Brestan and Eyberg, 1998). By applying criteria established by the APA Task Force to all studies, just two treatments met criteria for well-established treatment (success in reducing problem behaviours), and ten for probably efficacious treatment. These treatments were (1) a parent-training programme based on the manual, 'Living with Children' (Bernal et al., 1980) and (2) a videotape modelling parent training (Carey, 2002).

It is important to diagnose and treat mental disorders in children at the earliest opportunity. Kim-Cohen et al. (2003), in a prospective study, followed a cohort of 1,000 children in New Zealand from the ages of 11 to 26. They found that 75 per cent of those with an adult disorder at age 26 had received a diagnosis before the age of 18, and 60 per cent before the age of 15. Common among them were histories of conduct and/or oppositional defiant disorder, and of juvenile anxiety. Kumpulainen et al. (2000) studied 1,268 children in Finland from age 7 to 15. Problems noted by health professionals (problems in growth, somatic diseases, emotional/behavioural problems of the child, psychosocial problems of the family) before school age were related to future deviance. Emotional/behavioural problems and problems in psychomotor development before school were likely to remain at the age of 15. The authors concluded that psychiatric deviance is persistent over several years in children.

Genetic indicators that predict adult violent behaviour

Several studies have been published about the gene MAO-A; its low-activity version has been linked to aggressive behaviour. The gene is involved in the production of monoamine-oxidase A. This enzyme breaks down several neurotransmitters such as serotonin and dopamine; the low-activity version leads to increased tissue levels of these transmitters. One-third of all men have this version. It is rare among women. A study in New Zealand (Carey, 2002), of 1,037 men aged 30, showed that the low-activity gene alone was not linked to antisocial behaviour. Only those men with a combination of the gene variation and moderate or severe child abuse were more likely to commit crimes. That group made up 12 per cent of the study group, but was responsible for 44 per cent of all crimes. As adults, 85 per cent of those who had been severely mal-treated as children (sexual abuse, physical abuse and frequent changes of care-giver or rejection by the mother) had the gene version for low MAO-A activity (Carey, 2002). A 2006 meta-analysis confirms these findings (Kim-Cohen et al., 2006).

Examinations of genes alone will not reveal enough information; gene expression (penetrance) has to be studied: the process indicating that genetic information actively directs the structures and functions of a living cell. Although all the body cells have the same genes, the special-ized cells have selective DNA expression through the RNA. The regulation of RNA synthesis may be influenced by hormones.

Differences in gene expression may explain why some genes – which supposedly would be markers for violence – are also found in ordinary non-violent persons. It is likely that research related to hidden informa-tion encoded by cellular chromatin might serve better to explain the role and extent of gene expression.

Another technique for studying genetic influence is twin studies. A 2005 publication by Viding et al. has shown that individuals with early warning signs of lifelong psychopathy – callous unemotional traits (CU) and high levels of antisocial behaviour (AB) – can be identified among 7-year-old children. In their study, schoolteachers provided ratings at the end of the first school year for 3,687 same-sex twin pairs. The authors analysed a sub-group of 612 monozygotic twins with extreme CU, many in combination with extreme AB. The CU among monozygotic co-twins were similar in 73 per cent; a group of dizygotic co-twins were similar only in 39 per cent. Two-thirds of the difference between the extreme CU children and the population is explained genetically. Out of 3,687 twin pairs, 459 pairs (12.5 per cent) showed extreme CU and 364 pairs (9.9 per cent) showed extreme AB. Assessments of AB in the absence of concomitant CU showed no genetic influence. For the sub-group of children with AB (and in the absence of CU) the authors recommend preventive action. These children are 'probably amenable to traditional interventions aimed at improving family, school, and neighbourhood conditions'. The fact that antisocial behaviour can be identified at the age of 7 gives opportunities for early detection and targeted interventions. The authors are following up the children in their study group at the age of 9. In another twin study, Kim-Cohen et al. (2005) found that children of depressed mothers have elevated conduct problems, one-third of which is explained by genetic factors.

Kaufman et al. (2007) studied 109 maltreated and 87 non-maltreated comparison subjects. Their study included measures of psychiatric symptoms and social supports using standard research instruments, and of serotonin transporter (5-HTTLPR) (locus SLC6A4) as well as brain-derived neurotrophic factor (BDNF) (variant val66met) genotypes. Children with the met allele of the BDNF gene and two short alleles of 5-HTTLPR had the highest depression scores, but the vulnerability associated with these two genotypes was only evident in the maltreated children. A significant four-way interaction also emerged, with social supports found to further moderate risk for depression. Protective social supports ameliorate the genetic and environmental risks.

The present genetic evidence is likely to grow with more research; until now it has been shown that environmental factors modulate gene expression, thus the sharp distinction between nature and nurture is no longer tenable (Kim-Cohen et al., 2006; Moffitt, 2005; Rutter, 2006).

Health-related causes appearing in adulthood

Gender distribution

As discussed in Chapters 7 and 8, most perpetrators of abuse are the child's parents. The gender distribution is discussed by some authors. Newton (2001) claims that males and females perpetrate physical abuse against their own children at surprisingly similar rates:

> Among all abused children, those abused by their birth parents were about equally likely to have been abused by mothers as by fathers (50% and 58%, respectively), but those abused by step-parents, parent-substitutes, or other non-parental perpetrators were much more likely to be abused by males (80% to 90% by males versus 14% to 15% by females).

Newton's conclusions only relate to physical abuse, and it is mothers who usually punish children aged under 7. A study of a group of female sexual abusers has been published by Bader et al. (2007). The victims of the women who were convicted were mainly extra-familial males aged 13–19.

The high percentage of female offenders quoted above is unfair because it includes child neglect, in which mothers are named at absurd rates, given that women accused of child neglect in the USA are almost always single mothers. The fathers who abandon their children are almost never convicted of child neglect.

Other evidence would support the opinion that males are more abusive and violent than females. Most intimate partner abuse is perpetrated by men. In fifty population studies Heise et al. (2002) have shown that such abuse is experienced annually by 10–70 per cent of the women interviewed. About ten times more men than women are in prison because of child abuse. Men are responsible for most sexual abuse, assault and coercion of underage boys and girls, with reported prevalence rates sometimes exceeding 40 per cent. Men are overwhelmingly the clients of underage female and male prostitutes. Eighty-nine per cent of those who abuse disabled children are men. Most child murderers are men. War violence, riots, uprisings, and related mass killings of children and rapes of women are the acts of men. It would appear justified to assume that between 60 per cent and 75 per cent of the perpetrators are males.

Antisocial personality disorder (ASPD)

Personality disorders are a group of serious mental disorders that according to DSM-IV lead to a long-term pattern of inner experience and behaviour deviating markedly from the expectations of the culture of the individual who exhibits it. To be diagnosed as a personality disorder, a behavioural pattern must cause significant distress or impairment in personal, social, and/or occupational situations (DSM-IV, 1994).

(i) Diagnosis and prevalence

DSM-IV has formulated the following criteria:

> Diagnostic criteria for ASPD (which includes psychopathy) include a pervasive pattern of disregard for and violation of the rights of others and inability or unwillingness to conform to what is considered the norms of society. The disorder involves a history of chronic antisocial behaviour starting before age 15 and continuing into adulthood. The person affected shows irresponsible and antisocial behaviour, indicated by academic failure, poor job performance, illegal activities, recklessness, and impulsive behaviour. Symptoms may include dysphoria, inability to tolerate boredom, feeling victimized, and a diminished capacity for intimacy.
>
> ASPD, also known as psychopathic personality or sociopathic personality often brings a person into conflict with society because of amoral and unethical behaviour. Complications from ASPD include frequent imprisonment for unlawful behaviour, alcoholism, and drug abuse. People with this disorder may appear charming on the surface, but they are likely to be aggressive and irritable as well as irresponsible across all areas. They may have numerous somatic

complaints and possibly attempt suicide, but due to their use of manipulative behaviour, it is difficult to separate what is true and what is not.

A study of a representative US sample revealed that 51 per cent of 1,422 ASPD respondents lacked remorse (Goldstein et al., 2006). DSM-IV estimates the prevalence of ASPD in the USA to be about 3 per cent of men and 1 per cent of women. In the USA, some 80 per cent of all prisoners have ASPD (Hart and Hare, 1996). Coercive and precocious sexuality are fundamental aspects of psychopathy (Harris et al., 2007).

(ii) Aetiology

The aetiology of ASPD is disputed. It would be reasonable to assume that adverse childhood experiences play a significant role. Other ASPDs appear to have the same aetiology as those mentioned for conduct disorder above.

(iii) Treatment

Goldstein et al. (2006) report:

> Persons with ASPD are highly unresponsive to any form of treatment, in part because they rarely seek treatment voluntarily. If they do seek help, it is usually in an attempt to find relief from depression or emotional distress. Although there are medications that are effective in treating some of the symptoms of the disorder, non-compliance with medication regimens or abuse of the drugs prevents the widespread use of these medications. The most successful treatment programs for ASPD are long-term structured residential settings in which the patient systematically earns privileges as he or she modifies behaviour. In other words, if an ASPD person is placed in an environment in which they cannot victimize others, their behaviour may improve. It is unlikely, however, that they would maintain good behaviour if they left the disciplined environment.

Paedophilia

(i) Diagnosis and prevalence

Paedophilia is the preference for repetitive sexual activity with pre-pubescent children. (For persons sexually interested in pubescent children the term 'hebephilia' is used; the term 'paraphilia' refers to a larger group of sexually related disorders.)

The DSM-IV diagnostic criteria are:

- A. Over a period of at least six months, recurrent, intense sexually arousing fantasies, sexual urges, or behaviors involving sexual activity with a prepubescent child or children (generally age 13 years or younger);
- B. The person has acted on these sexual urges, or the sexual urges or fantasies cause marked distress or interpersonal difficulty;
- C. The person is at least age 16 years and at least 5 years older than the child or children in Criterion A.

Paedophilia has been seen by some as an 'orientation', not necessarily leading to criminal child abuse. But it is common now to use the term for a group of male abusers who seek pre-pubescent victims. The prevalence of paedophilic orientation is not known through any large population studies. Biere and Runtz (1989) surveyed 1,923 male undergraduate students regarding their sexual interest in children: 21 per cent of subjects reported sexual attraction to small children; 9 per cent described sexual fantasies involving children; and 7 per cent indicated some likelihood of having sex with a child if they could avoid detection and punishment. Smiljanich and Briere (1996) surveyed 180 female and 99 male university students: 22 per cent of males reported sexual attraction to children versus 3 per cent of females.

Much of what is described in this book about sexual abuse of young children are paedophilic acts; 80–90 per cent of the victims are boys; their mean age is 11 years. The mean age of the convicted paedophiles is the mid-20s, most have a low IQ and are poorly educated (Hughes, 2007). But that ignores the fact that those who do not get caught may be quite well educated and successful in their careers and some belong to the upper classes. Some travel to developing countries to avoid attention. Quite a few seek jobs where they have direct contact with children. Their acts are criminal and cause extensive damage to the children.

(ii) Aetiology

Hughes (2007) has published an extensive review of 554 papers on paedophilia. A causative factor that has been mentioned is child abuse, but the prevalence difference between paedophiles and non-paedophiles is small (Freund et al., 1990). Another factor is insecure attachment, but this is also common among non-abusive persons (see p. 152). Galli et al. (1999) studied twenty-two boys aged 13–17 years who had molested a younger child at least once. All met the lifetime criteria for paedophilia, twenty-one had two or more paraphilias, eighteen had a mood disorder, twelve a bipolar disorder, twelve an anxiety disorder, eleven substance abuse, and twelve an impulse-control disorder. Twelve of seventeen subjects who were further examined had ADHD and sixteen had conduct disorder. Perez-Albeniz (2003) compared a group of thirty-six adult high-risk parents with thirty-eight matched low-risk (for child abuse) parents. The high-risk parents showed higher deficit in dispositional empathy, less feelings of warmth and compassion, and more anxiety. Keenan and Ward (2000) suggest that the intimacy deficits, empathy deficits and cognitive distortions seen among sexual offenders point to a lack of awareness of other people's beliefs, desirable perspectives and needs. Kafka and Hennen (2002) found among eighty out-patient paraphilic males: mood disorders (72 per cent), anxiety disorders (38 per cent), especially social phobia (22 per cent), psychoactive substance abuse (41 per cent), especially alcohol abuse (30 per cent), and attention deficit hyperactivity disorder (ADHD) (36 per cent). Dunsieth et al. (2004) studied 113 convicted male sex offenders. They displayed high rates of mental illness, substance abuse, paraphilias, personality disorders, and co-morbidity among these conditions. Sex offenders with paraphilias have significantly higher rates of certain types of mental illness and avoidant personality disorder. It is not known whether these mental disorders are the primary causes of paedophilic behaviour, or whether they are secondary consequences of the behaviour. Studies of genetic factors among sexual offenders have not yielded any conclusive results.

(iii) Treatment

Hughes (2007) has made a thorough review of the options for treatment. Behaviour therapy and neurosurgery have not been effective, but four different anti-androgenic medicines have been helpful, if the paedophile agrees to take them. Mental disorders with high prevalence, long duration and co-morbidity – such as those described above – are usually therapy-resistant. Changes in the brain biochemistry and anatomy (see pp. 147–8) may reduce the prospects for curative treatment.

Maladaptive alcohol use

(i) Diagnosis and prevalence

DSM-IV (1994) classifies alcohol abuse as a maladaptive pattern of substance use leading to clinically significant impairment or distress, manifested by at least one of the following recurrent problems:

(a) failure to fulfil major role obligations at work, school and home;
(b) use in situations in which it is physically hazardous;

(c) alcohol-related legal problems;
(d) continued use despite having persistent or recurrent social or interpersonal problems caused or exacerbated by the effects of alcohol.

Over time, abuse may progress to dependence. Some users abuse alcohol for long periods without developing dependence. Dependence is
suspected when alcohol use is accompanied by signs of the following:
(i) abuse, (ii) compulsive drinking behaviour, (iii) higher than normal
tolerance, and (iv) withdrawal.

Alcohol is implicated in child violence. Many perpetrators act under
the acute or chronic influence of drinking. Some perpetrators may qual-
ify as alcohol abusers, and some as alcohol dependent. But for others,
their use of alcohol in the context of child abuse may be occasional.
The interim term 'maladaptive alcohol use' is proposed to include all
alternatives.

A US study (Langhinrichsen-Rohling, 2005) showed that alcohol facilitates violence: the odds of physical aggression were eight to eleven times
higher on drinking days for men in domestic violence treatment programmes. Alcohol is implicated in many crimes. Alcohol abuse also leads
to many health problems: brain damage, memory defects, liver cirrho-
sis, heart disease, arteriosclerosis, poor nutrition, injuries, and co-morbid
mental disorders.

Alcoholic drinks are available everywhere even where alcohol is a
taboo, for example in Hindu and Muslim areas. They are used by increasing numbers of people. In developing countries alcoholic drinks are made
from palm wine, sorghum, bananas, corn malt or sugar cane. There,
local beers and country liquor (such as akpetshie, chibuku, enguli, ton-
ton omwenge and waragi) are found almost everywhere. Local herbs are
often added; several of these are known to contain alkaloids, which cause
mental disturbance so severe they may result in temporary psychosis
and aggression, including murders. The brewers are mostly women.
Some products are distilled; many of these are toxic; some contain
methanol which causes blindness, brain damage, and sometimes death.
Drunken men fight with knives, machetes and guns; they rape, commit
incest, some kill. Community permissiveness of alcohol abuse appears to
increase with poverty: drinking makes the poor man forget his worries –
that there is no food in the house; that he cannot pay his children's
school fees or for their health care; that his self-esteem is gone or that he
is oppressed. Five examples from different parts of the world follow.

United States. In the USA (Bridget, 1998) 5.6 per cent of the population
are assessed to be chronic alcoholics. In 1998, there were 10.4 million
drinkers aged 12–20. Of these, 5.1 million were binge drinkers (drank five

or more drinks on at least one occasion in the month before the survey). Two million were heavy drinkers: binge drinking at least five times that month. The average age when young people first try alcohol is 11 years for boys and 13 years for girls. According to research by the National Institute on Alcohol Abuse and Alcoholism, adolescents who begin drinking before the age of 15 are four times more likely to develop alcohol dependence than those who begin drinking at the age of 21. Data from a 1999 US National Household Survey indicate that while 915,000 young people aged 12–20 reported alcohol dependence in the past year, only 16 per cent of them received treatment. Several large-scale school surveys suggest that 4–20 per cent of teenagers have either a current or past diagnosis of alcohol abuse or alcohol dependence (Chung et al., 1998). Five million alcoholic parents have at least one child at home under the age of 18. Of these children 58 per cent smoke cigarettes and 35 per cent use illicit drugs (US Department of Health and Human Services, 2004).

India. Gupta et al. (2003) carried out a study in Mumbai, India. Fifty thousand men from lower and lower-middle society were interviewed. The study included only urban men aged 45+, had an attrition rate of 50 per cent, and excluded people from higher social groups. Nineteen per cent were currently consuming alcoholic beverages; 75 per cent of these could be characterized as heavy drinkers. These findings are lower than the 25–50 per cent found among men (vs.10 per cent among women) in other Indian surveys. Most alcohol beverages are home-made: beer and distilled country liquor. The percentage of Christians who had any experience of alcohol was 61 per cent, 59 per cent among the Buddhists, 26 per cent among the Hindus, and 9 per cent among the Muslims. The prevalence of experience of alcohol was 27 per cent among the illiterates and 18 per cent among the college educated. Another Indian study confirmed that drinking and alcohol-related problems are higher among the poor (Chakravarthy, 1990). Prohibition has a limited effect in India, as alcoholic beverages are mostly home-produced and difficult to control (Rahman, 2003). Alcohol consumption per capita in the South Asia sub-continent increased by 50 per cent from 1980 to 2000 (Butchart and Poznyak, 2005).

Russia. Nicholson et al. (2005) report from Russia (in a study of 10,475 male and 3,128 females) that of the 61 per cent responders, 14 per cent of the men never drank, 41 per cent were occasional drinkers, and 13 per cent frequent binge drinkers; among women the numbers were 54 per cent, 5 per cent and 17 per cent, respectively. Eighty per cent of all alcohol consumed is vodka; a considerable proportion comes from illicit production.

Chile. Of Chile's adolescents 22 per cent aged 10–19 have consumed alcohol at least once in the past year, and 30 per cent of high-school seniors drink alcohol frequently (Naveillan and Vargas, 1989). Very young children in Chile are given alcoholic drinks and may suffer neurological and mental damage. It is known that the police arrest drunken children in the street as young as 8 years old. Children who regularly become drunk are often violent. Some are street children, but others live in 'ordinary families'. The Chilean government declared in 2006 that dealing with child alcohol use was a national priority.[16]

South Africa. Indicators point to the widespread maladaptive use of alcohol (Parry, 2002). In 2000, patients in trauma units often tested positive for alcohol, ranging from 40.3 per cent (Durban) to 91.8 per cent (Port Elizabeth). Persons who died in these hospitals often tested positive for alcohol, ranging from 40.3 per cent (Durban) to 67.2 per cent (Port Elizabeth). Alcohol misuse occurs among all sectors. School surveys reflect harmful drinking patterns among students, with 53.3 per cent and 36.5 per cent of male students in Durban and Cape Town, respectively, reporting heavy-drinking episodes by Grade 11 (aged about 16–17 years).

(ii) Relations between childhood violence and alcohol

Butchart and Poznyak (2005) state that:

> In the USA, 35% of parental child abusers had consumed either alcohol or drugs at the time of the incident. In Germany, 32% of fatal child abusers were under the influence of alcohol at the time of the crime, and 37% of the offenders suffered from chronic alcoholism. In Canada, alcohol or drug use was reported in 34% of child welfare investigations. In Australia, alcohol or drug use was a contributing factor in 57% of child out-of-home care applications. In London, England, parental substance use was present in 52% of families on the child protection register, with alcohol the principal substance used.
>
> A wide range of alcohol-related risk factors have been identified that increase a child's risk of being maltreated. These include: having young, poor, unemployed or socially isolated parents; having a history of domestic violence in the home; living in a single parent family, and living in an overcrowded household. Having a parent with a history of harmful or hazardous alcohol use increases the risk of childhood violence. When both parents experience problems with alcohol, the risk of child violence is even greater. In addition to being a high grade marker for the parent's emotional turmoil, alcohol has a significant disinhibiting effect that often worsens an already bad

situation. Adolescents with low parental involvement, or who report physical or sexual abuse, are more likely to be influenced by social pressures, including parental example, to drink alcohol and are at greater risk of regular drinking because of their need for the anti-anxiety effects of alcohol. Such frequent drinking by adolescents is linked to problems such as truancy, poor school performance, and delinquent behaviour; these can further increase the risk of physical abuse by a parent. Children who have experienced violence are more likely to drink heavily as adults, and have higher potential for physically abusing their own children in later life.

This is further confirmed by other studies, where the victims reveal that sexual assault, rape and physical abuse of children and adolescents are often carried out by drunken, disinhibited aggressors often attempting to intoxicate the victim also.

(iii) Treatment

The effectiveness of treating alcoholics is disputed. Several million alcoholics all over the world receive alcoholism treatment on any given day. The techniques of therapy for alcoholics have traditionally been based on clinical intuition, with little rigorous validation of their effectiveness. Only a minority of alcoholics report abstinent one year after treatment; many have dry periods alternating with wet relapses. Most are unable to stop drinking totally. However, few programmes attempt to deal with the psychodynamic issues underlying alcoholism. A key feature of Alcoholics Anonymous is the group support and acceptance that supplies a key childhood life experience missing in the lives of most of its members.

Aston (1999) presented the largest study ever made of the effectiveness of treating alcoholism. Project MATCH was carried out in the United States from 1989–97. It was a multi-site clinical trial of alcohol dependent volunteers (n = 1,726). The participants were offered three different twelve-week, high-quality outpatient programmes: (a) a twelve-step self-help programme (twelve sessions); (b) motivational enhancement therapy (four sessions); and (c) cognitive behaviour therapy (twelve sessions).

The patients' participation was excellent and 90 per cent were followed up over a fifteen-month period. The patients in all three groups showed major improvements: (a) the number of drinking days diminished from 25 per month to 6 per month; (b) the volume of drinking decreased from an average of 15 drinks per day to 3 per day; (c) there were significant decreases in the use of other drugs, and improvements in liver function. There were few significant outcome differences between the three treatments.

There was, however, one surprising feature: the patients' improvements took place during the first week, and then remained more or less on the same level, apparently uninfluenced by the therapies. Also, a group of 100 drop-outs from the programme, who had no treatments, reached positive results of about the same size. The conclusion was that the patients selected for treatment were extremely well motivated.

Enrolling in this study suggests that the alcoholic had crystallized a decision to reduce or abstain from drinking (Naveillan and Vargas, 1989). Topping the list of client characteristics linked to treatment success – and even more important than the initial severity of their alcohol problems – was their readiness to change behaviour. Over three years on, this still had a profound impact on abstinence and restraint when drinking (Aston, 1999).

The magnitude of positive results of the MATCH study is explained by Aston (1999) as follows:

> the exclusion of young people under the age of 18, of those who were drug dependent, of recent injectors, of the psychotic, of the potentially violent, of the socially isolated or homeless and of those currently under justice supervision. There were very few highly disturbed outpatients. The study thus can only afford limited clues about how to handle the most disturbed and violent drinkers and those ordered into treatment by the courts.

Those mentioned are the alcoholics with the most pronounced problems: poor motivation and the experiences of treating them are rather negative. It is among these that we will unfortunately find some of the violent child abusers; we should, however, also realize that adverse childhood experiences contribute 65 per cent to the population risk for alcoholism (Felitti and Anda, 2003).

Disorders among care-givers: mental disorders

(i) Diagnosis and prevalence

Diagnoses of mental disorders are often carried out using the Composite International Diagnostic Interview (CIDI). The prevalence throughout a person's lifetime of any mental disorder in community-based samples is high: for example 48 per cent in the USA (Kessler et al., 1994); 41.2 per cent in the Netherlands (Biji et al., 1998) and 47.5 per cent in Brazil

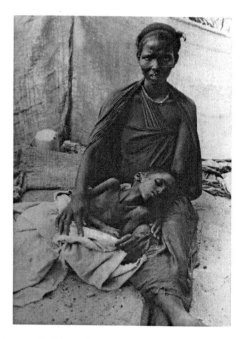

Photo 16.   **Mother and child.** *This mother's child is dying. There is no help and no health services in her village. In many poor countries like hers between 10% and 20% of the children die, a very traumatic event, causing depressive disorder, anxiety and stress to the mother, who does not know what will happen next to her family. Her health condition is further impaired by her own malnutrition and anaemia.* © *World Health Organization.*

(Santos et al., 2006). Prevalence rates are higher for women than for men. The most common of these disorders among women are anxiety (about 33 per cent) and mood disorders (about 20 per cent).

  The conclusion is that close to every other person during their life-time is affected by a mental disorder. That disorder may occur when that person is the care-giver of a child. About one-third to one-half of those affected had a period of mental disorder during the last twelve months, and through the duration of the disorder about 70 per cent of them expe-rienced role impairment at home, at work, in relationships and socially (Kessler et al., 1994). Care-givers, mothers and fathers, carry out the physical and psychological punishment of their children. The presence of mental disorders among them significantly contributes to their own behaviour towards their children and may cause persisting behaviour problems among the children (Mash and Johnston, 1983; Mezey et al., 2005).

(ii) Aetiology

Many ecological factors contribute: poverty, lack of education, spouse abuse (in many populations affecting 40–70 per cent of all women), poor marital relations, daily stress, diseases and death among close family members and friends, low levels of social and emotional support, poor parental competence, growing up with abusive and neglectful parents, alcohol abuse, and lack of medical care and other community services. Other causes are related to post-partum depression among women, and general tiredness because of work overload in combination with anaemia and malnutrition. The children's behaviour also contributes, and it is common to see that leading to their punishment.

(iii) Treatment

Treatments are available in developed countries, and will reduce the mental symptoms over time, but will not be very effective as long as the root causes prevail. In the developing countries, mental health care, except for the well-to-do, is insufficient or non-existent, and the root causes are more difficult to resolve as many are based in poverty and hunger.

Disorders among care-givers: foetal abuse and neglect

Some mothers use alcohol and drugs during their pregnancy. Relevant scientific studies mostly deal with their alcohol and illicit drug use which damages the foetus. Alcohol is a leading teratogen; the incidence of foetal alcohol spectrum disorder (FASD) in the USA is 2.2 per 1,000 live births (Wattendorf and Muenke, 2005). In Italy, the prevalence is 3.7 to 7.4 per 1,000 schoolchildren. (May et al., 2006). The highest prevalence of FASD worldwide is reported among first-grade children in a wine-growing region in the Western Cape province of South Africa: 40.5 to 46.4 per 1,000 children aged 5–9 years (May et al., 2000). Prevalence rates of FASD probably underestimate its incidence, as some of these children meet an early death. The main complication is brain damage. The disorder may lead to neurological, cardiac, facial and joint deformities, stunted physical and emotional development, mental retardation, memory and attention deficits, a tendency to impulsive behaviour, inability to reason from cause to effect, a failure to comprehend the concept of time, difficulty telling fantasy from reality, inability to control sexual impulses, and an apparent lack of remorse. Among babies born to cocaine/crack-using mothers, the frequency of mental retardation is high. Smoking during pregnancy may delay foetus growth and intellectual development, and cause behaviour disturbances. Children with foetal neglect symptoms are exposed to very disturbed meso-systems and for many there will be no willing substitute families.

Neurobiological correlates of violent behaviour

It would seem reasonable to assume a priori that serious pathological behaviour would be reflected in neurobiological correlates, and indeed scientific evidence supports this hypothesis. Neurobiological correlates – biochemical, hormonal, physiological and anatomical aberrations – are found among violent offenders. These changes can be explained in three ways:

(a) *downstream*: the neurobiological aberrations are primary and lead to the aggressive behaviour (the causes could be genetic, prenatal or perinatal, or post-natal brain damage through infections, direct trauma or thrombosis);

(b) *upstream*: the perpetrator's behaviour (related to his/her abuse of others, lifestyle problems such as chronic drug abuse, including amphetamine; Rogers et al., 1999) induces secondary changes in the brain;

(c) *a combination*: the violent person may have been a victim of child violence causing upstream neurobiological effects, and when acting violently the upstream damage is enforced and further increases downstream aggressive behaviour.

These questions are ethically important. Hart and Hare (1996) support the primary downstream hypothesis – the brain-based aetiology. They found no convincing evidence that psychopathy is the direct result of early social or environmental factors. If the causes of violent action are only seen as downstream, does this imply that these individuals are predisposed to become criminals and does this therefore excuse them from legal and moral responsibility (Popma and Raine, 2006)? Among them are some who have committed horrible crimes against children, including murder. Responsible or not, the conclusion is that they should be locked up; the public needs to be protected, especially from callous repeaters.

A number of recent neurobiological studies show that significant aberrations have been identified also among psychopaths. LaPierre et al. (1995) made comparisons between a group of criminal psychopaths and criminal non-psychopaths. The psychopaths differed in having impairments in the orbito-frontal-ventral part of the brain, which is involved in instrumental learning and response reversal. Raine et al. (2003) found that the corpus callosum had a larger than normal volume, which indicated either an atypical neurodevelopmental process with a deficit of axonal pruning, or increased white myelination. Kiehl et al. (2004, 2006) have in separate studies of psychopaths shown temporal lobe and limbic abnormalities, which are involved in semantic processing. Tiihonen et al. (2000) identified amygdaloid loss, which appears to explain the psychopaths' lack of remorse. Early damage to the prefrontal cortex impairs social and moral behaviour (Soderstrom et al., 2000) and in non-psychotic violent offenders, regional blood flow to the prefrontal cortex is reduced. Birbaumer et al. (2005), using magnetic resonance imaging, revealed that while healthy controls showed enhanced differential activation in the limbic circuit during acquisition of fear, the psychopaths displayed no such activity in the circuit.

The *Canadian Psychiatric Journal* published an article in 2001 on the neuropsychopharmacology of criminality and aggression. A summary follows:

> About 40% of the propensity toward antisocial behaviour may be attributable to heredity, specifically violent impulsive behaviour. Impulsive violent offenders have diminished serotonergic function. In addition to genetic factors, the serotonergic system is influenced by environmental factors; this influence is complex. Some of it may occur during developmental phases, such as birth complications and maternal rejection which are associated with early onset violent behaviour. Serotonin may be one of the mediators of environmental influence on the brain. Changes in serotonin function in humans may relate to socio-economic status, sustained childhood abuse, and histories of impulsive aggressive behaviour.
>
> Hypoglycemia has been associated with aggression; it is thought to lead to impaired cognitive processes and judgement, which may increase the risk of aggression or impulsivity. A study of impulsive violent offenders with APD and offenders with intermittent explosive disorder were shown to have lower glucose nadir after glucose challenge, compared with normal volunteers. Heritability was suggested by the finding that impulsive violent offenders with criminal fathers had lower glucose nadirs than those without criminal fathers.
>
> The role of testosterone in impulsive aggression is well documented in animal studies, but the role of testosterone in human aggression

is less clear. Violent aggression in men, on the whole, seems more correlated with abnormalities of serotonergic function. The serotonin function may be modulated by sex hormones.

Positron emission spectroscopy was carried out to study brain activity in forty-one murderers pleading not guilty by reason of insanity. It was found that murderers had reduced metabolism in the prefrontal cortex, superior parietal gyros, left angular gyros, and in the corpus callosum. Asymmetry was also noted in the amygdala, thalamus, and medial temporal lobe. Looking specifically at impulsive aggression in subjects with personality disorder, six impulsive-aggressive patients were compared with five healthy volunteers. Patients with impulsive aggression showed significantly blunted metabolic responses in orbital frontal, adjacent ventral medial, and cingulate cortex, but not in the inferior parietal lobe. The highly serotonergically innervated prefrontal cortex may be involved in the regulation of impulsive aggression. In this sense, a theory of serotonergically mediated inhibition of impulsive aggression is not biologically deterministic because the influence of environmental variables as a modulator of serotonergic function is significant from moment to moment as well as over a lifetime and serotonin's role in behaviour is only in the context of the complicated relationship between brain, mind, and environment.

Oxytocin and vasopressin are two neuropeptides released into the blood from the pituitary gland, and from centrally projecting oxytocin neurons. It is the latter, and the oxytocin receptors in the brain, that are responsible for their behaviour effects (De Weid et al., 1991). These peptides have been intensively studied since the 1950s. Many results confirm their involvement in emotional processes. Oxytocin facilitates attachment between offspring and parents and between males and females, whereas vasopressin is involved in aggressive behaviour. The attachment process is built on social recognition formation and the formation of social memories, mediated by these neuropeptides. Oxytocin and vasopressin are important in the modulation of anxiety, and may be involved in antidepressive-like effects. Vasopressin facilitates memory processing. Oxytocin acts as a natural amnestic agent by impairing memory consolidation and retrieval (Caldwell and Young, 2006; Takayanagi et al., 2005).

Studies of the neurobiology of paedophiles have been carried out. Maes et al. (2001a, 2001b) have shown that paedophilic men have elevated plasma epinephrine and norepinephrine, and abnormal cortisol and luteinizing hormone reactions. In response to stress, the hypothalamus produces corticotrophin-releasing hormone, which depresses the reproductive system. It prevents the release of gonadotropin that regulates reproduction and sexual behaviour. Glucocorticoids also inhibit the production of testosterone, estrogen and progesterone and of the luteinizing hormone that prompts the production of ovulation and sperm. Schiltz et al. (2007) studied the brain pathology in fifteen paedophilic perpetrators in comparison with normal subjects. The paedophiles had a significant decrease of right amygdala volume compared with healthy controls, reduced grey matter in the right amygdala, hypothalamus (bilaterally), septal regions, substantial innominata, and bed nucleus of the striae terminalis. In eight of the fifteen perpetrators, enlargement of the anterior temporal horn of the right lateral ventricle that adjoins the amygdala could be recognized by routine qualitative clinical assessment. Smaller right amygdala volumes were correlated with the propensity to commit uniform paedophilic sexual offences. Cantor et al. (2008) using MRI showed significant negative associations between paedophilia and white matter volumes of the temporal and parietal lobes bilaterally. The regions of lower white matter volumes were limited to two major fibre bundles: the superior fronto-occipital fasciculus and the right arcuate fasciculus. No significant differences were found in grey matter. Because these fasciculi connect the cortical regions that respond to sexual cues, these results suggest (1) that those cortical regions operate as a network for recognizing sexually relevant stimuli, and (2) that paedophilia results from a partial disconnection within that network.

Among violent offenders there is a 'cascade' of complex, interrelated brain changes that damage its biochemical and hormonal regulation, and which are reflected in significant anatomical, metabolic and circulatory disturbances. Some of these changes appear to be attributable to genetic factors in combination with the perpetrator's own experiences of childhood violence. The perpetrators' behaviour is anchored in an organic context. The lack of effectiveness of therapeutic interventions in many clients with personality disorders may depend on an irreversible fixation of these neurobiological alterations. Furthermore, neuropharmaca are most often limited to influencing only single biochemical brain pathways, such as serotonin uptake. In view of the cascade of changes that take place, such medication is unlikely to exert more than minor effects. Thus, large-scale violence prevention programmes cannot build on presently available methods for therapeutic interventions to 'correct' the behaviour of the perpetrators.

Conclusions regarding health-related causes of child violence

Health-related causes of child violence are important. Severe personality disorders explain some of the worst instances of extreme cruelty to children by perpetrators with callous and unemotional traits. These people are responsible for much of the long-lasting and high recurrence rates of child abuse. They lack remorse. Some may be members of the 'upper classes' and have important jobs, while their abuse of children remains hidden. I find it difficult to accept the DSM-IV's proposed low prevalence of ASPD, especially as Viding et al. (2005) revealed a prevalence of 12.5 per cent extremely callous unemotional behaviour (CU) among 7-year-old children, whom Viding et al. then did not even consider treating. The very high prevalence of extreme CU shows that it is urgent to identify the means to cure it. Although there are some effective methods to treat children with conduct disorder, the treatments for ASPD do not appear to be effective. The reason for this is their fixed, irreversible neurobiological impairments.

Maladaptive alcohol use is one of the most common contributors to child abuse. Alcohol makes people – who in a sober situation control their aggression – lose their inhibitions and become violent. It has proved difficult to reduce alcohol consumption in the general population, and binge drinking among the young. It is urgent to stop women from consuming alcohol while they are pregnant. More research is needed concerning the groups of unmotivated alcoholics who were not included in the MATCH study. Mental disorders, some temporary, among care-givers are very common and often related to environmental factors (poor marital relations, daily stress, somatic diseases, poverty and hunger, and so on). These will for most continue as long as the root factors remain unresolved; they have negative effects on the children.

The social system

Family malfunction related to incompetent and ignorant parenting

The most important cause of childhood violence is the malfunction of families. Parents are the main group of perpetrators. The most important cause of childhood violence is abusive, incompetent and ignorant parenting, not only in poor families, but also in affluent ones.

The most common form is neglect. Parents do not provide food, education, health care, acceptable lodging, security, and so on. Even worse, many parents do not care about these problems. Spouse abuse is common and creates an atmosphere of fear. Criminality and substance abuse further complicate the problems. In such families it is common to see that the essential emotional contacts between parents and children have been neglected right from the beginning, so there is no bonding and no creation of empathy. In abusive families, many children lose their perception of identity (Bastian, 1994):

> The children who could not cope with life in whatever setting were those who did not understand who they were, why they were there and what was happening to them.

Another common form of abuse is emotional: yelling, screaming and cursing, scolding, name-calling, humiliation, threats to throw the child out of the house, locking out the child, threats with magic and evil spirits or sheer terrorizing. Ineffective family child-rearing practices increase risk for child behaviour problems. One example is in China (Li et al., 2001) where these problems were prevalent in children aged 2–6 in a rural area: 71 per cent had temper tantrums; 48 per cent were swearing; 30 per cent were disobedient; 30 per cent had difficulty initiating sleep; and 17 per cent were picky eaters. In Finland, Räikkönen and Keltikangas-Järvinen (1992) examined 924 mothers who use hostile child-rearing practices (i.e. they ignore the child, are punitive and irritable, and perceive the child as a burden). These children exhibit high levels of inattention, impatience, anger and aggression.

This is often combined with physical abuse, which in many cultures is seen as positive for character-building. All parents know that sexual abuse is legally forbidden and a taboo, yet one-third of them get involved in such abuse. Skute et al. (1998) revealed that exposure to intra-familial violence is a risk factor for the development of sexually abusive behaviour. Boys who are victims of sexual abuse are more likely to become abusers of other children in their early adolescence if they have experienced or witnessed intra-familial violence (odds ratio 39.7). Marital violence impacts on the emotional and behavioural development of children. In some families, the contacts between 15-year-old children and their parents seem distant (see Box 9.1, adapted from Ngwudike, 2005).

The most common recommendations for preventing family malfunction are: family life preparations supported by pre-parental education and home visits, as described in Chapter 14.

Box 9.1:   Child–parent relations in the USA

The Program for International Student Assessment 2000 by the OECD revealed the following about child–parent relations in the USA; students were 15 years old. (a) Students eating dinner with parents around a table: 8 per cent never, 8 per cent a few times a year, 5 per cent once a month, 11 per cent several times a month, 23 per cent several times a week, and 37 per cent every day; (b) parents discussing their schoolwork: 3 per cent never, 6 per cent a few times a year, 8 per cent once a month, 15 per cent several times a month, 21 per cent several times a week, and 41 per cent every day; (c) parents discussing books, films or television programmes with them: 12 per cent never, 15 per cent a few times a year, 12 per cent once a month, 20 per cent several times a month, 19 per cent several times a week, and 16 per cent every day; (d) how often their mothers worked with them on homework: 33 per cent never, 19 per cent a few times a year, 12 per cent once a month, 13 per cent several times a month, 11 per cent several times a week, and 6 per cent every day; (e) how often their fathers worked with them on homework: 45 per cent never, 17 per cent a few times a year, 11 per cent once a month, 10 per cent several times a month, 7 per cent several times a week, and 3 per cent every day.

A detailed review of violence prevention was published in 2004 by WHO. The strategies are arranged by age group and demonstrated effectiveness, built on US studies:

Children aged 0–3: Home visiting services; parenting training, therapeutic foster care.

Children aged 3–11: Social development training; pre-school enrichment.

Children aged 12–19: Social development training, educational incentives for at-risk and for disadvantaged high school students: school-based dating violence prevention programmes, academic enrichment programmes, mentoring, family therapy.

Preventive research has centred on poor, undereducated or disadvantaged families. There are clear links between violence against children and the social malfunctioning of families, institutions and services in the community and in the society at large. Such interventions are often called 'social engineering'. In the welfare statistics, a few categories of vulnerable children in disadvantaged families dominate; they are the ones most often targeted by 'engineering' programmes:

1. children with parents abusing alcohol or illicit drugs, or who have a mental disorder, or are criminal;
2. when there is abuse or neglect at home, for instance reported by neighbours or teachers;
3. children reported by teachers for mental disorders;
4. children with a disability;
5. children with serious relationship problems (for instance, with foreign roots, of different ethnicity, religion or culture, with language barriers);
6. children in conflict with the law.

However, the concentration on these groups tends to neglect the fact that abusers are everywhere (Box 9.2).

Box 9.2: Child abuse among the upper and middle classes

In the large 2007 India study of child abuse Kacker states that the prevalence of sexual abuse in the upper and upper middle classes was proportionally higher than in the lower and lower middle classes. As Holla and Gupta (2005) describe from India: 'A 5-year-old boy from a well-to-do family was brought by his father and stepmother with fracture of right tibia, severe malnutrition, multiple abrasions, bruises, scars, hemiparesis, psychomotor retardation, and old fractures in both ulnas and right humerus. Skeletal survey showed 15 fractures involving ribs, metacarpals, mandible, ulnas, right humerus and right tibia and old subdural hematomas. Brittle bones and neuropathy were excluded. The child was moved to the grandparents. A medico-legal report and involvement of social organizations yielded no action.'

Exposure to domestic violence

Exposure to domestic violence is traumatic to children. Such violence is common, especially for the female partner. The World Health Organization (2002) reviewed data from a large number of population studies (six countries in Africa, thirteen in America, nine in Asia, six in Europe and one in Oceania). Such abuse is experienced annually by 10–70 per cent of the women interviewed. A recent US study (Thompson et al., 2006) of 3,429 women found 44 per cent lifetime intimate partner abuse. Experiencing such abuse has serious consequences for children. McGuigan and Pratt (2001) studied a sample of 2,544 at-risk mothers with first-born children participating in a home-visiting child abuse prevention programme. They investigated the effect of domestic violence during the first six months of child rearing on confirmed physical child abuse, psychological child abuse, and child neglect, and then followed the child's first five years. Domestic violence occurred in 38 per cent of the 155 cases of confirmed maltreatment. Domestic violence preceded child maltreatment in 78 per cent of the 59 cases of co-occurrence. Domestic violence during the first six months of child rearing was significantly related to all three types of child maltreatment up to the child's fifth year. McFarlane et al. (2003) studied children aged 6–18 years to 258 abused mothers: these children exhibited significantly more internalizing, externalizing and total behaviour problems than children of the same age and sex of non-abused mothers. Similar results were reported by Kernic et al. (2003). Family violence during the last year had been experienced by 71 per cent in China and by 69 per cent of the children in Korea (Kim et al., 2000). Koenen et al. (2003), based on a population sample of 1,116 monozygotic and dizygotic 5-year-old twin pairs in England, concluded that children exposed to high levels of domestic violence had IQs that were, on average, eight points lower than unexposed children. The findings are consistent with animal experiments and human studies documenting the harmful effects of extreme stress on brain development. Programmes that successfully reduce domestic violence therefore should also have beneficial effects on children's cognitive development.

Identification of future perpetrators using social methods

Table 9.1 lists some social predictors of aggression and violent crimes published by several authors from developed countries. They mainly concern young boys, the main group showing criminal behaviour as adolescents or adults – an important target group for prevention.

A set of recommendations for the USA was drafted in the Summary Chapter of the 1999 San Diego Child Maltreatment Conference (Sadler et al., 1999). Because the problems of child maltreatment have existed for many centuries, many have estimated that it will take 100 years to eradicate it (Chadwick, 1999). This may reflect these authors' views of the past: cannibalism, ritual human sacrifice and the practice of suttee took a long time to eliminate. Not until 180 years after Jenner's introduction of

Table 9.1 Examples of studies of factors related to aggression and violent crimes

Factors	Symptoms	Comments/source
Individual	Early aggressiveness	Schoolboys aged 10–13 were rated by teachers for aggression. Two-thirds with high scores had been arrested for violent offences by age 26. In a control group with low scores the arrest rate was one sixth (Stattin and Magnusson, 1989, Sweden).
Family	Parental criminality/ antisocial behaviour	Risk for violent criminality increases 3.8 times compared to a group with non-criminal parents (Baker and Mednick, 1985, USA).
	Childhood violence	Physically abused or neglected children are more likely than others to commit violent crimes as adults (Smith and Thornberry, 1995, USA).
	Inconsistent discipline and low level of parent involvement	Boys with overly strict parents reported the highest rate of subsequent violence; boys with overly permissive parents reported the second highest level of violence. Least violence found among boys not belonging to these groups (Park and Comstock, 1994, USA).
School	Poor academic results	Academic failure predicts later violent behaviour (Maguin and Loeber, 1996, USA).
	Truancy	Pupils with high truancy rates at ages 12–14 more likely to show future violent behaviour (Wells and Rankin, 1988, USA).
Peer relations	Delinquent siblings or peers	Having delinquent siblings by age 10 predicts convictions for violence (Farrington, 1989, USA).
	Gang membership	Delinquent adolescent peers, including gang members, have a negative influence (Moffitt, 2001, USA).
Community factors	Poverty	Boys raised in poverty have higher criminality. Self-reported felony assault and robbery were twice as common among young people brought up in poverty compared to controls from the middle class (Elliott et al., 1989, USA).
	Neighbourhood disorganization	High presence of criminals, drug-sellers, gangs, availability of drugs and weapons and poor housing are predictors of violence at age 18 (Maguin et al., 1995, USA).

the smallpox vaccine in 1796 was the disease finally eradicated. We are still struggling with efforts to eliminate capital punishment of children and of persons with mental retardation, female sexual mutilation, the right to possess guns, illicit drug business inside the closed gates of prisons, and the abuse of children in government institutions. The 'partial' success with the stop-smoking evolution required 'a dogged, relentless campaign to communicate the database to the people, and consistent advocacy in the halls of government' (Garbarino, 1996).

Cultural and economic systems

Violence in the society

The individual's frustrations in daily life

One of the explanations proposed for 'understanding' why interpersonal violence is so common is the frustrating economic and physical insecurity that appears to be part of our everyday life. In 2005, community violence exploded in the suburbs of many French cities: over twenty-one nights, more than 10,000 vehicles were burnt, 200 public buildings destroyed, 1,300 policemen injured, 3,200 persons arrested, and 400 offenders sentenced to prison terms. A US study (Rapp et al., 1986) showed that teenagers experienced 40 per cent of all robberies and 36 per cent of all personal attacks against them while at school (where they spend about 25 per cent of their time). A Danish study (Balvig, 1999) of 1,270 eighth-grade (mean age 14) students from three different regions of the country found that 44 per cent had experienced a theft, 16 per cent had been beaten and 36 per cent threatened with violence within a period of twelve months. Twenty-six per cent of them came from a split home.

There are many factors that suggest that violence is even more common in developing countries than in the industrialized ones: the high number of fist and knife fights; the more widespread abuse and neglect of women and children; the greater degree of frustrating poverty and the lack of political clout among the poor; the hierarchical power system that does not allow those of 'lower rank' to comment on or to contradict what 'elders and leaders' say and do; the insufficiency, unreliability and corruption of the police, security and judicial systems; the non-compliance with UN Human Rights; the oppressive education system with abusive teachers; civil unrest and local wars; and the fact that 85 per cent of all natural disasters occur in developing countries. Among the many problems are the increasing levels of alcoholism and use of drugs, such as heroin, cocaine, amphetamines, hallucinogens, and qat.

The culture of violence

The so-called 'weapons culture' accounts for a very large part of the avalanche of violence. Oxfam estimated in 2003 that 639 million hand-guns are in the hands of 'ordinary people', one for each fourth man aged over the age of 15. In a US study Mocan and Tekin (2006) showed that having a gun at home increases the propensity to commit crime by 30 per cent among adolescents. Duggan (2001) reports that decreases in gun ownership during the 1990s explains about one-third of the decrease of crimes during that period. Other private weapons for stabbing (knives, machetes, daggers) are impossible to count; nor is their use restricted only to men – women and children also use them.

Another part of the violence culture appears in the products of the entertainment industry. Many children are exposed to emotional, psy-chological, sexual and physical violence on television. 'Soap operas', action movies, songs, video clips and computer games for children are often soaked in violence. A 6-year-old child playing his games can be seen to 'kill' several hundred 'virtual persons' a day; the quicker the bet-ter. Developing countries are increasingly invaded by these products of foreign cultures. Violence attracts people's attention and produces strong emotional reactions that enforce desire. Marketers call this 'arousal': it helps to sell the 'merchandise'. It may also be addictive, which could explain why, during the last decades, the media have gradually increased the doses of graphic violence. Several meta-analyses indicate that expo-sure to media violence increases short-term aggressive behaviour towards both friends and strangers but may not lead to increases of homicides or physical assaults (Park and Comstock, 1994; Wood et al., 1991). Anderson and Bushman (2001) state that:

- media violence increases the likelihood of aggressive and violent behaviour in the immediate situation and over time;
- research evidence is consistent, clear and conclusive;
- negative effects of media violence are large enough to warrant serious concern;
- most parents seriously underestimate the long-term impact of media violence;
- violent video games are likely to be more harmful than violent movies or television;
- self-imposed regulation is not working.

Media exposure to violence is still relatively uncommon among the poorest people in the developing countries. In the future, however, it will be increasingly difficult for them to escape. Mitchell et al. (2007) studied a US national sample of 1,501 youth internet users (aged 10–17 years); 57 per cent reported some form of offline interpersonal victimization (e.g. bullying, sexual abuse), and 23 per cent reported an online interpersonal victimization (i.e. sexual solicitation and harassment) in the past year. Seventy-three per cent of those reporting an online victimization also reported an offline victimization. Both types of such victimization were related to depression, delinquent behaviour and substance use.

Risk factors

The US Department of Justice brought together a group of twenty-two researchers to analyse current research on risk and protective factors and the development of serious and violent offending careers (Table 9.2) and this has resulted in a comparative ranking of 'malleable' predictors of violent or serious delinquency at ages 15–25 (Hawkins et al., 2000).

The breeding of criminal behaviour

Not all violence is criminal; some exceptions, for instance, include some levels of physical abuse of family members or of schoolchildren, and – most important – collective violence: wars, occupation and action by armies, police and security forces in many countries. Most crimes are non-violent, but violent perpetrators are frequently involved in stealing (Canter and Kirby, 1995), vandalism (Mitchell and Rosa, 1979) and drug selling (Maguin et al., 1995). In self-reporting questionnaires, they admit to a high frequency of participation in non-violent crimes (Farrington, 1989). Criminologists tell us that criminal behaviour is an adaptation to the perpetrator's social environment (Giddens, 2001; Hirschi, 1969; Merton, 1968).

Violent crime has many explanations; some are one-dimensional, some multi-dimensional. Many theories have been published, and continue to appear (De Keseredy and Perry, 2006). Some criminologists tell us that the theory of 'differential association' suggests that criminal behaviour is learned from other criminal persons. The more the individual is exposed to unlawful persons, the more likely he/she will learn and adopt their values as the basis for his/her own 'behaviour'. It is important not to be in the wrong place at the wrong time with the wrong persons. According to Laws and Marshall (1990), 'Deviant sexual interests may be learned through the same mechanisms by which conventional sexuality is learned … maladaptive behaviour can result from quantitative and qualitative combinations of processes that are themselves intrinsically orderly, strictly determined, and normal in origin.'

Table 9.2 Predictors of violent or serious delinquency by age group

Ranking of ages 6–11 and ages 12–14 predictors of violent or serious delinquency at ages 15–25. Correlations between the predictor and the outcome

Predictors at ages 6–11	Predictors at ages 12–14
Rank 1 Group	
General offences (.38) Substance abuse (.30)	Social ties (.39) Antisocial peers (.37)
Rank 2 Group	
Gender (male) (.26) Family socio-economic status (.24) Antisocial parents (.23)	General offences (.26)
Rank 3 Group	
Aggression (.21) Ethnicity (.20)	Aggression (.19) School attitude/performance (.19) Psychological condition (.19) Parent–child relations (.19) Gender (male) (.19) Physical violence (.18)
Rank 4 Group	
Psychological condition (.15) Parent–child relations (.15) Social ties (.15) Problem behaviour (.13) School attitude/performance (.13) Medical/physical characteristics (.12) IQ (.12) Other family characteristics (.12)	Antisocial parents (.16) Person crimes (.14) Problem behaviour (.12) IQ (.11)
Rank 5 Group	
Broken home (.09) Abusive parents (.07) Antisocial peers (.04)	Broken home (.10) Family socio-economic status (.10) Abusive parents (.09) Other family characteristics (.08) Substance abuse (.06) Ethnicity (.04)

Ward and Keenan (1999) state that 'child molesters' cognitive distortions are generated by maladaptive implicit theories concerning the nature of victims (children as sexual objects), the offender (entitlement), and the world (uncontrollability and nature of harm)'.

A criminal individual often gangs up with a social group of persons that shares his/her attitudes and behaviour. Gangs breed and attract crime

(Shaw and McKay, 1972). There is evidence of an inter-generational disposition to mete out corporal punishment, supporting the theory of 'social learning' (Muller et al., 1995), while other studies concerning transmission of sexual abuse indicate that such transmission may have other causes (Mahlangu and Sibindi, 1995; Collin-Vézina and Cyr, 2003). One-third of sexually abusive men and half of the mothers of sexually abused children mention that they were sexually abused during their childhood.

Merton's (1968) theory of anomie proposes that criminality is a result of the perpetrator's inability to identify any legally acceptable means to reach the individual goals that society expects, including the unreachable success goals some parents seek for their children. Therefore, the perpetrator – seeking escape from frustrating realities – decides to use socially unacceptable means. Other criminologists (Giddens, 2001) portray the delinquent as an individual who subscribes generally to the morals of society but who is able to justify to himself particular forms of delinquent behaviour by a process of 'neutralization', in which the behaviour is redefined in moral terms to make it acceptable. To give an example using the self-perception theory (Bem, 1972): a young girl who has learned that abortion is 'unacceptable' finds herself pregnant and then decides to have an abortion. Then, she changes her opinion: abortion is now 'acceptable as an ultimate solution'. Other examples are the members of terrorist groups, who have been co-opted to work in the name of a political or religious creed. Such groups may resort to violence in all forms and even take pride in claiming responsibility for atrocious acts: killing innocent people, raping women, and torturing and murdering their victims. Illicit drugs and alcohol contribute to weaken any 'moral' inhibitions the individual might have learned previously.

Some criminologists blame delinquency not on the individual but on the political and legal systems in the society (Giddens, 2001): 'The law is seen as an instrument by which the powerful and affluent maintain their position and coerce the poor into patterns of behaviour that preserve the status quo.'

The theory of 'differential association', learning violence from others, would apply to many violent perpetrators. How do perpetrators learn? Most abuse starts early in life with the parents administering physical punishment, an intimidating experience for all small children, who quickly understand that human power is exercised by the use of brutal physical force. Although 'learning' appears to be the preferred theory to explain the development of interpersonal violence, we should not exclude looking into other 'mechanisms' that are discussed: genetic factors and neurobiological changes.

Passive bystanders play a role. When a brutal father abuses the child in the presence of the mother, is there any reaction from her to stop the violence? Do bystanders encourage the act by complete agreement or by passive acceptance? Or is the mother just another victim, too frightened to interfere because she is subjugated by the offender? (Slaby et al., 1995).

Zingraff et al. (2005) showed that in a representative sample of 4,293 children aged 12–15 in Canada self-reports revealed a criminality rate of 43 per cent among the boys, and 36 per cent among the girls. Among the younger children, these were mostly petty crimes, but with increasing age the seriousness of the crimes increased. It was shown in Chapter 8 that victims of childhood violence commit twice as many crimes as non-abused children.

Adolescents aged 13–17 commit a substantial proportion of sex crimes. In the USA, in 2003, 17 per cent of all arrests for sex crimes and about one-third of all sex offences against children were by this group, and almost all the perpetrators were males (National Center on Sexual Behaviour of Youth, 2003). Many of them self-report high rates of sexual victimization; Weinrott (1998) states that it may reach as high as 50 per cent. Adolescent sex offenders are different from adult sex offenders; they have lower recidivism rates, engage in less abusive behaviour over shorter times, and exhibit less aggressive sexual behaviour. These findings support Moffitt's (2001) theory of two different types of anti-social behaviour: (a) the adolescence-limited and (b) the life-course-persistent. The adolescence-limited antisocial behaviour is caused by temporary maturity gaps encouraging teenagers to mimic antisocial behaviour in ways that are normative and adjustive. In the case of the life-course-persistent group, children's neurobiological problems interact cumulatively with their criminogenic environments during their entire development, culminating in a pathological personality. The antisocial behaviour of the first group is temporary, situational and less extreme than that of the second group, represented mostly by males whose problems are more pronounced and persistent over the life-course.

Paedophile activism

We must not underestimate how insidious activists for child abuse can be. Among them are some organized groups. Modern activism origi-nated in the 1930s in the Netherlands and was then focused on Western Europe (Thomasson, 2006; Wikipedia: Paedophilia, 2007). The Dutch psychologist Bernard published *Sex met kinderen* (Sex with Children) in 1972, laying the foundation for the activism movement, first in Western Europe, then in Northern America. In 1979, the Dutch Parliament received a demand for the decriminalization of sexual activities between children and paedophile adults. This petition was authored by the Dutch Society for Sexual Reform, which reported a membership of 240,000. It was supported among others by: all leading politicians in the country, the General Teachers Association, a large number of university professors, physicians, psychiatrists and psychologists, and some more or less famous private people. Alarmed by the success of the petition, the section of child and youth psychiatry of The Netherlands Society for Psychiatry publicly opposed the demands for decriminalization (Thomason, 2006).

In 1981, the Dutch Protestant Foundation for Responsible Family Development sold and distributed to Dutch elementary schools tens of thousands of copies of a book entitled *Pedophilia*, illustrated with photos. In one passage it states that:

> far from all sexual contacts or sexual relations between a child and an adult imply sexual abuse. Many sexual contacts between adults and children do not have to result in any damage, and there are also sexual contacts which are pleasant and valued by the child ... the present laws are meant to protect children ... in reality they do more harm than good. Advice to parents: Friendship between a pedophile and a child is no reason for panic or fear. Nor is there any reason for this, even if sexual contact is a part of the relationship.
>
> (Protestantse Stichting voor
> Verantwoorde Gezinsvorming, 1981)

In 2006, a Dutch political party (PNVD) founded by three activists demanded the decriminalization of adult sexual activities with children aged 12–16. They proposed the legalization of child pornography and of the practice of human sex with animals, and the screening of pornographic films on daytime television. The party was legalized by a Dutch tribunal based on 'the pillars of states with democratic rights'.

In 1994 the United Nations granted consultative UN status to a number of paedophilic non-governmental organizations, among them: the US North American Man/Boy Love Association (NAMBLA) and Project TRUTH, the Dutch Martijn, and the German Association for Sexual Equality. The paedophile promotion activities of these cannot have been unknown to the UN; many NAMBLA members have been arrested by the FBI for child molestation. Under pressure from the USA, the UN soon after suspended these organizations' consultative status (Thomason, 2006).

Social expenditures diminish child poverty

Malfunctioning in society, especially in the developing countries, is also linked to social, cultural, educational and economic factors (among them, poverty and hunger). In these countries, many of the consequences of social malfunctioning are swept under the carpet into oblivion. Often, ignorant or insensitive politicians, or their economic advisers, allocate budgets to the 'social' ministries that are far from commensurate with the needs.

Increasing social, public expenditure for children will diminish their violent treatments. Poverty and hunger are associated with child violence. Although children bear no responsibility for living in poverty, they are penalized not only in childhood but later in life if their health or education suffers from a lack of resources. All economies face the trade-off between how much money should be spent and what level of childhood poverty is acceptable.

The data in Figure 9.1 compare social economic expenditures and child poverty rates of the rich, industrialized countries that belong to the Organization for Economic Co-operation and Development OECD. This

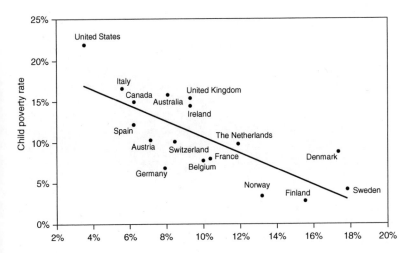

Figure 9.1 Social expenditures as a percentage of GDP and child poverty in the OECD

comparison provides a yardstick for gauging the commitment of the US government to reducing child poverty and its lifelong effects. Countries with higher social expenditures – as a percentage of their gross domestic products – have dramatically lower poverty rates among children. The line in the figure shows the correlation between expenditures and child poverty rates for all countries. Individually, the Nordic countries – Sweden, Norway and Finland – stand out, with child poverty rates between 2.8 per cent and 4.2 per cent. The United States has the lowest expenditures and the highest child poverty rate – five times as much as the Nordics. The paucity of social expenditures addressing high poverty rates in the United States is not due to a lack of resources – high per capita income and high productivity make it possible for the United States to afford much greater social welfare spending. In spite of this, in 2007 the US President vetoed the State Children's Health Insurance Program, which provides 6 million of the poorest children in the country with free health insurance, a scheme that had started in 1997 (Iglehart, 2007). Moreover, 'other OECD countries that spend more on both poverty reduction and family-friendly policies have done so while maintaining competitive rates of productivity and income growth' (OECD, 2004).

Increases in national income combined with growing inequality are not correlated with better social health. Figure 9.2 illustrates the relationship between social health indicators and national income in the United

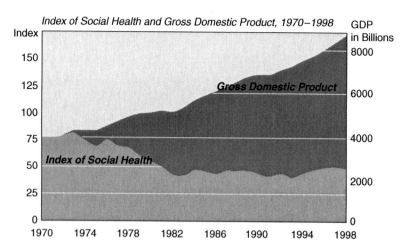

Figure 9.2   Social health does not increase when the GDP goes up
Source: Fordham Institute for Innovation in Social Policy.

States (Fordham Index). The Fordham Index of Social Health is based on sixteen social indicators. Since 1970 five of these have improved: infant mortality, high-school drop-outs, poverty among the elderly, homicides, and alcohol-related traffic fatalities; the remaining eleven have worsened: child abuse, child poverty, teenage suicide, teenage drug abuse, unemployment, average weekly wages, health insurance coverage, out-of-pocket health costs among the elderly, food stamp coverage, access to affordable housing, and income inequality. Between 1973 and 2005, the Index declined from 74 to 53. Although the national per capita income more than doubled during the period 1970–2005, the overall well-being of the US population decreased (Miringhoff, 1996; Miringhoff et al., 1999). There appears to be a relation between what is illustrated in Figure 9.1 and in Figure 9.2: insufficient (and short-sighted) levels of social expenditure lead to decreasing social health; this certainly affects the children.

The impact of poverty in the developing countries

The situation in many developing countries is complex. Half of the children live in poverty, many affected by diseases and malnutrition (see Chapters 12 and 13). Poverty is traumatic and under the WHO definition can be seen as maltreatment as it causes 'actual or potential harm to health, survival, development or dignity'. Many developing nations lack policies and plans to guide efforts to prevent childhood violence.

Child murder rates in poor and middle-income countries are two to three times higher than in the richer countries; in Africa these rates are about seven times higher. In many poor countries violence is aggravated by wars, civil unrest, criminal gangs and mafias. Local conflicts and efforts to repress them by police brutality mostly lead to an escalation of the already high levels of violence, fear and insecurity. Violence is known for its contagion; when the conflict is 'over', subsequent rates of counter-violence and revenge crimes remain elevated.

Analysing the potential for prevention

Most of this chapter has analysed the perpetrators of child violence – who they are and what are the most common explanations for their behaviour – and has reviewed the evidence of the effectiveness of what is or may be done to prevent their aggression and violence. The important role of our social institutions has also been reviewed. One of the limitations for our conclusions is that most published evidence has originated from the developed countries, especially the United States, and not enough from the developing countries.

A very large number of different actions can be taken to prevent child violence. The judgement on what to prioritize is difficult. In spite of several decades of research, we have neither quantitative data nor enough broad-based experience of interventions in different cultures to make the necessary cost-effectiveness calculations to assist our decision-making. Lacking these, in Table 9.3 I have cautiously assessed what we know about the relative prevalence of the twelve major causes of childhood violence described in this chapter: which of them have low prevalence, which are more common and which have the highest prevalence. This is followed by estimates of the potential effectiveness of primary prevention for each of them.

Table 9.3   Relative prevalence and potential primary prevention effectiveness of some major causes of childhood violence

Causes	Relative prevalence	Potential effectiveness of primary prevention
Health-related causes appearing in childhood		
Pregnancy and delivery complications	Moderate	Moderate
Conduct disorder	Moderate	Low
Genetic factors	Moderate	Low
Health-related causes appearing in adulthood		
Antisocial personality disorder	Rare to moderate	Low
Maladaptive alcohol use	High	Moderate
Paedophilia	Moderate	Low
Mental disorders among care-givers	Moderate	Moderate
Social factors		
Family malfunction	Very high	High
Domestic violence	Very high	High
Cultural and economic factors		
Violence in the society	High	Moderate
Lack of child support and services	High	High
Poverty	Very high	High

It would be reasonable to give priority to the primary prevention of the causes with highest prevalence and then to choose to assign priority to those which have a combination of very high or high prevalence with the highest potential effectiveness. These are: family malfunction, lack of child support and poverty. It should be remarked that the estimated 'high' potential for poverty prevention depends on international support; it is analysed in Chapters 12 and 13.

There are two main options for how to carry out primary prevention of childhood violence:

(a) The *targeted prevention* of violence, which builds on the following assumptions:
   1. That those persons or groups with a risk of becoming perpetrators can be identified at an early stage, using methods that are reliable, easy to apply and affordable (especially in the developing countries) on a large scale.
   2. That programmes (applied to the individuals identified) exist that will eliminate or reduce in a measurable way the root factors which cause people to maltreat children; the expectation is that these interventions will lead to a decrease of the identified persons' abusive or neglectful behaviour, and that as a result the general level of abuse and neglect will diminish.

      In spite of the impressive research on neurobiological 'markers', however, there are as yet few reliable methods of identifying and 'curing' high-risk future offenders while they are still very young. It is unlikely (see Chapter 10) that diagnostic and curative methods will be available in the near future that can be applied on a large scale in the developing countries, where 85 per cent of all violent offenders live. This is why targeted prevention has critical limits. These limits can be reduced by more research.
(b) The *universal prevention* of violence is the option that aims at generating broad societal changes, using general population education and development programmes aimed at preventing violence. It implies that children everywhere, irrespective of their social status (avoiding the present bias targeting mainly poor, disadvantaged families) should be raised in a benign and supportive manner so that they might fully develop their potential as non-violent, altruistic and generous human beings.

In the choice between these two, one has to consider the very high prevalence of perpetrators and victims. This supports the proposal that the *first line of defence* of violence towards children should be community-based primary prevention programmes (this option is described in Chapter 14). The *second level of defence* should be directed towards solving the problems that remain in spite of primary prevention, and those that are too severe to be dealt with at the community level. For this, professional personnel working in a referral system are required. More clinical research is needed to clarify many of the causes and treatments mentioned above, among others: pregnancy disorders, conduct disorder, callous unemotional behaviour, antisocial behaviour disorder, paedophilia and maladaptive alcohol use. Methods should be found to reduce the high level of community and media violence, and to increase the technical and economic support for children. Research programmes should be set up and funded in developing countries, where there is a dearth of professionals.

10
Human Services for the Child Victims: Care of Somatic and Mental Disorders and Rehabilitation

Providing services for the child victims is the responsibility of the exo- and macro-systems: the community and the governments. The sheer numbers of clients for treatment, however, appear to be beyond the capacity of all existing health care systems. The service needs for the victims are not only for acute problems, but also for long-term chronic disorders (Felitti et al., 1991, 1998), and for psychosocial support and rehabilitation programmes. The term 'human services' is employed here to indicate the wide range and inclusive nature of the interventions required. One group of US paediatricians (Adams et al., 2007), for example, has issued guidelines for the medical care of children who may have been sexually abused.

Treatments

When assessing the availability of treatments for the victims of child-hood violence, we need to look at the larger picture of the world's health expenditure. In 2004, that expenditure was US$4.1 trillion. The world's thirty richest countries (the members of OECD) which make up 20 per cent of the world's population spent 90 per cent of this expenditure; this equals US$3,170 per capita. In Africa and South-East Asia, with 37 per cent of the world's population, they spend 2 per cent (US$36 per capita) of the global health resources (WHO, 2007b).

Treatment of somatic consequences

Somatic sequels to child violence are common. Medical resources to repair acute injuries are required for simple wounds, burns, spinal cord injury, brain damage, complicated fractures, and so on. Adverse child-hood experiences increase the prevalence of some important somatic diseases appearing in adulthood, for which curative health care should be available. In developing countries, simple tasks are carried out by the primary health care (PHC) system, but for 750 million poor people there is no PHC yet. To the extent that they exist, hospitals in these countries assist with treatment for acute injuries. Care for chronic sequels such as extensive burns, spinal cord injury, brain damage or complicated fractures is not widely available.

Furthermore, the health personnel in these countries are rarely aware of the 'hidden' causes of child trauma and seldom initiate follow-ups to protect children from further abuse and neglect. Some patients with somatic sequels cannot be cured by medical interventions: among them the millions of sexually mutilated women. Infectious diseases, such as HIV/AIDS, may spread to children by sexual abuse, and for this disease medicines are insufficiently available. Poverty-related protein-calorie malnutrition and avitaminosis affect hundreds of millions of neglected children. When they have grown up many have stunted growth, reduced muscular strength, and low physical energy and fitness; this makes them less fit for jobs that require physical strength and endurance. Malaria and tuberculosis are common among neglected children in the developing countries (see pp. 239–40).

Treatment of mental consequences

Mental health problems are exacerbated by the worldwide lack of psychiatric care. WHO (2001a) states that between 36 per cent and 50 per cent of all serious cases of mental disorder (such as psychoses) do not now receive treatment in the developed countries; for the developing ones, the corresponding rates are 77–85 per cent. The WHO survey of 192 countries showed that worldwide there were about four psychiatrists for 100,000 people: the distribution varied from 9.8 in Europe to 0.04 in Africa.

Given the high prevalence of stress and co-morbid mental disorders, it is important that clear guidelines on how to treat these disorders are available. The most recent review of the results of the available treatment, entitled 'Practice guidelines for the treatment of patients with acute stress disorder (ASD) and post-traumatic stress disorder (PTSD)', was issued by American Psychiatric Association (APA) in 2004. The guidelines are very carefully formulated; the text gives 284 references. However, the experts' conclusion is 'there are limited data to guide the clinician'. 'The first interventions consist of stabilizing and supportive medical care and supportive psychiatric care and assessment.' This process should 'include functional assessment, determining the availability of basic care resources (e.g. safe housing, social support network, companion care, food, and clothing), identifying previous traumatic experiences and co-morbid physical or psychiatric disorders'. It is recommended to 'ensure physical and psychological safety, required medical care' and to evaluate the 'risk for suicide and potential harm to others'. The specific treatment strategies consist of psychopharmacology and psychotherapeutic interventions. The present evidence of pharmacological treatment is, however, 'limited and preliminary'. Selective serotonin reuptake inhibitors are recommended as first-line treatment for PTSD. Cognitive behaviour therapy given over a few sessions, beginning two to three weeks after trauma exposure 'may speed recovery and prevent PTSD. In contrast, psychological debriefings or single-session techniques are not recommended, as they may increase symptoms in some settings and appear to be ineffective in treating individuals with ASD and preventing PTSD.'

These guidelines are carefully formulated, and conclude that the evidence of treatment efficacy is still thin. The factors that appear to facilitate resilience in the USA (see p. 151) – which some recommend for general use as therapy – would appear culturally difficult to apply in many developing countries. In most such countries, for an individual to share openly her/his experience of sexual and other abuse with outsiders is often culturally constrained. Some researchers state that psychiatric therapeutic interventions for maltreated children have no effect. Tebbutt et al. (1997), for example, carried out a five-year follow-up of sixty-eight (out of an initial eighty-four) abused children and found that, over these years, there were no significant changes in low self-esteem (43 per cent), depression (43 per cent) and behavioural dysfunction (46 per cent). Some had improved during that period, while others had deteriorated; as Tebutt sums up: the treatments had no effect.

At present, the efficacy of psychiatric treatment of post-traumatic stress disorder for the victims of child violence does not appear convincing in the eyes of the leading experts. A possible explanation of the lack of therapeutic efficacy is that the already existing anatomical, biochemical and hormonal alterations and brain changes, which remain organically fixed and permanent, may no longer be influenced by therapy using existing technology. If so, this would support the clinical experience that early intervention is crucial when attempting to break the cycle of neurobiological damage before it has become fixed. However, early reporting is often prevented due to reluctance on the part of the victim or due to threats or other interference by the offender. Victims need easier local access to an authority or to the social system or to a non-governmental organization.

Some recent studies have focused on neurobiological processes aimed at extinguishing the intrusive and malignant memories of past abuse. A challenging question is: can a 'retrograde, targeted amnesia' be generated? Loss of consciousness during a traumatic event creates retrograde amnesia that protects against PTSD (O'Brien and Nutt, 1998). It should be easier to extinguish memories immediately after the abusive event, rather than trying to eliminate the 'engraved' memories of victimization that took place years ago, especially if the abuse was often repeated and if the victim was a child at the time of the abuse. Recent studies by Strange et al. (2003) and Pitman et al. (2002) of the effects of the β-blocker propranolol showed that it blocks the stress hormones released after a traumatic event. Early administration of this drug may decrease the intensity of the memories. A series of profound, interrelated biochemical processes are involved in memory extinction. To 'cure' victims of PTSD innovative techniques have to be invented, such as interfering with gene expression and protein synthesis in the hippocampus (Vianna et al., 2004). Present pharmacotherapy is moderately effective but far from ideally targeted (Hageman et al., 2001). Present knowledge is built on research in developed countries, mainly the USA. It might not be applicable in countries with other cultures, especially if their child-rearing customs are different.

Many children from the high-risk groups are substance abusers. While staying in an institution they may have been overdosed with sedatives, street children may have been sniffing glue or chemical solvents, or others again may have used alcohol, cocaine, heroin or some local addictive drug while they were soldiers or child prostitutes. Immediate steps have to be taken to deal with the addiction.

Social support and rehabilitation

There are many guidelines and practical books about how to work with abused children (Doyle, 2006); in the following a short resumé is presented. Hall and Williams (2008) prefer to use the term 'safeguarding', a more inclusive concept than child protection which emphasizes not only the diagnosis and management of child abuse as conventionally understood, but also the importance of recognizing children in distress and intervening where possible to prevent a range of adverse outcomes. Achieving these goals will depend in part on greater awareness and more extensive training in psychosocial issues and the mental health of children and young people, and their parents.

First contact

All child victims of violence need personalized support in an environ-ment that creates a feeling of warmth, security, empathy and stability. The first-contact person may be a social worker, a psychologist, a doctor or a police officer. That person should listen to what the victim says about the trauma and give all the time needed to understand. If appropriate, contacts should be sought with the perpetrator, or persons who can con-firm the violence. There may be a lot of immediate practical problems, such as money, clothes, personal hygiene and lodging.

Removal of an abused child

There is a lot a debate regarding the removal of children from their birth families (see Chapter 6). Doyle (2006) explains that the notion of 'blood-tie' has been important in practice and policy and that the belief is common that (Colwell Report, 1976):

> there is a strong physical tie between a child and his parent by virtue of his physical inheritance and the fact of conception and child-bearing. The term 'natural parent' somehow implies that any kind of substitute for the parent is to a degree 'unnatural'.

Some countries allow continued contact between a removed child liv-ing with the foster family and the birth parents; the hope among the latter is that the child will be returned to them. In some circumstances, this might be possible, for example if the reason is temporary disease or if the abusive parent has been removed. On the other hand, the sys-tem to continue contact with the birth family is criticized because of common disputes between them and the foster parents, and because the child is disturbed by 'not knowing where it belongs'. Efforts have been made to increase the parenting skills and improve behaviour among abu-sive parents, but a recent meta-analysis (Barlow et al., 2006) failed to reveal any effectiveness of parenting programmes for physically abusive or neglectful parents. This failure may depend on the irreversible fixa-tion of neurobiological damage, described in the previous chapter, or continuing alcoholism and/or criminality. If the child has been abused over a long period, or if the abuse has revealed serious cruelty or lack of remorse in the perpetrator, continued contacts with the birth family are usually seen as inappropriate.

For older children there are alternatives to foster families, such as shel-ters organized by local, non-governmental organizations. If the child or adolescent was involved with a gang or an armed group, disengaging from that gang/group may expose them to threats. Therefore, their shelter should be located away from the gang's or group's territory.

Psychosocial rehabilitation

After the acute period, the victims should be offered long-term, supervised multi-sectoral services, palliative and supportive interventions, commonly referred to as 'psychosocial rehabilitation'. These include education, vocational training, assistance for employment, and provision of permanent lodging and security. Skills training programmes exist to prevent revictimization of sexual abuse survivors (Cloitre, 1998).

The reintegration of the survivors of violence

How will the abused child be integrated into the community? Some children from 'bad families' may be rejected by others. Greater community awareness is needed to make its members sensitive to the need for human contact for the children who have lived their lives unprotected and been abused. In some developed countries, there are support groups of families offering their homes for visits (sometimes called solidarity families) and young people's friendship groups have successfully been initiated in many places.

In developing countries, the difficulties may be close to insurmountable; for the victims there is nowhere to escape to and no resources for removal; they will remain among the people and families that abused them. Some abused children will run away to urban areas, and we find them on the streets, away from their family tormentors, still exposed to the risk of continued abuse. Several social researchers have presented some experiences from developing countries.

Das et al. (2001) point out that in communities where people by necessity continue to live with murderers who killed their family members, or with rapists, torturers and abusers:

> no glib appeal to 'our common humanity' can restore the confidence to inhabit each other's lives again. Instead it is by first reformulating their notions of 'normality' as a changing norm, much as the experience of a disease changes our expectations of health, that communities can respond to the destruction of trust in their everyday lives ... At the level of the ordinary, the everyday social realities, states of rebuilding and accommodation are as complex as are the networks of individual lives of victims, perpetrators, victim-perpetrators, internal resisters, and critics and witnesses.

Perera (2001) describes:

culturally authorized forms providing a coping strategy by which survivors of civil conflict continue to live in the midst of torturers and
murderers, long after mass violence has ended but in settings in which
there is official silence, a state compliant with offenders, and no judicial ways of seeking justice . . . The situation may look normal from the
outside, but this is mere seeming. Memories of terror continue, as does
the desire for witnessing and for a response to deep grievances. Story-
telling, ritual, and possession – all symbolic means embedded in old
religions – provide ways by which the traumatized continue to find
meaning in their suffering, to exist and to rebuild their relationships.

Mehta and Chatterji (2001) state that:

The altered everyday is marked by a new knowledge and memory
of loss, but also a practical wisdom of negotiating this loss. It tells us
that reparation cannot take the form of justice; co-existence is possible
only if the acts are deliberately set aside.

Is there a way to negotiate a community and family 'healing process'?
The present evidence as to the effectiveness of such projects is as yet very
thin; very often the victims face memories of a reality that cannot easily
be swept under the carpet. It would seem irrational to apply forgiveness
to cruel, violent criminals; it may just encourage them and others to
continue. The proposal of forgiveness neglects the fact that poor people
are deprived of their legal rights and have no political clout.

Child abuse and neglect are important public health problems. Very
few of the victims are at present receiving competent help. To supply
this will require much more resources than are now available, and that
includes more research to improve the efficacy both of presently available
therapeutic interventions and of primary prevention. The cost to society
of perpetuating the present indifference to vulnerable and defenceless
children will not only cause suffering, but also economic losses that
substantially exceed the cost of interventions.

Part V

The Global System: Perspectives of Human Rights, Evolution, Development and Progress

11
Human Rights and Human Wrongs

At its inception in 1948 the United Nations proclaimed a legal code of conduct for all its member states: the Universal Declaration of Human Rights (UDHR). Following this, an extensive system of international treaties, Covenants and Conventions has been built up by the United Nations and its High Commissioner for Human Rights. The idea was that UN basic principles of justice – the international law – would be part of all national laws. The legal international treaties – Covenants and Conventions – were designed to bind all nations to a framework of citizens' rights under the control of the UN Human Rights Commission.

In this chapter the questions are:

1. What is the intended role of international laws in the life of children?
2. Are these legal treaties fully accepted by all countries – the macro-systems of the human ecology? (Office of the United Nations High Commissioner for Human Rights, 2006)
3. Globally, to what extent are children legally protected from violence; or using the formulation in UDHR, 'cruel, inhuman and degrading treatment and punishment'?
4. What are the ethical rules for health personnel, and are they followed?

Human rights issues have always been controversial. It took twenty years – until 1966 – of wrangling between the UN member states to agree to the formulations of the first Covenants: one about economic, social and cultural rights (ICESCR), the second about civil and political rights (ICCPR). Then it took another ten years before they came into force (1976). Both were binding upon ratification, but governments had the right to refuse ratification and by 2006, thirty-six and thirty-four governments, respectively, had still not ratified these basic international

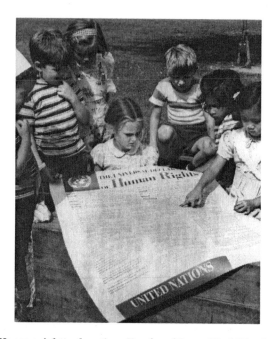

Photo 17. **Human rights education**. *Very few of the world's children have ever heard about Human Rights – their rights. The texts of the United Nations' many Declarations, Covenants and Conventions are rarely available to them. Also, the legal texts are often written in a language unfamiliar to children. The UN launched the Decade for Human Rights Education 1995–2004. The photo shows the efforts to include human rights education in all schools. © World Health Organization.*

treaties.[17,18] This reflects no doubt a high degree of political dissonance, and reluctance among many governments to accept even a minimum of legal obligations to their own peoples. The Covenants are of specific interest to children, as they contain clear statements about the responsibility of governments to protect children from 'cruel, inhuman and degrading treatment and punishment' and to 'accord the family the widest possible protection and assistance', further specifying that 'special measures should be taken on behalf of children and young persons' and to 'recognize the right of everyone to education'. The ICCPR Covenant did not allow the Human Rights Commission to 'receive and consider, communications from individuals claiming to be victims of violations of any of the rights set forth in the Covenant'. ICCPR, however, has an Optional Protocol which 'enables the Human Rights Committee to receive and consider such communications'. Eighty-nine countries with combined populations of 4.7 billion (with close to 2 billion children) have not ratified this Protocol (among them Japan, the United States and the United Kingdom). Thus, from almost 80 per cent of the world's population there will be no communications about violence towards children received by the Committee.

The Covenants were followed by more detailed Conventions. From 1966 to 2006 forty-one Conventions, Protocols and Optional Protocols were accepted by the UN General Assembly.[19] The UN Conventions are only part of a much larger non-UN framework of international treaties, for example the Hague Convention on adoptions.[20]

In the context of this book the *UN Convention on the Rights of the Child* (CRC) and the *UN Convention Against Torture and Other Cruel, Inhuman or Degrading Treatment or Punishment* (CAT) are the most important. Below are some excerpts from the CRC articles:

Article 3. States Parties shall ensure that the institutions, services and facilities responsible for the care or protection of children shall conform with the standards established by competent authorities...as well as competent supervision.

Article 6. States Parties recognize that every child has the inherent right to life. States Parties shall ensure to the maximum extent possible the survival and development of the child.

Article 19. States Parties shall take all appropriate legislative, administrative, social and educational measures to protect the child from all forms of physical or mental violence, injury or abuse, neglect or negligent treatment, maltreatment or exploitation, including sexual abuse, while in the care of parent(s), legal guardian(s) or any other person who has the care of the child. Protective measures...include effective...social programmes to provide necessary support for the child and for those who have the care of the child, as well as for other forms of prevention and for identification, reporting, referral, investigation, treatment and follow-up of instances of child maltreatment described heretofore, and, as appropriate, for judicial involvement.

Article 23. States Parties recognize that a mentally or physically disabled child should enjoy a full and decent life, in conditions which ensure dignity, promote self-reliance and facilitate the child's active participation in the community.

Article 28. States Parties recognize the right of the child to education and with a view to achieving this right progressively and on the basis of equal opportunity, they shall, in particular: (a) Make primary education compulsory and available free to all...(e) Take measures to encourage regular attendance at schools and the reduction of drop-out rates.

Article 37. States Parties shall ensure that no child shall be subjected to torture or other cruel, inhuman or degrading treatment or punishment.

Article 39. States Parties shall…promote physical and psychological recovery and social reintegration of a child victim of: any form of neglect, exploitation, or abuse; torture or any other form of cruel, inhuman or degrading treatment or punishment; or armed conflicts. Such recovery and reintegration shall take place in an environment which fosters the health, self-respect and dignity of the child.

The CRC has been ratified by all countries, except Somalia (which has no government) and the USA. Many states do not comply as they should with these articles; some disregard them on a massive scale.

The UN Geneva-based Committee on the Rights of the Child is the body of independent representatives that monitors the country implementation of the CRC. All states are obliged to submit regular reports (every five years) to the Committee on how the rights are being implemented. The Committee examines each report and addresses its concerns and recommendations to the state party in the form of 'concluding observations'. The Committee cannot consider complaints from individuals; these may be raised before other committees with appropriate competence. States who disregard their obligations receive no punishment or sanctions. Legal means to enforce this Convention are not used.

A common excuse for states to delay action to meet the needs of vulnerable children is that resources are not available. Lack of resources is the excuse for the understaffing of residential institutions, neglecting community child defence and support programmes, and efforts to halt child abandonment and to care for social orphans. Regarding this restriction, the UN Human Rights Commission states:

even in times of severe resources constraint…the vulnerable members of society can and indeed must be protected by the adoption of relatively low-cost targeted programmes. States' obligations are not exhausted until all appropriate measures have been taken to ensure the realization of a right. Such measures include, *inter alia*, administrative, financial, educational and social measures. If a State claims that it is unable to meet even its minimum obligations because of lack of resources, it must be at least able to demonstrate that every effort has been made to use all resources that are at its disposal in an effort to satisfy, as a matter of priority, these minimum obligations.

In September 2000, the Commission had a general discussion about violence suffered by children living in institutions managed, licensed or supervised by states. The Commission recommended urgent attention to ensure the establishment and effective functioning of systems to monitor the treatment received by children deprived of a family.

In the context of this book, the second most important UN Convention is that Against Torture and Other Cruel, Inhuman or Degrading Treatment or Punishment (CAT). Article 19 of the CRC (see above) defined exactly what cruel, inhuman and degrading treatment and punishment means. The following CAT article explains the states' responsibilities:

> *Article 16.* Each State Party shall undertake to prevent in any territory under its jurisdiction other acts of cruel, inhuman or degrading treatment or punishment...when such acts are committed by or at the instigation of or with the consent or acquiescence of a public official or other person acting in an official capacity. In particular, the obligations contained in Articles 10, 11, 12 and 13 shall apply with the substitution for references to torture of references to other forms of cruel, inhuman or degrading treatment or punishment.

This article is unambiguous, but there are two major problems. The first is that by June 2006, fifty-two countries had not ratified the CAT. Another fifty-six have used the option to opt out of all their responsibilities related to CAT.[21] This is possible and completely legal:

> No action can be taken by the Human Rights Commission unless the States Parties also make the declaration mentioned in Article 22 paragraph 1. That Article states: A State Party to this Convention may at any time declare under this article that it recognizes the competence of the Committee to receive and consider communications from or on behalf of individuals subject to its jurisdiction who claim to be victims of a violation by a State Party of the provisions of the Convention. The Committee shall receive no communication if it concerns a State Party which has not made such a declaration.

Out of 195 UN member states, only 66 were on 31 May 2007 in full compliance with the CAT. As shown above, the ICCPR has similar restrictions. Combining the countries that have not ratified the ICCPR protocol number 1 with those who did not sign the CAT article 22.1, the total comes to 140 countries. These do not allow the UN's Human Rights Commission either to receive information or to take any action to protect their populations from 'cruel, inhuman and degrading treatment and punishment'. These countries have a combined population of over 5 billion, of whom some 2.1 billion are children. The legal and moral vacuum affects 80 per cent of the global population, and 90 per cent of all its children; the massive refusal by the UN member states to accept the international law makes the efforts by the Geneva Commission for Human Rights to protect children inoperable.

The next problem is the constraints on enforcing UNHCR inspections (United Nations Human Rights Fact Sheet). These are allowed only on invitation by the government of the nation in question, and often there is a delay of several months between the request and the government agreement, giving governments the opportunity not only to 'clean up' sub-standard practices but also to move away abused persons that they want to hide. Governments have a right to refuse the setting up of a national UN Human Rights office, to refuse accreditation for a country Representative, and, if granted, to restrict his/her entrance to the institutions in question and his/her asking questions to be answered by alleged victims. In short, governments have made a mockery of the international inspection system. The governments referred to above behave in conflict with the human rights priorities of the United Nations organization they have joined; they are filtering information that would reveal conflicts with these priorities, involving themselves in massive, systematic cognitive dissonance.

Several hundred million children experience cruel, inhuman and degrading treatment. There does not seem to be much public reaction, perhaps because most abuse is hidden and the victims silenced. The macro-systems of justice do little in 143 countries to protect their own abused children. A few local organizations may represent these countries' 2 billion children's interests, but the victims are often without the judicial means of seeking local help. Pressures have been applied to change what is criminal behaviour on a large scale, but these have made little impact. Poor people everywhere have little trust in the fairness of the police, the prosecutors and the courts.

In March 2005, the Secretary-General of the United Nations, in a report (*In Larger Freedom*) confirming the concerns in this chapter, stated:

> The Human Rights Commission's capacity to perform its tasks has been increasingly undermined by its declining credibility and professionalism. In particular, States have sought membership of the Commission not to strengthen Human Rights, but to protect themselves against criticism or to criticize others. As a result a credibility

deficit has developed, which casts a shadow on the reputation of the UN system as a whole.

The Secretary-General proposed to replace the Commission – which does not 'meet the expectations of men and women everywhere' – with a UN Human Rights Council, directly elected by the General Assembly, 'which should work in a more professional way, with the Councillors taking their responsibilities more seriously'. These changes started in mid-2006.[22] It is doubtful, however, whether the non-compliance can be reduced if it is not supervised and enforced by courts rather than by the voting members of a commission or a council.

The failures to implement the international law at the levels of the global and of the macro-system have had downstream consequences for children's human ecology. Human Rights are unknown by most 'ordinary people' in the developing countries, and in some it might be safer not to mention them. The legal means to protect children are poorly implemented; consequently, many suffer 'cruel, inhuman and degrading treatment and punishment'. The effects of the international rights described in this chapter, when effectively applied, should be important and should reduce the levels of child violence.

Legal obligations of medical personnel

Regrettably, some of the macro-system's guardians – such as doctors, whose influence could transform the treatment of children in institutions, for example – fail to take action. Most ethical rules for medical personnel are built on the Hippocratic Oath. This Oath is an ethical code or ideal, an appeal for right conduct. In one or other of its many versions, it has guided the practice of medicine throughout the world for more than 2,000 years.

The World Medical Association (WMA) was set up in 1948 as a reaction to the atrocities committed during and after the war by members of the medical profession in Europe. The WMA promotes policies in accord with the Hippocratic tradition, first represented in modern form in the Geneva Convention, 1948 (Bloch, 1997). Since 1975, many declarations have been made by the WMA, the WHO and the UN on the role of the physician in protecting human rights of those who are in their care. The following undertakings are from universally adopted declarations:[23]

(a) The physician shall not countenance, condone or participate in the practice of torture in any situation. (Tokyo Declaration, WMA, 1975)

(b) The physician shall not provide any premises or knowledge to facilitate the practice of torture. (Tokyo Declaration)

(c) The physician shall not be present during any procedure related to torture, cruel, inhumane or degrading treatment. (Tokyo Declaration)

(d) Unjustified medications, abuse by other patients, by staff or other acts causing mental distress or discomfort are not allowed. (UN Principles on the Protection of Persons with Mental Illness, 1991)

(e) Seclusion and physical restraints are forbidden (except when it is the only means available to prevent immediate or imminent harm to the patient or others). (UN Principles)

(f) Sterilization is prohibited; psychosurgery or other irreversible treatment or other experimental treatments without informed consent are forbidden. (UN Principles)

These policies reflect the obligations the medical profession imposes upon itself in any bioethical analysis. These initiatives were taken because many psychiatrists have pointed out that psychiatry 'lost its anchor' when its professionals agreed to take part in the euthanasia programme in Nazi Germany, and in the suppression of political dissent in the Soviet Union and other communist countries, and in human experiments and brainwashing of prisoners carried out in many other places, including the USA and Canada.

The rules are not followed by large numbers of physicians and other medical personnel. This is matter of great concern, especially when the victims are defenceless, downtrodden, or vulnerable children. It is particularly deplorable that those who are directly responsible for breaking or allowing others to break these rules enjoy virtual impunity. It is a fact that the homes – described in this book – in which inert, traumatized children are stored have not received the necessary supervision and support from the medical establishment.

When it comes to the examples of violence and cruel treatment in institutions or other settings described in this book, how can we explain the active participation and complicity of so many apparently decent and well-meaning people? How can the atrocities described just continue? We may consider five factors:

- Obedience to authority. Experiments on obedience were made by the US psychologist Stanley Milgram in the 1960s (Milgram, 1974). His conclusions apply to the situation of many children in institutions: ordinary, decent and law-abiding people (including doctors)

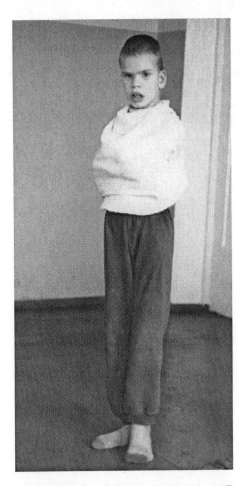

Photo 18. **Boy in a straitjacket.** *With arms and hands totally constrained by a straitjacket, this boy is left alone without supervision in a room empty of furniture. He has no shoes, no proper clothes, no activities, and no contact, except when he is spoon-fed and has to be cleaned: he is doubly incontinent. Such treatment is cruel, inhumane and degrading, and forbidden. This institution's head is a medical doctor totally non-compliant with his professional obligations. Credit: Star of Hope, Sweden.*

are willing to inflict severe and brutal pain on others if they are given an order by an authoritative person (such a person may even be a doctor). Human nature cannot be counted on to insulate citizens from brutality and inhumane treatment at the direction of malevolent authority.

- Social group conformity, pressure from peer groups.
- The acquired pattern of denigrating myths about the victims of the cruel and uncaring conduct.
- Bureaucratic behaviour distancing basic personnel from the decision-makers.
- Compliance with the obligations of medical personnel has to be better enforced. Children living in their micro-systems are in many countries poorly protected against cruel, inhumane and degrading treatment and punishment.

12
Poverty, Inequality and Solidarity

Poverty

This and the next chapter deal with the situation of the poor in the world. They investigate the role of the international community in the present, massive structural neglect of over one billion children. In 2005 there were about 2,140 million children in the developing countries aged 0–18, or slightly more than 40 per cent of their population. In very poor countries, about 50 per cent are children. About half of all these children are affected by poverty. The World Bank[24] describes the situation for poor people in the developing world; for each problem between 40 per cent and 50 per cent of those affected are children:

- 800 million people go hungry.
- 750 million people do not have access to primary health care.
- 2.4 billion people lack basic sanitation and 1 billion lack access to safe, clean water.
- A number of diseases, both communicable and non-communicable, are more common among the poor in the developing countries than they are in developed ones. About 45 million people are infected by HIV/AIDS and its incidence is growing. 250 million people are estimated to have malaria annually worldwide and 1.1 million to die annually from that disease. 1.5 million die annually from tuberculosis.
- The mean survival age in poor developing countries is 49 years, 77 years in the developed ones. The under-5 mortality rate is 84/1,000; 11 million children die each year from preventable diseases.
- 130 million children of school age (21 per cent) in 1998 had no access to basic education, and millions more received sub-standard education resulting in little learning. An estimated 900 million people,

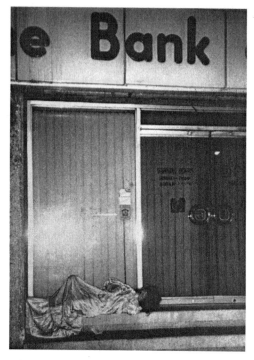

Photo 19.   **Homeless child.** *The bank houses the money of the few; its entrance offers a place to sleep for one of the many with no house and no money.* © *World Health Organization.*

especially girls and women, today are functionally illiterate because they have been denied education as children. Insufficient degrees of literacy lead to limitations in adaptive skills and to dependency on others for support.

Poverty, states United Nations Development Programme (1997):

> is a complex and multidimensional phenomenon. It is not simply a matter of incomes that are too low to meet basic subsistence needs. It is a symptom of imbedded structural imbalances, which mani- fest themselves in all realms of human existence ... highly correlated with social exclusion, marginalization, vulnerability, powerlessness, isolation ... is reflected in malnutrition, poor health, low literacy, inadequate housing and living conditions ... no access to basic infra- structure and services ... lack of access to land, credit, technology

and institutions... productive assets and resources needed to ensure sustainable livelihoods... people in poverty are deprived of legal rights and political clout to make their collective voice heard... the power differential helps to keep people in poverty invisible, isolated, marginalized and vulnerable.

To this description, we need to add the pervasive violence. Poverty is a 'culture'; to change it is not a question of money alone. A person's capacity to break out of poverty is reduced when he/she goes to bed and wakes up every morning hungry and with little or no reserves to draw upon. Poverty is an evil circle; it is mentally and physically traumatic, and will require generations to alleviate. For a child to grow up in a poor family that lacks almost everything is harrowing.

Regarding the number of the poor, for the developing nations the World Bank defines those who live on less than US$2 a day as poor, and as absolutely poor those who live on less than US$1 a day. The measurements are based on the individual's consumption and not on his/her income. The World Bank's dollar-a-day poverty line is a PPP (purchasing power parity) dollar poverty line (see note 30 below). About 80 per cent of the poor live in Asia. In 2004, the number of people living in absolute poverty was estimated at about 1 billion; those living in poverty were 2.6 billion. The developing countries in 2004 had 5.1 billion people, thus close to three-quarters of them (72 per cent) were under the poverty level. The arbitrary choice of US$1 and US$2 converted to PPPs has been criticized. In some countries health care is free, in others education is free. Thus, when official income levels increase over the US$2 level, while at the same time public services disappear or are reduced, a part of the population seen as escaping poverty will in reality remain as poor as before; one such example is China (*The Economist*, 2007; see also pp. 235–6 for more recent and much higher prevalence data).

In developed countries the 'poverty lines' for a person are higher; an amount often used is '60 per cent of the minimum salary level'. In the USA, in 2005, it was US$14.40 per day per person: the USA had 37 million people living in poverty (13 per cent of the population) including 13 million children (US Accountability Office, 2007). In Russia, the poverty level was US$4; at that level, 60 per cent of the children in Russia were below the poverty level in 2001. In the European Union (fifteen countries) there were, in 1997, 57 million poor (17 per cent of households, 20 per cent of children). In Eastern and Central Europe poverty increased from 4 per cent of the population in 1988 to 32 per cent in 1994; the number of poor people from 14 to 119 million (about one-third of whom were

---

Box 12.1:   The poorest among the poor

*'A list of some criteria used by local people in "ill-being" grouping and
ranking: sources in Asia and sub-Saharan Africa. Those at the top are seen
as worst off by fellow community members:*

(1) Disabled (e.g. blind, crippled, mentally impaired, chronically
     sick)
(2) Widowed
(3) Lacking land, livestock, farm equipment, grinding mill
(4) Cannot send children to school
(5) Having more mouths-to-feed, fewer hands to help
(6) Lacking able-bodied members who can fend for their families
     in the event of crisis
(7) With bad housing
(8) Having vices (e.g. alcoholism)
(9) Being "poor in people"; lacking social supports
(10) Having to put children in employment
(11) Single parents
(12) Having to accept demeaning or low status work
(13) Having food security for only a few months each year
(14) Being dependent on common property resources.'

---

children). Chambers (1995) published a list of the poorest among the
poor (Box 12.1). In these poor families, children share the deprivation.

The Sri Lanka Ministry of Social Welfare (2003) published a study of
poverty among adult disabled persons. Almost all fell below the poverty
line of US$2 per day and 60 per cent below US$1 per day. The national
employment rate in 2003 was about 90 per cent, but only 15 per cent
of the disabled persons had a job. Primary schooling is obligatory in Sri
Lanka, but only 61 per cent of the disabled children started school at all
and their drop-out rate was high.

Concerning widows (about 7–8 per cent of the population) poverty is
common (Owen, 1996). Thousands of them are still young, and have
children. They are often blamed for the death of the husband. Many
are humiliated, hounded from their homes and denied access to essential resources such as shelter and land to grow food. Their children are
sometimes taken away and maltreated in the substitute families. There
are many irrevocable long-term implications for the future well-being of
these children.

To be landless or to have to share common land or other resources is a fate experienced by many hundred millions. Those families who use land 'by tradition' rarely have legal title to it, and for that reason they seldom have access to bank loans to buy better seeds, fertilizers, machines, and other equipment that would help them to increase their farming outputs. Successful programmes to assist landless people exist, but help only a small proportion of them. Poor families do not always have food for their children, and cannot afford to send them to school because there are school fees (some illegal) to be paid, and the children may not have clothes. Chambers' list represents some 75 per cent of all absolutely – and it seems at present chronically – poor. To provide them with a way out of poverty is a major challenge.

Another group of very poor people – without development programmes – consists of 350 million indigenous people living in seventy countries, half of them children. They account for an astonishing diversity of cultures, and have a vast and irreplaceable amount of knowledge, skills and ways of understanding and relating to the world. For them, political and cultural violence is a devastating reality (International Work Group for Indigenous Affairs, 2004).

Inequality

The economic inequalities between countries and between individuals in countries are pronounced. Table 12.1 shows the 'official' world macroeconomic data (UNCTAD, 2007).

Table 12.1 shows the enormous inequalities between countries (column six). Similarly, the individual differences are very large and increasing: the world's richest 1 per cent receives as much income as the poorest 57 per cent, and the richest 2 per cent own 50 per cent of all the assets in the world. The combined incomes of the richest 25 million Americans (USA) equal those of almost 2 billion poor people. More money, when unequally distributed, does not seem to solve social problems (see p. 198). Neither is money the best indicator of happiness (Easterlin, 1995, 2003).

The reasons for the increasing inequalities and persistence of poverty are many and some are disputed. Some of the issues are: The policies of the rich countries to alleviate poverty have proven ineffective. Some urgent actions, such as attention to family planning, to the malfunctioning judicial systems, to human rights and to violence prevention, have been sidelined. The planning processes among the donor organizations are poor,[25] and the outcome evaluations are built on unreliable

Table 12.1   World official macroeconomic data, 2005 (market exchange rates)

Region	Population millions	% of world total population	GDP total US$ billions	GDP/ capita/ year US$	GDP/ capita/ day US$	% of world GDP
Whole world	6,515	100.0	44,475	6,827	**18.7**	100.0
Developed countries	971	14.9	33,782	34,791	**95.3**	76.0
Developing countries	5,212	80.0	9,963	1,912	**5.2**	22.4
Transition economies	332	5.1	1,198	3,372	**9.2**	2.7
USA*	304	4.7	12,542	41,257	**113.0**	28.2
25 EU countries*	463	7.1	13,443	29,035	**79.5**	30.2
China*	1,296	19.9	1,980	1,528	**4.2**	4.5
India*	1,134	17.4	801	706	**1.9**	1.8

* USA and the European Union countries are also included in developed market economy countries, total. China and India are also included in developing countries.

data collection.[26] The rich industrialized countries have not been suffi-ciently helpful; some experts claim that more is needed to motivate the richpopulations to show more generosity, and pay better attention to the targeting, management and evaluation of donor inputs. Others consider the whole approach as misdirected (Easterly, 2005).

The failure is also attributed to the recipient countries: corruption, internal power struggles, large-scale insecurity, government incompe-tence, instability and community violence. The governments of most poor countries have given insufficient attention to the quality of edu-cation, the development of managerial skills, the importance of using community mobilization programmes and providing the poor with legal security through an expanded judicial system. They have remained overly dependent on the production of commodities; their problems are compounded by regulatory problems, and a lack of measures to encour-age industrial and services development and to protect investments. They have been unable to benefit from the enormous technological evo-lution, as their citizens lack the education and the skills required to use the new methods.

The obvious question is: knowing the problem, why have the donor countries during fifty years of assistance neglected the management

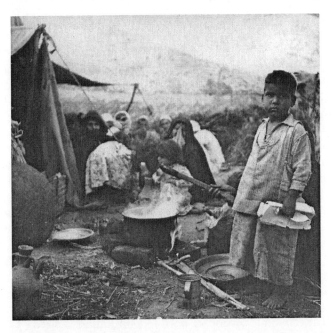

Photo 20. **Gypsy camp in Egypt.** *The people who live here have never heard of international aid. Here is poverty at its lowest level. Will these children ever see a better future?* © *World Health Organization.*

training of civil servants and political leaders? Why have they not created sufficient numbers of national and regional schools for public adminis-tration? Why, for example, are not more of the 13,000 employees at the World Bank in Washington working in the field?

The World Bank has introduced pro-poor polices. These are built on the finding that rapid growth, combined with low initial inequality and pro-poor distributional change, could significantly reduce poverty. Growth is less efficient in lowering poverty levels in countries with high ini-tial inequality or in which the distributional pattern of growth favours the non-poor (Bourguignon, 2004; Ravallion, 1997, 2004). In the late 1990s the term *pro-poor growth* became popular as economists recognized that accelerating poverty reduction required both more rapid growth and lower inequality (Aghion et al., 1999). High initial inequality is a brake on poverty reduction. Asset inequality predicts lower future growth rates. Income redistribution accelerates the rate of poverty reduction (World Bank, 2007).

Solidarity

The origins of international development aid

To understand better the implications of international development aid
for the lives of the world's children a short summary of its origins follows.
The first large-scale programme for development was the Marshall Plan
(1948–52) to assist the rebuilding of Europe after the Second World War
(Arkes, 1972) (see note 15). Aid was offered to all of Europe, including
the Soviet bloc, but Stalin refused and denounced the plan as a capitalist
plot. During the last decades, the achievements of the Marshall Plan
have been re-evaluated: in reality its effects were mixed (OEEC Report,
1948; Kostrzewa, 1990; Cowen, 1985). The European economic growth
started some years later and was related to the introduction of free market
policies: a major step forward was the creation of the European Economic
Community in 1957.

The fact that Western Europe was rebuilt and its economy functioning
well ten to fifteen years after the devastating world war encouraged the
idea that a similar development could be achieved in the poor developing
countries, for instance, in double that time. There emerged a conviction that economic planning, careful identification of needs, followed
by some economic aid for implementation were all that was necessary
to close the gap between the rich and the poor countries. These plans
met early opposition from many economists, including Peter Bauer and
Milton Friedman who in the 1960s argued that aid would not work. Nevertheless, development programmes started and have been maintained
for about fifty years. They turned out to be a technocratic fantasy.

Any 'analogy' between the Marshall Plan for Europe and the aid to
developing countries is misconceived. The Marshall aid was targeted only
at some 300 million Europeans. Europe had existing institutions (public
administration, education, health care, judiciary, transportation, and so
on) and an educated population, industries, services and banks. Developing countries lacked functioning institutions, public administration,
managerial capacity and infrastructures – for many even tax collection
systems. In these countries – in the late 1950s – illiteracy was widespread,
primary health care virtually non-existent, the judiciary system (where it
existed) under-funded and biased, and corruption was seen at all levels.
In the developing countries, the type and size of the needs were infinitely
different from those in Europe, and their combined populations were at
that time already seven times larger than those of Europe and rapidly
growing.

Table 12.2 Official development aid (ODA) in % of donor countries' GDP

Year	ODA US$ million	ODA, % of donor countries' gross national income	Population, less developed regions, millions	ODA US$/person of less developed regions (gross)
1956	3.3	n.a.	1,937	1.6
1960	4.7	0.51	2,109	2.2
1965	6.5	0.48	2,371	2.7
1970	5.4	0.33	2,688	2.5
1975	13.3	0.34	3,027	4.4
1980	26.2	0.35	3,360	7.8
1985	28.8	0.33	3,729	7.7
1990	52.7	0.33	4,131	12.8
1995	58.8	0.26	4,518	13.0
2000	53.7	0.22	4,892	10.9
2005	104.8*	0.33*	5,253	20.3*
2006	103.9*	0.30*	5,330	19.5*

* These numbers are not comparable with the others as they include very large amounts of funds for debt relief and for natural disasters.

Development contributions

The size of the official development aid (OECD, 2007) is shown in Table 12.2. Support for development programmes (after adjustment for inflation) has not increased from 1990 to 2006, except for the amounts for Afghanistan (US$2.2 billion) and Iraq (US$21.4 billion); the 2005 increase is also explained by large allocations for debt relief and emergencies (US$36 billion); these contributions are helpful, but they will not assist long-term economic development (World Bank, 2006). The development programme aid has remained at the level of some US$50–65 billion from 1990–2006, which equals about US$12–14 (gross amount) per person in the developing countries per year. ODA in 2006 fell 5.1 per cent and is expected to fall further in 2007. According to the World Bank, the expansion of global aid through 2006 has stalled despite donor promises at several international meetings, and disbursements have fallen (World Bank, 2007).

If we take a longer perspective, we will find that in 1960 ODA per capita amounted to US$61 and in 2002 it was US$67 (adjusted for inflation). During the same period the income of donor countries went from US$11,308 per capita to US$28,500, thus the ODA increased 10 per cent and the donors' income increased by 152 per cent (Global Health Watch, 2005–6).

Only part of the development aid is spent in the 'recipient countries' and even less will reach poor children. Firstly, the administrative costs of the donors have to be deducted.[27] Secondly, the recipient governments have to cover their administrative costs.[28] Some of the grants are used for the purchase of industrial equipment and services from the donor country, although they often may be purchased at lower prices from other sources. Many ministerial cars, computers and other office equipment are bought using the foreign donations. In addition there is the corruption factor.[29] It is easy to see why the proportion of development aid sent to a recipient country that will reach the children is going to be small. It seems reasonable to assume that the bilateral and multilateral aid available for 'benefiting the poor' would be equivalent to *about US$4–6 per person per year* (net amount), annually equivalent to two to three days' average consumption by the poor. However, even these small amounts do not trickle down much; the trickle-down economic theory was never much more than a belief, an 'article of faith', unsupported by any research (Stiglitz, 2002). What is being done is welcome. I have seen both well-administered, good quality development programmes (most of them small) and others (often with large budgets) in which the funds have been squandered.

Will present methods for development aid reduce poverty?

The effects of external economic aid on the economic development of the poor nations are disputed. Burnside and Dollar (2000) and Easterly et al. (2004) – economists at the World Bank – carried out studies for the period 1970–97. The conclusion (made by Easterly) was that there is 'no evidence that aid promotes growth even in good policy environments'. Figure 12.1 (Rozenblat, 2002) confirms that the main income growth has been among the richest third of the recipient populations.

Development assistance has been ineffective as a means to reduce poverty, although it certainly has had some small-scale results. Some experts claim that because of the insufficient amounts provided and because of the management problems described (see notes 25 and 26), the early expectations of international aid have not materialized: these proponents argue for very large increases in international aid. Others point to the fact that 'spending $2.3 trillion (measured in today's dollars) in aid over the past five decades has left the most aid-intensive regions, like Africa, wallowing in continued stagnation; it's fair to say this approach has not been a great success' (Easterly, 2005). Children in developing countries have seen little action, and during these years

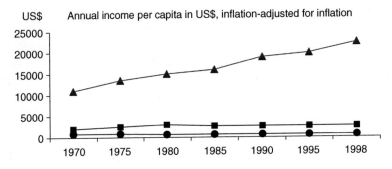

Figure 12.1   Comparative changes in income 1970–1998
The lines on the chart show the average annual income levels, adjusted for inflation, in three groups of nations. The lower line represents the income level in the one-third poorest countries in the world, the intermediate line the average income in the one-third group of middle-income countries, and the upper line the income in the one-third richest countries. The populations of the richest one-third of these countries (top line) have seen their average annual income double from about US$11,000 to about US$22,000 over the last thirty years. The lowest two lines, representing the poorer two-thirds of the world's countries, have remained for the last thirty years at approximately the same levels of poverty. The efforts to increase the income for the least affluent two-thirds of the world's populations have failed. Credit: Céline Rozenblat.

their numbers have more than doubled and childhood violence is growing. Is the international community capable of reducing these levels, to prevent the causes of violence and to help the victims? Or should we look for other approaches, such as piecemeal reforms and using small-scale community-based programmes? In the following chapter, we will examine the activities of the United Nations Millennium Development Programme, the largest effort ever to address the main economic, health and social problems in the developing countries.

13
The Sacrifice of the Poor

The United Nations declaration of the Millennium Development Programme

The latest international efforts to advance economic and social development – to 'eradicate poverty' – are described in the Millennium Development Programme and its Millennium Development Goals (MDGs) which were adopted in 2000 by the largest summit of Heads of States and Governments ever seen in New York. It was made retroactive to 1990. The Programme has eight MDGs, eighteen targets and forty-eight indicators. The Programme was to meet all its targets by 2015; it may be noted that during the Programme period 1990–2015, the world's population will grow by 2 billion people, and this increase will be concentrated in the Programme's target countries.

The Millennium Plan was formulated and supported by the United Nations and six of its specialized agencies: the Word Bank, the International Monetary Fund, the Organization for Economic Co-operation and Development (OECD), the United Nations Development Programme, UNICEF, and some large, non-governmental organizations. It was built on the separate concerns of the summits of the 1990s and of the major specialized agencies, arranged as a concerted, holistic Plan. The traditions of the 'individual' prescriptions included in the Plan were already many decades long; the extent to which they have succeeded or failed in the past often had more to do with national efforts than with the international donor inputs.

We are now just seven years away from the end-point of the twenty-five-year Millennium Programme. Before reviewing the official data, we must realize that there are problems with the official numbers used in poverty measurements,[30] population size,[31] number of children,[32] morbidity and mortality[33] and literacy.[34] The evaluation of Millennium Development Goals includes information of variable accuracy from some 200 nations and territories, collected by multiple organizations over a period of twenty-five years. Few surveyors will remain with the MDG during the entire period. Thousands of individual surveyors have been instructed separately, sometimes inadequately. They do not reliably apply the same standard criteria for consumption assessments, seriousness and diagnostic criteria of health problems and hunger, and checking of education, literacy and employment. The data are therefore of highly varying quality, such that their use in assessing the Millennium Goals is of uncertain reliability. Indeed, some insiders wonder if positive outcomes may at times be the result of invented data. We also need to remind ourselves that the collection of basic data should begin in the communities of the developing countries, many of which do not have the resources to undertake these tasks systematically and reliably.

The World Bank (see note 24) has always reminded its personnel that missing data, unclear application of indicators, and lack of reliable statistics limit its ability to monitor progress. The review below will examine the implications for the world's children of the present results of the Millennium Programme. The data below, unless specified otherwise, are from the World Bank.

Goal 1: Eradicate extreme poverty and hunger

Target 1: Halve, between 1990 and 2015, the proportion of people whose income is less than $1 a day.
This poverty goal implies a reduction, from 29 per cent to 14.5 per cent, of the proportion of people living on less than one dollar a day. According to the World Bank people living on less than US$1 a day in 1990 amounted to 1,276 million; in 2004 this figure was assessed to have fallen by 290 million to 986 million, of whom about 40 per cent are children. China alone reported a fall of 246 million, implying that elsewhere the number of people living in extreme poverty had hardly changed. In sub-Saharan Africa there was an increase of 58 million poor people. In 1990, 2.7 billion people in the world were living on less than US$2 a day; in 2004, the estimate was 2.6 billion.

Experts have been hoping that the economic poverty reduction goals for 2015 would be reached globally, largely due to the strong economic growth in China and India. In China, according to the World Bank, in 2005 there were 593 million people (UNDP has 422 million for 2005) under the poverty level of US$2 a day, and in India, there were 807 million (total for both countries, 1.4 billion under US$2 a day). In 2005 there were 202 million (16.1 per cent) in China (UNDP has 120 billion for 2005) and 350 million (34.7 per cent) in India living on less than US$1 per day (total for both countries, 552 million).

The outcomes of poverty alleviation in China and India are important, but the levels of the past estimates are incorrect. Recent estimates by the Asian Development Bank have revised upwards the number of US$1 per day poor in China to 500 million and in India to 800 million (Keidel, 2007). Thus, the World Bank's miscalculations in just two developing countries – out of some 150 – amount to about 800 million. This alone almost doubles the Bank's 2005 global estimate of 986 million US$1 per day poor people, *raising the inevitable question of the trustworthiness of all poverty data*. The new data will also have an effect on the estimate of the US$2 per day poor, which is likely to increase to between 3.6 and 4 billion.

Experts generally do not expect the poverty-reduction goals to be reached in most other regions, particularly not in sub-Saharan Africa, where GDP per capita shrank 14 per cent, and poverty rose from 41 per cent in 1981 to 46 per cent in 2001, adding 150 million people living in extreme poverty. Without the financial resources needed, and with about 1.7 billion more people added (1990–2015) to the populations in the developing countries, by 2015 it is likely that there will be more poor people in absolute numbers (with somewhat less in relative numbers). Although the Least Developing Countries (LDCs) have higher rates of economic growth than in the past, this is not yet translating into poverty reduction and improved human well-being.

Target 2: Halve, between 1990 and 2015, the proportion of people who suffer from hunger.
According to the World Food Programme, in 1997–9 there were some 815 million undernourished people in the world; 40 per cent of these were children. Poor or insufficient nutrition has caused impaired growth among some 226 million children. In addition, over 2 billion people worldwide, many of them children, suffer from micro-nutrient malnutrition. Their diets supply inadequate amounts of vitamins and minerals such as vitamin A, iron, iodine, zinc, and vitamin C. Micro-nutrients are essential for human growth and development, especially for children. Because of hunger, millions of people, including 6 million children under the age of 5, die each year. Most are dying because they lack adequate food and essential nutrients, which leaves them weak, underweight and vulnerable to infections. Chronic undernutrition in childhood is linked to slower cognitive development which affects learning at school,

and produces serious health impairments later in life that reduce their economic productivity. Undernourished infants lose their curiosity, motivation and even the will to play. Millions leave school prematurely. All too often, child hunger is trans-generational: 17 million children are born underweight annually, the result of their mothers' malnutrition before and during pregnancy.

After decreasing by 37 million during the first half of the 1990s, the number of hungry people in developing countries increased by 18 million in the second half. Overall, from 1990 to 2003, the number of hungry decreased insignificantly from 823 to 820 million. One recognizes that the reduction of hunger foreseen in the Millennium Programme is not taking place: the goal of reducing by half the undernourished people by 2015 cannot be reached.

The UN agencies and the NGOs that distribute food to the hungry are seriously underfinanced. From a record of almost 17 million tonnes in 1993, global food aid fell to 9.9 million tonnes in 1995, 7.6 million

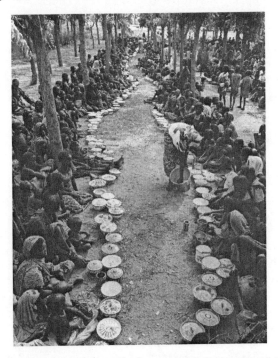

Photo 21. **Feeding the hungry.** *Here, food is distributed to families in the Sahel but, as desert areas increase and the population grows, their chance of escaping hunger is nil.* © *World Health Organization.*

tonnes in 1996, and 5.1 million tonnes in 2004. The World Food Programme delivers food to 77 million people in 82 countries; its deliveries – which are almost 50 per cent of all global food deliveries – have been hit by increasing food prices and costs for transportation; its budget has not kept pace with these increases.

Goal 2: Achieve universal primary education

Target 3: Ensure that, by 2015, children everywhere, boys and girls alike, will be able to complete a full course of primary schooling.

Attaining this goal would require enrolling some 200 million more children in primary school than there are today, an increase of 41 per cent over current levels. However, from 2000 to 2006 just an additional 35 million children were completing primary school. The World Bank calculations do not make it clear that for 200 million additional children aged 5–14, with a teacher to pupil ratio of 1 to 50, some 4 million teachers need to be added quickly. According to a World Bank study, only thirty-seven of 155 developing countries analysed had by 2004 achieved universal primary completion. Based on trends in the 1990s, another thirty-two are likely to achieve that goal. But seventy countries risk not reaching the goal. In several of them, completion rates have stagnated or even fallen in recent years. If current trends persist, children in more than half of developing countries will not complete a full course of primary education by 2015. An important but insufficiently addressed question is whether the quality of education is maintained as the number of schoolchildren increases: most poor children who attend primary school in the developing world learn shockingly little. More efforts are needed to monitor outcomes and to understand what students are actually learning and retaining.

Goal 3: Promote gender equality and empower women

Target 4: Eliminate gender disparity in primary and secondary education, preferably by 2005 and in all levels of education no later than 2015.

Progress in gender equality and women's empowerment has been uneven. Concerted national efforts have helped raise girls' enrolments in the past decade so that gender parity for primary school enrolments has been reached in 83 of 106 reporting countries. Yet, in the same period, the increase in women's participation in the economy and in political decision-making has been modest at best. According to the World Bank, the results of gender equality programmes at all levels of education are less than comforting.

Goal 4: Reduce child mortality

Target 5: Reduce by two-thirds, between 1990 and 2015, the under-5 mortality rate.

Goal 5: Improve maternal health

Target 6: Reduce by three-quarters, between 1990 and 2015, the maternal mortality.

The prospects in the health sector are grave. The clear impression is that we do not really know how much of existing state health programmes reach the poor. The same problem is shared with the civil society projects. Only sixty-four countries, mostly those with high incomes, have complete mortality data (see note 33). Thus, no developing country has reliable information about Goals 4 and 5; the following statistics are rough estimates only. Infant mortality rates in low- and middle-income countries may have fallen from 86 per 1,000 live births in 1980 to 60 in 2002. Forty-six countries, however, still have under-5 mortality rates between 100 and 280 per 1,000 (WHO, World Health Report 2005) while, as an example, Sweden has an infant mortality rate of 3 per 1,000, and other high-income countries have rates of 5 per 1,000.

In the forty-two countries that account for 90 per cent of child deaths, 80 per cent of children are not given oral rehydration therapy when needed; 61 per cent of children under six months are not exclusively breastfed; 60 per cent do not receive treatment for acute respiratory infections; and 45 per cent do not get vitamin A supplements. The gap in survival between the richest and poorest children in the world is increasing. The well-off are improving, while survival of the poorest is worsening.

The maternal mortality rate may also have diminished during the same period but is still assessed at 684 per 100,000 births in low- and middle-income countries as against 14 per 100,000 in the high-income countries. The highest registered is in Afghanistan: 1,600 per 100,000 (Ahmad, 2004). An estimated 529,000 women die in pregnancy and childbirth each year, 99 per cent of them in developing countries. The Millennium Programme's goal of reducing child and maternal mortality will not be achieved because only 15–20 per cent of all countries are on track.

Goal 6: Combat HIV/AIDS, malaria and other diseases

Target 7: Have halted by 2015 and begun to reverse the spread of HIV/AIDS.

Target 8: Have halted by 2015 and begun to reverse the incidence of malaria and other major diseases.

The worldwide incidence of HIV is rising. The number of people living with HIV has gone up from some 30 million in 2000 to 40 million in 2006 (WHO, 2007b). The annual global numbers of deaths from HIV/AIDS are projected to increase from 2.8 million in 2002 to 6.5 million in 2030. The situation is catastrophic, and not simply a result of better reporting.

In 2004, 107 countries reported malaria transmission risks. To diagnose malaria a microscopic examination of blood films or an antigen detection test is needed. These require specialized laboratories which are rare in developing countries. Precise statistics are unknown because many cases occur in rural areas where people do not have access to health care. Consequently, the majority of cases are undocumented. What follows are 'guesstimates': about 350–500 million cases of malaria occur annually; each year, approximately 50 million women living in malaria-endemic countries become pregnant, over half in tropical Africa. An estimated 10,000 of these women and 200,000 of their infants die because of malaria during pregnancy. In Africa, one in twenty children dies of malaria before the age of 5. In children who survive, malarial anaemia is common. The number of people living in malaria-exposed areas has increased since the 1980s; the severity of infection and the number of deaths will indeed continue to increase (Hay et al., 2004; WHO, 2007b).

In 2005, there were 8.8 million new cases of tuberculosis. The total numbers of newly detected cases are increasing. WHO (2007b) concludes that the '1990s prevalence and mortality rates will not have been halved by 2015'.

Goal 7: Ensure environmental sustainability

Target 10: Halve by 2015 the proportion of people without sustainable access to safe drinking water.
This implies providing another 1.5 billon people with water and 2 billion with sanitation. The rate of progress of this Millennium Goal is only half of what is needed. At the current rate of development, only 20 per cent of all countries will achieve the goal; in the low-income countries, only 10 per cent will do so. Nearly 80 per cent of all child deaths in the developing countries are caused by contaminated water (WHO and UNICEF, 2000).

Target 11: Have achieved by 2020 a significant improvement in the lives of at least 100 million slum dwellers.
This goal mainly refers to the provision of safe water and sanitation in slums. Half of the world's population is urbanized; most live in slums. The size of their living quarters is very small – with little space for

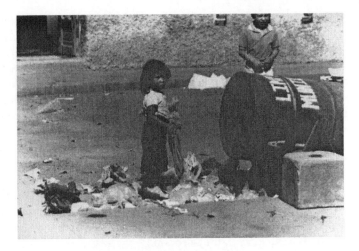

Photo 22. **Slum children.** © *World Health Organization.*

children – and there is a lack of public facilities: water, sewers, electricity and toilets. Schools and health services may be missing. Violence and aggression are common. Massive investments are needed to provide decent living conditions; poor countries do not have the means. Not much improvement in Target 11 can be expected to occur during the remaining seven years of the underfinanced Millennium Programme.

Goal 8: Develop a global partnership for development

Target 12: Develop further an open, rule-based, predictable, non-discriminatory trading and financial system (includes a commitment to good governance, development, and poverty reduction – both nationally and internationally).

The commitment to good governance

The World Bank concluded that efforts to improve the quality of governance were important for the overall development process. In the mid-1990s, it created a new group for Worldwide Governance Indicators (WGI) (Kaufmann and Kraay, 2007). The initiative came from Mr James Wolfensohn, at that time the World Bank President, who had reacted to the finding that the Bank's control over the use of its fund was insufficient; some of it 'appeared' to have gone to corruption, a phenomenon he called 'the cancer of corruption'. The Bank introduced six 'dimensions' to measure the quality of governments; the indicators of these are based on several hundred individual variables measuring governance, drawn from thirty-seven separate data sources constructed by thirty-one different organizations. Based on the indicators, each of the six dimensions is rated from 0 to 100; the higher the better. Results covering 213 countries and territories from 1996–2006 were presented in a paper by the World Bank in 2007 and on its internet site (World Bank, 2007). The Governance group 'supports the collection, rigorous analysis, careful interpretation, and transparent dissemination of data for empirical research, capacity-building, and learning programs'. The WGI group is very clear about the difficulties in making the measurements, and presents the margins of error of its data. The indicators are:

1. *Voice and accountability* includes a number of indicators measuring various aspects of the political process, civil liberties, political and human rights, and measuring the extent to which citizens of a country are able to participate in the selection of governments.
2. *Political stability and absence of violence* combines several indicators, which measure perceptions of the likelihood that the government in power will be destabilized or overthrown by possibly unconstitutional and/or violent means, including domestic violence and terrorism.
3. *Government effectiveness* combines responses on the quality of public service provision, the quality of the bureaucracy, the competence of civil servants, the independence of the civil service from political pressures, and the credibility of the government's commitment to policies.
4. *Regulatory quality* focuses more on the policies themselves, including measures of the incidence of market-unfriendly policies such as price controls or inadequate bank supervision, as well as perceptions of the burdens imposed by excessive regulation in areas such as foreign trade and business development.
5. *Rule of law* includes several indicators which measure the extent to which agents have confidence in and abide by the rules of society. These include perceptions of the incidence of crime, the effectiveness and predictability of the judiciary, and the enforceability of contracts.
6. *Control of corruption* is a measure of the extent of corruption, conventionally defined as the exercise of public power for private gain. It is based on scores of variables from polls of experts and surveys.

All of these dimensions are of direct importance to children's lives. The first mentions the compliance with 'human rights'; the second takes up 'domestic violence'; the third the 'quality of public services' (such as health care and education) and the 'governments' commitment to policies' (such as child support and alleviation of poverty); the fourth is an 'instrument for reducing opportunities for corruption'; the fifth 'the incidence of crimes' (such as child abuse) and 'the effectiveness and predictability of the judiciary' (related to the failure to convict child abusers and the impunity the perpetrators enjoy including government employees who commit child abuse); and the sixth 'corruption' (which robs the poor).

The WGI Group presents its results mainly country by country. In the context of this book, it appeared to be of great interest to evaluate this component of the global ecology system. What quality of governance is experienced by our children and their families and what are the implications? A presentation based on the World Bank's original data follows.

Table 13.1 shows the combined governance performance calculations from the twenty-one most populated developing countries: Argentina, Bangladesh, Brazil, China, Colombia, Democratic Republic of Congo, Egypt, Ethiopia, India, Indonesia, Iran, Mexico, Myanmar, Nigeria, Pakistan, Philippines, Republic of Korea, South Africa, Sudan, Thailand and Vietnam. By 1996, each of these countries had populations exceeding 30 million. In 2006, their combined populations were 4,177 million people, close to 80 per cent of the developing world's total population of 5,300 million (US Census Bureau, 2007). The WGI percentile rates for each of the six dimensions were multiplied by the population numbers separately for each country in 1996 and 2006; thus, the results from the twenty-one countries were weighted individually, the larger the population the higher the weight. The combined weights of the twenty-one countries were then added and divided by their combined populations (in 1996 and 2006); the dimension score averages appear in Table 13.1.

The average percentile ranks were already low in 1996: these countries had large governance problems. Since 1996, four of the six dimensions of governance performance showed negative changes, and the average for all six has been reduced by 5.4%.

In Table 13.1 'Voice and accountability' shows a small increase in democracy, but is still unacceptably low. Even lower is 'Political stability and absence of violence'; it reminds us of the many failed and still failing states, and of past and present violence; of the haunted world which since 1945 has experienced some 150 wars and civil uprisings; killed hundreds of millions and sent an equal number to refugee camps. Interpersonal violence, large proportions of which are against women and children, is also growing. The 'Regulatory' quality is seen by the WGI as an 'instrument for reducing opportunities for corruption – for example in tax, customs, permits and licensing, and inspections'. It is

Table 13.1 Changes from 1996 to 2006 of the six World Bank dimensions for government performance in the twenty-one most populated developing countries

WGI government performance dimensions	Combined government performance indicators of WGI dimensions, 1996	Combined government performance indicators of WGI dimensions, 2006	Difference: absolute value
Voice and accountability	27.8	30.6	+2.8
Political stability and absence of violence	24.2	25.1	+0.9
Government effectiveness	53.0	50.1	−2.9
Regulatory quality	47.7	43.6	−4.1
Rule of law	46.3	42.4	−4.1
Control of corruption	41.9	38.2	−3.7
Average	40.2	38.3	−1.9 (−5.4%)
Population million	3,653	4,177	+524

disappointing to see that this dimension, together with 'Rule of law' and 'Control of corruption', are those showing the highest decline, an unwelcome indication of the growing 'cancer of corruption'.

Combined scores of the six dimensions are available from the WGI Group for the forty-eight countries of sub-Saharan Africa and for the countries of the former Soviet Union. These are reproduced in Table 13.2 together with a few selected large countries as comparisons, including the five permanent members of the UN Security Council (China is also included in Table 13.1), and two economically important countries: Japan and Germany.

The countries of the former Soviet Union have the lowest scores on the WGI dimensions, even lower than sub-Saharan Africa. Even several developed countries show negative changes.

The results are that during the last ten years the quality of governance has declined for three major groups accounted for in Tables 13.1 and 13.2: 4,177 million in twenty-one developing countries, 318 million in sub-Saharan Africa (not already included in Table 13.1) and 283 million in the countries of the former Soviet Union; the total is 4,858 million,

Table 13.2 Analysis of the changes from 1996 to 2006 of the average performance on World Bank dimensions for government performance in selected countries

Region/ country	Average gov. performance indicators of WGI dimensions, 1996	Average gov. performance indicators of WGI dimensions, 2006	Difference absolute value 1996–2006	Population million 2006
Sub-Saharan Africa, average	31.1	30.3	−0.8	751 (353 included in Table 13.1)
Former Soviet Union	23.0	20.9	−2.1	283
China	44.1	37.2	−6.9	1,321
France	84.9	83.9	−1.0	64
Russia	25.8	27.1	+1.3	141
United Kingdom	90.3	88.9	−1.4	61
United States	91.2	84.9	−6.3	302
Japan	79.9	86.1	+6.2	128
Germany	93.1	90.0	−3.1	82

76 per cent of the world's population. Governance is a very important part of children's quality of life. Violence related to the lack of rule of law is growing. The conclusion of this analysis is that – having considered the margins of error – *during the last ten years the quality of governance has declined or been halted for three-quarters of the world's population.*

Whatever the World Bank and other organizations have attempted to implement, the efforts to raise the quality of governance have yet to succeed. It is interesting to reflect on a disclaimer which appears on the published documents produced by the World Bank's staff: *'The data and research reported here do not reflect the official views of the World Bank, its Executive Directors, or the countries they represent. The Worldwide Governance Indicators (WGI) are not used by the World Bank Group to allocate resources or for any other official purpose.'* Were the results of the Bank's own governance study an embarrassment?

The World Bank's board management insists that huge amounts of funds will continue to be transferred even to countries in which corruption is common. It should not surprise anybody that some of its loans will end up in the wrong pockets. A report from January 2008 made by the Bank's internal auditor concluded that over US$500 million worth of contracts in India had been tainted by 'significant indicators of fraud and corruption' such as 'collusive behaviours, bid rigging, bribery and manipulated bid prices' (*The Economist*, 22 March 2008). The World Bank has a Department of Institutional Integrity, which investigates allegations of misconduct, fraud and corruption at the Bank, and designs anti-corruption measures to safeguard Bank resources. Recently it decided to suppress the results of an investigation of corruption in three World Bank projects in the Democratic Republic of the Congo 'for political reasons', and regarding a project in Armenia it failed to investigate documented evidence of fraud, although the fraud was both extensive and ongoing.

Target 16: In co-operation with developing countries, develop and implement strategies for decent and productive work for youth.
Increasing the chances of young people finding and keeping decent work is critical to achieving the UN Millennium Development Goals (Somavia, 2004). Youth unemployment worldwide, however, is at an all-time high. Young people aged 15–24 represent nearly half the world's jobless although they are only 25 per cent of the global working age population. The number of unemployed youth increased by 27 per cent from 1993–2003 because this population grew 10.5 per cent during that period to some 1.1 billion in 2003, but youth employment grew only 0.2 per cent. An additional 1 billion youth will enter the global labour market in the next decade, mostly in developing countries – places where jobs are least likely to be found. Experts predict that only 300 million new jobs will be created over the same period, leaving an employment gap that is expected to exacerbate poverty, worsen public health, and dampen economic growth in countries already struggling to provide the basics to their citizens. Too few of the developing world's children will have any chance of finding a job when they grow up.

The Millennium Programme and its predecessors have not included action in three important areas affecting development:

1. *Family planning/birth control* programmes have met with resistance from religious and cultural groups in many countries. The populations of developing countries are predicted to grow from 6 billion (2000) to 9 billion (2050), yet the Millennium Development Goals do not include any targets for family planning/birth control. The overcrowding of the world is a serious ecological problem, and gains in MDGs may readily be offset by the population explosion. This bodes ill for the future of our children. The estimated cost of universal access to sexual and reproductive health services is US$23 billion for 2005. Donor nations thus have to triple their current financial commitments.

2. *A decentralized judicial system.* For the poor, the neglect and abuse of their legal rights is a clear reality. Their experience in seeking justice often leads them to give up; those in power will 'always win', by corruption or by the use of personal influence. The impunity enjoyed by those who misuse their authority and maltreat children also must end. In the tables above, the 'rule of law' has received low and decreasing scores. It is well known that the justice system is both severely under-dimensioned and malfunctioning in developing countries, yet the Millennium Programme does not address this blatant inequality. Support for the informal system in the developing countries through the training of lay judges could help.

3. *Prevention of violence.* In the 2000 Millennium Development Programme there is no single reference to violence or child abuse. By 2005, evidently under pressure (United Nations Millennium Programme, 2005), a few words were added with a recommendation to 'focus' on 'freedom from violence' as part of the women's and girls' health programme. This recommendation is welcome, but is vague and insufficient, given the magnitude of the problem. Although economic development is threatened by increasing violence, there are still no specific Millennium Goals about violence.

Conclusions and alternatives

The global neglect of children

The summary above shows the extent of global, structural child neglect. Over 1 billion children live in poverty, most of them in sub-standard housing, lacking clean water and sanitation. One-fifth of them do not even start school, and many of those who do double classes or drop out. What they find in school is mostly of poor quality. The school curriculum emphasizes mostly the basic skills and learning obedient behaviour, although these basic skills may soon be lost, because few of them have pen and paper at home, and reading materials are scarce. Insufficient attention is given to comprehension, critical analysis and conscientization. Development in these poor countries would be enhanced if the curriculum included learning progress-oriented knowledge and problem-solving skills. Parents' poor education leads to under-stimulation of their children. Health services do not exist for about one-quarter of the poor, and the quality is often insufficient, especially when it comes to curative services. Child nutrition is a large problem, both regarding protein-calorie and micro-nutrient supply. Millions of children continue to die, although almost all deaths could have been prevented.

In addition, the chances for a child of fully realizing its innate potential are impaired by a multitude of combined factors appearing during these periods:

1. *Pre-natal health conditions of pregnant mothers*: their under-nourishment leads to anaemia, inadequate supply of calories, vitamins and essential minerals, to which are added frequent infectious diseases, stress, marital conflicts, sexual, physical and emotional abuse during the pregnancy and mental disorders, all of which may contribute to negative effects for the foetus' neurobiological development. Foetal growth rate that slows brain growth in utero impairs the acquisition of some cognitive and academic abilities (measured at ages 7–9), even when followed by good catch-up head growth after birth, whereas poor brain growth in utero followed by little or no catch-up head growth results in widespread impairments (Frisk et al., 2002).

2. *Perinatal complications at childbirth and the high frequency of under-weight infants*: Poor growth after pre-term birth, particularly poor head growth, is associated with impaired neurodevelopmental outcome. Infants born to mothers living in poverty often have small head circumferences at birth; they will gain normal head size if given high energy nutrients (Brandt et al., 2003), but these are seldom available in developing countries.

3. *Post-natal factors*: poor nutrition, compounded by ignorant and incompetent parenting, poor schooling with insufficient cognitive and non-cognitive stimulation of the child during the early years.

   - A South African national food survey showed that for children as a whole, the intakes of energy, calcium, iron, zinc, selenium, vitamins A, C, D and E, riboflavin, niacin, vitamin B6 and folic acid were below two-thirds of the recommended dietary allowances. Of all children, 52 per cent experienced hunger, 23 per cent were at risk of hunger and only 25 per cent appeared food-secure. Energy deficit and micro-nutrient deficiencies were common, resulting in a high prevalence of stunting (Labadarios et al., 2005). Vomk et al. (1993) studied 515 5-year-old children in a rural area in Kenya and found 17 per cent with a head circumference reduction exceeding two standard deviations. Studies in Mauritius (Liu et al., 2003) showed that malnutrition at age 3 is associated with poor cognition at the age of 11 independent of psychosocial adversity. In 1998 Gray et al. began research of a population sample from three villages in Uganda. The study has involved some 1,500 children and their mothers and is still ongoing. In a sub-sample (Gray et al., 2008) of breastfed children aged 0–3 the authors made behavioural and nutritional observations, and anthropometric measurements, including head circumference. At the age of 3 years all children were below the third percentile for height and weight. Regarding head circumference, all children at the age of 12 months were under the fifteenth percentile, and during their second year of life – when healthy, well-nourished children show rapid growth of this measure, indicating ongoing major brain development – the Ugandan children showed no such growth.

- A study from Egypt (Shaaban et al., 2005) describes a random sample of 1,000 children aged 6–36 months from an area with high levels of malnutrition: 24 per cent had stunted growth. Underweight children had frequent chronic coughs, chronic and recurrent diarrhoea, and intestinal amoebas and worms. Serum haemoglobin, albumin and plasma pre-albumin levels were significantly lower in underweight children compared to normal children. All anthropometric measurements, including head circumference, were lower than normal in underweight subjects.
- Khor (2003), in a review of children in Asia, states that half of all pre-school children are malnourished. They also suffer from frequent micro-nutrient deficiency; iron deficiency anaemia affects close to half of pre-school and primary school children, and iron deficiency is very common.
- A Chilean review shows that undernutrition at an early age affects brain growth and IQ. Most students with the lowest scholastic achievement have sub-optimal head circumference and brain size. Considering that the absolute numbers of undernourished children have been increasing in the world, it is of major relevance to analyse the long-term effects of undernutrition at an early age. Nutritional problems affect the lowest socio-economic stratum with negative consequences manifested in school-age, in higher levels of school drop-out, learning problems and a low percentage of students enrolling into higher education. This limits the development of people; increasing adult productivity is a clear economic benefit for the whole country, and this can be achieved through successful prevention of childhood malnutrition (Leiva Plaza et al., 2001).
- Strathearn (2000), in a US prospective study, showed that childhood neglect is significantly associated with delayed cognitive development and head growth.

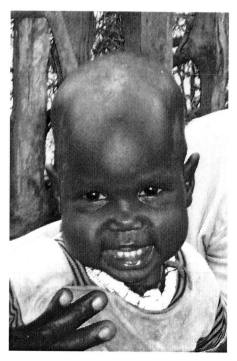

Photo 23.   **Child in Moroto District, Uganda**. *The child is twelve months old in the photo but at the time, her head circumference was in the lowest percentile of growth for children aged three months. Credit: Sandra Gray.*

It is difficult to escape the conclusion that structural neglect causes large-scale impairments, among them: low body weight and size, low muscular strength and endurance, and sub-optimal brain growth. The latter will at some point lead to lifelong neurobiological deficiencies, and reduced cognitive (IQ) and non-cognitive functions. The costs to the individuals and to the society are very high. The common wisdom is that there is enough food to feed the entire world's population, but the problem is the distribution of it. It is urgent to find a better solution to reach the children, especially those under the age of 5, when most of the brain development takes place. But what we find instead is that the World Food Programme and other donors and distributors of food to children see their resources decrease at the same time as the child population grows.

Who is responsible for this large-scale neglect? The primary care-givers – mostly the family – cannot be blamed for circumstances over which they have no power. *The responsibility lies in the functioning of poor countries' macro-institutions and in the lack of appropriate development assistance. The structures of the macro- and global systems have failed to provide what is needed to prevent massive child neglect leading to the destruction of the potential of the victims' lives, for some even before they are born.*

The outcome of the Millennium Programme

Close to three-quarters of the time between 1990 and 2015 has now passed, and for many nations, the results of the MDGs related to children are still insufficient and do not appear promising. Added to the problem is the insufficient quality of information provided by the institutions under the leadership of the World Bank, so we may never know the real outcomes. The fact that most of the goals will not be reached is sad and discouraging. Rogerson et al. (2004) at the Overseas Development Institute in London sum up:

> many low-income countries have no realistic chance of meeting some, if not most, MDGs, virtually regardless of their efforts, or of the size and quality of outside support in the intervening period. The intermediate group, where greater efforts now could yet tip the balance, will shrink quickly – well before 2010 and probably much earlier. During the period of 2005–2010, therefore, and perhaps already by 2005–6, the MDGs will probably cease to be an effective reference point both for very successful and very unsuccessful countries, and may lose their potency for most of the undecided category.

The Millennium Declaration promised: 'We will spare no efforts to free our fellow men, women and children from the abject and dehumanising conditions of extreme poverty, to which more than a billion of them are currently subjected.' At the 2000 Summit the public was told to expect rapid improvements. It is now evident that the Programme is in deep trouble. In spite of all the rhetoric, a large proportion of this generation of the poorest – including the children – in the developing countries is being sacrificed. Most of the destitute, the excluded, the vulnerable and downtrodden will – as in the past – continue to live a life without dignity and rights, without mercy, and they will die in misery under catastrophic and inhumane conditions.

Utopian ideas become dangerous and destabilizing when they succeed in eliciting enthusiasm, hopes and energies among the poor and oppressed for ends that will not be achieved. To convey hope and then to fail to deliver is cynical and immoral. Could this failure have been foreseen? Indeed, the World Bank, in its 1997 World Development Report – three years before the Millennium Declaration – stated:

> the notion that good advisers and technical experts would formulate good policies, which good governments would then implement for the good of society, was outdated: the institutional assumptions implicit in this world view were, as we all realize today, too simplistic... Governments embarked on fanciful schemes. Private investors, lacking confidence in public policies or in the steadfastness of leaders, held back. Powerful rulers acted arbitrarily. Corruption became endemic. Development faltered, and poverty endured.

One undisputed effect of the monolithic economic order is the growing inequality – described in Chapter 12 – showing that the world's richest 1 per cent receives as much income as the poorest 57 per cent; the richest 2 per cent own 50 per cent of all the assets in the world; and the combined incomes of the richest 25 million Americans (USA) equal those of almost 2 billion poor people. This outcome of the Western world's concept of progress can only be described as a colossal failure.

The reasons for this are debated, but there is certainly an institutional and academic imbalance between economic and social domains. Enormously increased resources were given to economists after the Bretton Woods agreements, creating two citadels of world power – the International Monetary Fund and the World Bank – and then further enhancing their clout by the creation in 1969 of a special new Nobel prize in economics, until now received by no less than 61 laureates. Social science and policy were never given comparable institutional counter-weights or publicity, and have had less recruitment attraction. Although some eminent economists have analysed social subjects, the imbalance has remained. The criticism started in the 1950s, and one of the most influential thinkers was the economist E. F. Schumacher, who in his book *Small is Beautiful: Economics as if People Mattered* (1973, republished in 1999) states that:

> the general evidence of material progress would suggest that the modern private enterprise system is – or has been – the most perfect instrument for the pursuit of personal enrichment. The modern private enterprise system ingeniously employs the human urges of greed and envy as its motive power, but manages to overcome the most blatant deficiencies of laissez-faire by means of Keynesian economic management, a bit of redistributive taxation, and the 'countervailing

power' of the trade unions. Can such a system conceivably deal with the problems we now have to face? The answer is self-evident: greed and envy demand continuous and limitless economic growth of a material kind, without proper regard for conservation, and this type of growth cannot possibly fit into a finite environment. We must therefore study the essential nature of the private enterprise system and the possibilities of evolving an alternative system which might fit the new situation . . . the vacuum of our minds may only too easily be filled by some big, fantastic notion – political or otherwise – which suddenly seems to illumine everything and to give meaning and purpose to our existence. It needs no emphasis that herein lies one of the great dangers of our time.

The many proposals of global action to correct the enormous inequalities in income and assets have not translated from rhetoric to positive changes; on the contrary, the inequalities are actually growing. The implications for most of the world's children, and hence for the future, are bleak.

Seeking a new focus

The time for rethinking is overdue; as Rogerson et al. (2004) suggested, it appears that now is the time to say goodbye to the Millennium Programme. International assistance has in the past had some successes, but too much has been a deception. This costly deception has been allowed to continue without proper attention to its actual results (see notes 25 and 26). The conclusion is that poor nations have to use their own strengths and learn how to mobilize their own populations to rectify their existing conditions to create a better future for their children. Some countries, such as China and India, have succeeded well almost without any outside help. Donors can contribute to children's programmes using a 'piecemeal reform' approach. Easterly (2005), a professor of economics at New York University and formerly an economist at the World Bank, proposes that the stakeholders should

> humbly acknowledge that nobody can fully grasp the complexity of the political, social, technological, ecological and economic systems that underlie poverty. It would eschew the arrogance that 'we' know exactly how to fix 'them'. It would shy away from the hubris of what [is labelled] the 'breathtaking opportunity' that 'we' have to spread democracy, technology, prosperity and perpetual peace to the entire

planet. Large-scale crash programs, especially by outsiders, often produce unintended consequences. The simple dreams at the top run afoul of insufficient knowledge of the complex realities at the bottom. The Big Plans are impossible to evaluate scientifically afterward. Nor can you hold any specific agency accountable for their success or failure. Piecemeal reform, by contrast, motivates specific actors to take small steps, one at a time, then tests whether that small step made poor people better off, holds accountable the agency that implemented the small step, and considers the next small step.

To sum up: children in the developing countries can be better helped in other ways than our present attempts to force large-scale programmes upon the global human ecological system. We might reconsider our present penchant for assisting governments of poor nations, which is related to the huge role that intergovernmental organizations have been given. As shown above, these governments have large governance problems which have not improved over the last decade. Instead, it might be better to try directly to reach people via the civil society. The complexity of poor countries' socio-cultural heritage, the importance of their human potential and the positive experience of community mobilization in these countries should no longer be ignored. Encouraging and assisting piecemeal, local projects by communities have proved effective. The author has observed and been involved in the setting up of hundreds of them in many countries (Helander, 1999, 2007). These work well because they build on new entry points: working directly with the people. Decentralization and empowerment of poor communities is a promising path for improving the future of our children.

Part VI

Primary Child Violence Prevention by Exo-systems

14
A Community-based Child Defence and Support (CDS) Programme

Introduction

There are 2.3 billion children in the world under the age of 18; about 2.1 billion live in developing countries. To prevent them from becoming victims of violence using a programme of defence and support is an enormous task. It will take a few generations to see real improvements.

In Chapter 9, the reasons were given for assigning priority to a universal programme: no child should be left behind. *The main objective of a universal programme is to reduce the rate of violence towards children.*

The focus of the actions described in this chapter is to:

(a) promote family life preparation;
(b) assist the family with guidance and support;
(c) create public awareness using media;
(d) to increase the protection of children through legislation that forbids all forms of abuse.

At the core of action is the fostering of caring adults, who will understand and provide the social, emotional, physical and cognitive needs of the growing child, and establish patterns of interaction, mutual trust and security in a spirit of love, empathy and fairness. The preparations need to start early in life.

The discussion below will mainly deal with these priorities. An obvious reason for the choice of primary prevention instead of secondary and tertiary is that the results of the latter are often less effective; this might be caused by the presence of the neurobiological changes described earlier (pp. 147–51, 180–5, 205, 248–50).

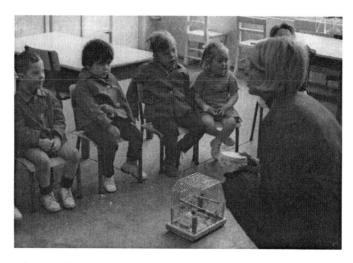

Photo 24. **Family preparation programme.** *It is easy to forget children with disabilities in family preparation programmes. The mentally retarded children seen here have the benefit of a modern approach: they learn to avoid strangers; they are normally very affectionate and will approach any unknown person without any hesitation. This increases their risk for abuse. © World Health Organization.*

Approaches to promote reduction of child violence

Effective child abuse prevention has over time tended to focus more and more on parent education and home visiting programmes. The four different strategies for coping with the problem of childhood violence will be discussed.

1. *Family life preparation*

The most commonly mentioned primary prevention programmes are known as pre-parent and parent education. The first major handbook on parent education was published in 1980 (Fine). The Council of Europe has recently published a book about parenting in contemporary Europe (Daly, 2007). In a meta-analysis McDermott (2002) cites no less than 142 articles and books describing twenty-four different approaches to parent and pre-parent education, most of which have been developed in North America. A few are reproduced in Table 14.1.

The education programmes listed in Table 14.1 include training in skills that go beyond those of 'primary child care'; and even include components of empowering adolescents. These aspects are valuable;

Table 14.1   Examples of approaches to parent and pre-parent education

Author	Type of intervention
Luster and Youatt, 1989, USA	High-school programme. Students interacting with children, in natural settings and observing patterns of parent–child interaction.
Webster-Stratton, 1994, Great Britain	Using videos for parents with conduct disorder children to learn model behaviour.
Brown et al., 1998, USA	Role-playing, coaching and modelling: practical exercises rather than theory or lessons or discussions. There should be early training of parents in simple, readily applicable skills so they can see changes in child behaviour quickly.
Taylor, 1997, USA	Student-centred training with role-play which allows them to express hidden feelings. Learning to estimate how the learner's behaviour affects others. Problem-solving exercises.
Tomison, 1998, Australia	Group work with students to discuss how they have been parented and how they want to be as parents.
Elias et al., 1986, USA	Developing parents' and children's competence in communication, teamwork and joint decision-making; understanding their own and others' needs, managing conflicts and disagreements.
Smith et al., 1994, USA	Learning to manage personal stress (for parents).
Chalk and King, 1998, USA	Groups of parents offered training in social skills and problem-solving. The resulting quality of parenting was better than just learning about child development.
Jaffe et al., 1992, USA	Letting teenagers participate in their family plans and activity decisions, developing skills to use when they become parents.

however, they amount to more than pre-parent or parental education. To include all of these, this book will use the term *family life preparation*.

2. Child community watch

Supervision – 'watch' – of children consists of visits to homes, and observations in schools and at leisure-time activities. The emphasis should be on supporting, not controlling, the meso-system, and preventing malfunction. Home visits bring services into the home; thus, families do not need to seek these outside, which may be inconvenient, and often requires long waiting times. During such visits observations can be made of the family's needs, modifications initiated and resources provided. The home visitor will be able to build a friendly relationship with the family. Home visits have in the past mostly been used for targeted families with social problems. It would be desirable to make these universal; firstly because half of all children are maltreated, and secondly because it will then be non-stigmatizing. It is, however, questionable whether this will be agreeable to everybody. If not, home visits can be replaced by observations in schools and in the community; these will be discussed below.

3. Publicity about the consequences of abuse, addressing widespread public ignorance

Wherever destructive child education practices exist, they have to be replaced. An anti-alcohol campaign is needed. Major media – where they exist – should be used: television, radio, press, posters, inclusion of aspects of child violence prevention in entertainment programmes and cinema films.

4. Introduction of laws

Sexual abuse is illegal everywhere, but in most countries laws do not forbid physical and emotional abuse of children. The Child Convention clearly forbids all types of abuse:

> States Parties shall take all appropriate legislative, administrative, social and educational measures to protect the child from all forms of physical or mental violence, injury or abuse, neglect or negligent treatment, maltreatment or exploitation, including sexual abuse, while in the care of parent(s), legal guardian(s) or any other person who has the care of the child. Protective measures ... include effective ... social programmes to provide necessary support for the child and for those who have the care of the child, as well as for other forms of prevention and for identification, reporting, referral, investigation, treatment and follow-up of instances of child maltreatment described heretofore, and, as appropriate, for judicial involvement (Article 19).

These four strategies will be more effective if operated in combination. Programmes can be communicated in many ways: by one-to-one education, in groups (such as in schools, at home with the family or in community programmes) and by using media, books and information campaigns.

Family life preparation

Before entering into the detailed analysis, it is proposed to look first at the semantics. What are the terms used for the methods that parents use to shape child behaviour? The most common term is 'discipline'; sometimes 'punishment', 'correction' or 'reform'. In people's minds these terms are associated with a negative view of child education: discipline is closely related to punishment using corporal and emotional abuse. Keeping the term 'discipline' will only prolong the misuse of parental authority, and thus the term cannot and should not be rescued even if it is renamed 'positive discipline'.

Socialization is the process by which human beings learn to adopt the behaviour patterns of the meso-, exo- and macro-systems in which they live. The most important time when socialization occurs is between the ages of 1 and 10. Socialization can be carried out without resorting to violence. The challenge is to establish a parental base of practical skills and knowledge to apply in childhood socialization. For many people that would imply a break with the parent behaviour inherited from our previous generations, or which is part of the 'culture'.

Parents', teachers' and peer groups' influence in child behaviour is a type of 'modulation'. To 'modulate an activity or process means to alter or adjust it in order to make it more suitable to a peculiar set of circumstances' (*Collins Dictionary*, 2002). Modulation – in our context – means educating children by guiding, using reasoning to explain why there are certain rules to follow, empowering and coaching them to success in their future life in the society of adults, while preserving their integrity, dignity, personality and creativity. Scientific studies of behaviour modulation have been published (MacPhail, 1990); these confirm the essential role in human behaviour both of the neurobiological system and of the modulatory effects of the environment.

Family life preparation programmes have been applied to different age groups:

(a) very young children, some starting already at the age of 3, fostering empathy and social skills;
(b) teenage children, including appropriate components described in Table 14.1;
(c) as an addition to pre-natal programmes for mothers pregnant with their first child;
(d) parents with one or several young children.

For each of these the activities are different. The programme seeks to develop the future or present parents' skills in child education, promoting a caring, consistent, supportive and safe environment for the child, while strengthening the bonding between parents and children. One of its most important objectives is to prevent domestic violence.

> All parent education programs are thought to assist families primarily by increasing parental knowledge and reducing parental stress. Parent education programs achieve these results by training parents in behavioural management techniques, problem solving and personal coping skills.
>
> (Garbarino, 1995)

Parenting style and its correlates

In all family life preparation programmes analyses of parenting style are important. How do parents behave while educating their children? Parental styles include the combination of two elements: parental responsiveness (warmth) and parental demandingness (behaviour control). Warmth and control can be either high or low; this creates four different combinations of parental styles: indulgent, authoritarian, authoritative and uninvolved (Baumrind, 1973, 1991). In the USA, parenting style has been found to predict child well-being in the domains of social competence, academic performance, psychosocial development and problem behaviour. A summary follows.

(1) Indulgent parents (permissive) are high in warmth and low in control. They are lenient, do not require mature behaviour, allow considerable self-regulation, and avoid confrontation. Children of permissive parents tend to be relatively immature. They have difficulty controlling their impulses, accepting responsibility for social actions, and acting independently. Adolescents from indulgent homes are more likely to be involved in problem behaviour and perform less well in school, but they have higher self-esteem, better social skills, and lower levels of depression. Baumrind (1973) observed that compared to authoritative and authoritarian parents, permissive parents were the most likely to report explosive attacks of rage in which they inflicted more pain or injury upon the child than they had intended. Permissive parents apparently became violent when they felt that they could neither control the child's behaviour nor tolerate its effect upon themselves.

(2) Authoritarian parents are high in control, but low in warmth. They are obedience- and status-oriented, and expect their orders to be obeyed without explanation. These parents provide well-ordered and structured environments with clearly stated rules. Authoritarian parents can be intrusive in their use of power. Children of authoritarian parents lack social skills with their peers. This is especially true for boys. They often withdraw from playful interactions and rarely initiate contact with other children. In situations of moral conflict, such as telling the truth, they tend to look to teachers and other outside authorities to decide what is right. These children seem to lack spontaneity and intellectual curiosity. Adolescents from authoritarian families tend to perform moderately well in school and be uninvolved in problem behaviour, but they have poorer social skills, lower self-esteem, and higher levels of depression.

(3) Authoritative parents are high in both warmth and control. They monitor and impart clear standards for their children's conduct. They are assertive, but not intrusive and restrictive. Their disciplinary methods are supportive, rather than punitive. They want their children to be assertive as well as socially responsible, and self-regulated as well as co-operative. Children of authoritative parents are able to do more for themselves, are more self-controlled, more willing to explore, and more content, compared to children of authoritarian or permissive parents. Girls in this group are especially independent and boys especially socially responsible. Probably as a result of having parents who explain things like rewards and punishments, children in this group understand and accept social rules. They rate as more socially and instrumentally competent than those whose parents are non-authoritative.

(4) Uninvolved (neglecting) parents are low in both responsiveness and demandingness. Some are even rejecting. Children and adolescents whose parents are uninvolved perform most poorly in all domains.

Parenting styles differ in the extent of psychological control: some intrude into the psychological and emotional development of the child through use of practices such as guilt induction, withdrawal of love or shaming. Authoritarian parents expect their children to accept their judgements, values and goals without questioning. In contrast, authoritative parents are more open to give and take with their children and make greater use of explanations.

Authoritative upbringing is associated with both instrumental and social competence and lower levels of problem behaviour in both boys and girls at all developmental stages. The benefits of authoritative parenting and the detrimental effects of uninvolved parenting are evident as early as in pre-school and continue into early adulthood. Just as authoritative parents appear to be able to balance their conformity demands with their respect for their children's individuality, so children from authoritative homes appear to be able to balance the claims of external conformity and achievement demands with their need for individuality and autonomy (Darling, 1999; Thurber, 2003).

One would expect that the risk for child abuse would be highest among the authoritarian parents, and child neglect highest among the uninvolved. Evidently, emphasis on authoritative skills should be part of the family life preparation. It should be recognized that parental styles are also influenced by the dyadic relations between child and parents. Lagace-Seguin and d'Entremont (2006), in a Canadian study of sixty-eight children (mean age 51 months) and their mothers and teachers, showed that less than optimal parenting (authoritarian parenting style and emotion dismissing emotional style) predicted maternal depression (see p. 177) over and above child transgressions (aggressive, asocial, excluding, anxious and hyperactive behaviours). Mothers who engage in less than optimal parenting strategies experience augmented levels of depression. Overall, mothers' parenting styles appear to be more salient in determining their negative moods than their children's transgressions.

The American Academy of Child and Adolescent Psychiatry in 2004 and the International Association for Childhood Education (Paintal) have issued recommendations to parents to adopt the authoritative style. Quotes follow from the latter:

- Set acceptable limits for behaviour. These should be firm, consistent, appropriate to the age of the child, and acceptable. For example, although a 5-year-old child may be able to resist the urge to touch things, it is not reasonable to expect that a 2-year-old will be able to follow such a rule. Therefore, parents may need to protect breakable items at home, and to keep children away from fireplaces, chemicals used at home or in agriculture, electrical outlets, and other dangerous objects. The parents should calmly explain to the child why these limits are needed.
- Teach children how to solve conflicts, for instance about toys or duties at home. They should learn to listen actively, speak clearly, show trust and be trustworthy, accept differences, set group goals, negotiate and mediate conflicts. They need to learn how to share, and to be fair and helpful at home.

Box 14.1: Parenting behaviours associated with risk for off-spring personality disorder during adulthood

Johnson et al. (2006) made a prospective study of a community-based sample of 593 families interviewed during childhood (mean age, 6 years), adolescence (mean ages, 14 and 16 years), emerging adulthood (mean age, 22 years), and adulthood (mean age, 33 years) of the offspring. Types of parenting behaviour during the child-rearing years were associated with elevated offspring risk for personality disorder during adulthood (assessed at ages 22 and 33 years) after controlling for childhood behavioural or emotional problems and parental psychiatric disorders. Risk for offspring personality disorder increased steadily as a function of the number of problematic parenting behaviours. Low parental affection or nurturing was significantly associated with elevated risk for offspring antisocial, avoidant, borderline, depressive, paranoid, schizoid, and schizotypal disorders. Aversive parental behaviour (e.g. harsh punishment) was significantly associated with elevated risk for offspring borderline, paranoid, passive-aggressive, and schizotypal disorders.

- Reason and talk with children in a simple way that is easily understood at the child's age. Such interactions will help the child to develop its intelligence.
- Be a role model of patience, kindness, empathy, and cooperation. Parents and teachers should be aware of the powerful influence their actions have on a child's or group's behaviour.
- When there is an opportunity, let the children practice rational problem solving. Encourage them to think about alternatives and the effect of each alternative.
- Encourage and praise children. A nonverbal response such as a smile or a nod, or a small word such as 'good' or 'right' is an incentive that builds children's confidence.
- Allow children to participate in setting rules – and identifying consequences for breaking them. It will make it easier for them to learn how to manage their own behaviour.
- As a parent or a teacher be consistent and predictable. Capriciousness scares children.
- Encourage children's autonomy – allow them to think for themselves, and to monitor their own behaviour and let their conscience guide them.

The parental style system has to a limited extent been studied in some developing countries; many different varieties of such styles exist, and sometimes older children take over the parental role. Whiting and Whiting (1975) studied six countries; an example follows:

> children in the Gusii tribe in Nyansongo, Kenya, exhibited more authoritarian and aggressive behaviour than did children in a small New England town. The authors guessed this was partly because older Gusii children were left at home to serve as substitute parents to the Gusii toddlers, while the mothers and fathers tended the fields. Perhaps Gusii children's cultural role as surrogate parents engendered more bossy behaviour. On the other hand, Gusii children also tended to be more nurturing and responsible than their US peers.

In developing countries, the authoritarian style appears to be very common: children are expected to obey without any explanations. The young poor do not have much opportunity to develop their full potential. It is difficult to overcome poverty and generate economic growth in the face of invariable discouragement and pervasive social control. Dwairy and Menshar (2006) report on a study of parenting styles in Egypt carried out among 351 adolescents:

> In rural communities, the authoritarian style was more predominant in the parenting of male adolescents, while the authoritative style was more predominant in the parenting of female adolescents. In urban communities, on the other hand, the authoritarian style was more predominant in the parenting of female adolescents. Female adolescents reported a higher frequency of psychological disorders. Mental health was associated with authoritative parenting, but not with authoritarian parenting. It seems that authoritarian parenting within an authoritarian culture is not as harmful as within a liberal culture

Box 14.2 describes the 'ideal' child education in China (Chao, 1995).

Needs of children and care-givers

As the risks for child violence are increased when parents lack knowledge of child development, have insufficient rearing skills and are under stress, a well-designed child violence prevention programme should include components addressing the needs of children and care-givers. These needs are not the same in all cultures or countries; studies of

Box 14.2:   The six liberations for children in China

The children should be set free in six respects. Their minds should be liberated, so that they think in a lively way and engage in innovative and creative thinking. Their eyes should be taught to read and observe, in order to widen their perspective. They should remove the plugs from their ears and listen to the songs of insects and birds in their natural surroundings, to fine music, and to moving tales. Their mouths should come unruffled, and they should be given more opportunity to express themselves through reciting, story-telling, participating in intellectual games, competitions and public speaking. Their hands should be unbound to enable them to do physical work and acquire skills in preparation for the future. Last but not least, their legs should be unshackled, to allow them to go into nature and society, to interact with people and make acquaintances. It is through these six liberations that they will acquire courage to engage in all sorts of social practice and build up their abilities.

needs – if not already known – should precede the initiation of preventive programmes. Programme content may have to be revised based on regular evaluations.

Attachment

The attachment process is important for improving the parents' attitudes to the child (it is reviewed in Chapter 8) and it is recommended as part of the Child Defence and Support Programme. A person's capability for attachment is defined as the lifelong ability to maintain emotional relations. Bonding is the process of forming an attachment. Such relations are a necessary part of human life to learn, to love, to survive and to procreate. Without emotional relationships the person will remain distant, isolated, self-absorbed and without close friends. Loving and caring relations make life a pleasure. The bonding process involves the human brain. Neurobiological processes take place, which have a lasting effect during adult life. Most bonding takes place early and will lead to the capacity in childhood to recognize close family members and friends, to develop love, sharing and empathy and to reduce aggression. Attachments formed by bonding will determine much of that individual's feelings of security throughout life.

A study in Ireland (Marsa et al., 2004), serves to illustrate the importance of bonding during early childhood. The authors compared four groups: twenty-nine child offenders, thirty violent offenders, thirty non-violent offenders and thirty community controls. A secure adult attachment style was four times less common in the child offender group than in any of the other three groups. Ninety-three per cent of the sex offenders had an insecure adult attachment style. The sex offenders group, when compared to the community group, reported significantly lower levels of maternal and parental care and significantly higher levels of maternal and pubertal overprotection during their childhood. Compared with all three comparison groups the sexual offenders reported significantly more emotional loneliness.

Fostering empathy

Programmes to foster empathy among very young children are based on the evidence that aggression and abusive parent behaviour is closely related to low levels of empathy. An example of a successful programme is Roots Of Empathy (ROE), initiated in 1981 in Canada by Mary Gordon. At present it is functioning in 1,141 classes with 28,525 children in Canada. So far, more than 67,000 children from kindergarten to grade 8 have taken part in the programme.

> As poor parenting and aggression cut across all socio-economic levels of the community, empathy needs to be fostered in all children. The Roots Of Empathy program teaches children as young as three years of age about the necessary affective side of parenting – empathy, and emotional literacy. Each class 'adopts' a baby who visits the classroom along with a parent and a trained instructor meeting the children for 27 sessions. Curricula are designed for four grade levels: Kindergarten, Grades 1–3, Grades 4–6, and Grades 7–8.
>
> During a family visit, the students observe, ask questions, discuss the baby's behaviour, the sounds she makes, and her temperament, gaining insights into the infant's growth and development and learning to respond appropriately to what the baby is trying to 'tell them' through physical cues. It increases students' knowledge of human development, learning, and infant safety, better preparing them to be responsible and responsive parents. Each level of the curriculum deepens the students' understanding of the tremendous amount of time, patience, love, and energy required to parent a child properly. Instructors work with the students to recognize the baby's emotions, and as they become more comfortable identifying and labeling the feelings of others, they are able to explore and discuss their own feelings. It helps them recognize the feelings of their peers and understand

how violent actions (like bullying) affect others. Children learn the importance of warm, responsive care which is a process of reading the baby's cues to respond to the baby's needs.

The results have been evaluated using pre-tests and post-tests in ROE classes and comparison non-ROE classes to determine:

(a) Increased emotion knowledge, social understanding and pro-social behaviour with peers
(b) Decreased aggression with peers and decreased proactive aggression (e.g. bullying)

The children showed significant improvements in all these categories . . . a decrease in average rating of proactive aggression, while the children in comparison classes showed an increase in average rating of proactive aggression. In ROE classrooms 88% of students who demonstrated some proactive aggression at pre-test showed a reduction at post-test.

(Gordon, 2005)

The earlier in life such preparation programmes start the better the results in cognitive functioning and socialization will be. Thus, the introduction of community pre-schools is important and the economic costs incurred have a very high rate of return (Heckman et al., 2006a, 2006b).

For older children there are many models of school programmes which offer a combination of interactive child contacts, observing and reflecting on patterns of child–parent interaction in natural settings, fostering empathic awareness, role-playing, acquiring negotiating skills, learning teamwork, and so on (see Table 14.1). Sexual education and sexual behaviour are subjects of importance in programmes for teenagers.

For adults, programmes have been offered in training in child care, social skills, flexible problem-solving and stress management. There are positive effects of activities that increase parents' capacity for empathic awareness: to recognize the emotions experienced by their children.

The experience of some large- and small-scale programmes at pre-school levels

The cognitive and social skills, and the motivation and stability of the adult population in the developing countries, should in principle augment considerably with increased pre-schools:

early experiences have a uniquely powerful influence on the development of cognitive and social skills, as well as on brain architecture and neurochemistry; both skill development and brain maturation are hierarchical processes in which higher level functions depend on, and build on, lower level functions. The capacity for change in the foundations of human skill development and neural circuitry is highest earlier in life and decreases over time.

(Knudsen et al., 2006)

Many pre-school programmes for poor and disadvantaged populations exist. They are – in relation to the needs – rare in many developing countries. In all Francophone African countries, French government assistance has been given to set up a model pre-school in the capital. Similar projects have been funded by many non-governmental organizations.

There are some large-scale, long-term programmes, such as the 1965 Head Start Programme in the USA (2006), and the 1975 Integrated Child Development Services (ICDS) programme in India (Gupta, 2001). These both continue, and have served millions of children. In the USA, there have been several small-scale research projects: among them the Early Training Programme for 92 children in 1962–4, the Perry pre-school programme in 1962–7 for 128 children, the Abecedarian Programme in 1972–7 for 111 children, and the Chicago Parent Centre Programme operating in the public schools since 1967; the last has an ongoing evaluation study for 1,539 children (Belfield, 2006).

The evaluation results of these programmes vary. The large-scale programmes have been seriously criticized. The US Department of Health and Human Services in 2003 issued a report about Head Start, describing:

the limited educational progress for the enrolled children and the problems resulting from a fragmented approach to early childhood programs and services ... most children enter and leave Head Start with below-average skill and knowledge levels.

The Indian ICDS:

promised to inexpensively increase the human capital of the nation and, thus, promote its rapid development. Investing in children, the logic went, was investing in the nation's future. Another, closely related payoff was its potential to bring down fertility rates. Better health, education, and increased rates of survival for children were expected to have long-term effects in slowing down population growth. The progress of ICDS has, however, been slow, there are budgetary constraints, and the bureaucracy manages these pro-grammes top-down, the anganwadi workers who run the programme at community level are bogged down with paperwork, and the absentee rates both of the staff and of the children are high.

(Gupta, 2001)

The US small-scale research projects have reported positive social results. The Perry School reported (Schweinhart, 2005) that at age 27 those who had participated in the programme during childhood had half as many criminal arrests, higher earnings and three times as many owned their home. There were many behavioural impacts; the Perry, Abecedarian and Chicago programmes reported the following gains (compared with control groups): teenage parent 13 per cent lower, single parent 14 per cent lower, abortion 22 per cent lower, drug user 21 per cent lower, adults needing treatment for drug or alcohol abuse 12 per cent lower (Belfield, 2006).

The conclusion is that large-scale programmes directly managed by governments do not work as well as small-scale ones based in communities.

Cost-effectiveness studies of child violence prevention

Several theoretical cost-effectiveness estimates of child violence pre-vention programmes have been made. Two examples are mentioned below.

1. *Colorado estimates* (Gould and O'Brien, 1995). In 1995, the State Uni-versity of Colorado made a cost-effectiveness study related to child maltreatment in that state. The authors concluded that maltreatment costs some US$400 million per year; preventive costs were US$24 mil-lion. Thus, if one were to prevent just 6 per cent of child maltreatment, this would offset the costs of prevention.
2. *Michigan estimates* (Caldwell, 1992). The annual costs for child abuse in Michigan were estimated at US$823 million in 1992; the costs of a prevention programme at US$43 million annually. The calculated cost advantage to prevention was 19 to 1.

In practice, it may turn out to be much more difficult and costly than estimated to implement such programmes, and their success rates are not exactly known from practice. Furthermore, there might be political problems, which will be described below.

Do family life preparation programmes work?

Holzer et al. (2006) evaluated twenty articles about parent education programmes in Australia, Canada and the USA. They all fulfilled scientific criteria for evaluation quality. Three were meta-analyses. Eighteen articles reported successful results following participation in a parent education programme. The results of the evaluations included:

1. Fewer incidents of child maltreatment (however, only a small number of studies directly measured this outcome);
2. A reduction in the prevalence of negative/unhelpful parenting attributions (for example, a parent attributing a child's behaviour to malicious intent);
3. A greater ability to use positive/productive discipline strategies rather than punitive strategies;
4. Increased parental competence and self-efficacy; and greater parental knowledge/awareness of child development, risk factors for maltreatment, and child outcomes following abuse and neglect.

When reviewing reports of parenting programmes that have failed, it is clear that those that start at a very early age are more successful than those which start later on; those provided to parents who are habitual abusers of their children have very limited value.

Community supervision: 'child watch'

Regarding home visitation, a 'classical' study by Olds et al. (1997, 2002) published research of 324 low-income, unmarried women (expecting their first child) with a follow-up over fifteen years. (Olds et al. first reported on home visiting in 1986.) A home visitation programme was set up with nurses (nine visits during pregnancy and twenty-three visits from the child's birthday until the age of 2 years). Comparisons were made with a matched group of women who did not receive any home visits. In the intervention group the incidence rate of child abuse and neglect was reduced by almost 50 per cent; the number of subsequent births went down from 1.6 to 1.3, with an increased spacing between the first and second child of 65 vs. 37 months. The use of welfare was reduced by one-third. Behavioural impairments due to the use of alcohol and other drugs went down by two-thirds and the number of police arrests by 75 per cent.

The experience of community visiting services to targeted risk families is positive. Such services have mainly been provided to those with low social status (poverty, unemployment, spouse abuse, alcohol and drug problems, delinquency or criminality). Child violence, however, also occurs among upper- and middle-class families, though under-reported and undetected unless revealed by the victim later in life. For this reason, universal home visits are desirable. At this point in time, however, the tasks (a)–(c) below might not be acceptable to everyone. Other components of a much wider community-based 'watch' pro-gramme may not pose many problems, such as those mentioned under points (d)–(o).

A person in charge of a 'child watch' programme could undertake these tasks:

(a) regular home visits to provide family support and advice, and hands-on guidance;

(b) inform the parents how they can follow the various stages of child development, and the importance of the bonding process;

(c) advise the family about how children are negatively influenced by parents' alcohol and drug abuse, and by violence and neglect at home; inform them of alternatives to spanking and emotional abuse;

(d) ensure that the children are benefiting from existing services: health, social and educational;

(e) observe children and parents at health controls; ensure that sick children and sick parents are treated;

(f) provide access to childcare day centres (if existing), and observe the children there, making sure that there are no symptoms of abuse or neglect among the children and that they are treated by the staff in a loving, nurturing and respectful way;

(g) help the community to set up pre-schools (if not existing), and fol-low the teachers' behaviour and the children's mental, physical and academic progress in these schools;

(h) brief the teachers on appropriate child education methods, and on how children's behaviour problems can be solved;

(i) regular visits, observations and teacher contacts at primary and secondary schools;

(j) organize and supervise community leisure activities;

(k) introduce family life preparation for all teenagers, who have not been reached by early childhood training programmes. This includes discussions about responsible sexual behaviour, intimate partner abuse, alcohol and illicit drugs;

(l) teach children about human rights and responsibilities;

(m) encourage teenagers' participation in family plans and activity decisions;

(n) assist needy families with direct economic help, provide food, clothes and improved housing;

(o) identify abandoned and run-away children living of the street, engaged in prostitution, and gang members, and initiate community arrangements for their living, daily needs and education.

It has been shown that programme quality outcomes increase (Olds, 2002) when

- services were delivered by more highly trained and qualified home visitors;
- home visitors were experienced in dealing with the complex needs of many 'at risk' clients;
- the programmes had long enough duration and visiting frequency to impact on risk factors that contribute to child violence;
- programmes were matched to the needs of the client group; and
- programmes focused on improving both maternal and child outcomes.

In home-visiting activities carried out in developing countries, existing groups of personnel can be used: teachers, health workers, social workers, and so on. Another option is to recruit purpose-motivated staff locally, including community volunteers (Barnet et al., 2002). All staff will need a training programme. Evidently, depending on the local communities' and their decision-makers' attitudes, programmes of 'child watch' will be designed to reflect their cultural values and build on analyses of the root causes of ongoing child violence.

Do home visiting programmes work?

In February 2002, the Centers for Disease Control and Prevention Task Force on Community Preventive Services concluded, 'there is strong evidence to recommend home visitation to reduce child maltreatment'. The group based this recommendation on a review of twenty-five studies that found an overall 39 per cent reduction of child maltreatment in high-risk families.

Higgins et al. (2006) have reviewed twelve articles on home visiting, all of which fulfilled scientific requirements on evaluation. These revealed:

1. There were fewer incidents of child maltreatment (when this outcome was directly measured);

2. Enhanced parental knowledge and parenting skills;
3. Improvements in children's cognitive and social development; and
4. Increased linking of parents to health care and other services.

In a randomized trial used trained community volunteers to provide parenting training, Barnet et al. (2002) noted a significant improvement in parent behaviour. It is concluded that targeted home visiting programmes are effective, although they have their political aspects.

Plummer (2001) reviewed eighty-seven home visitation programmes for the prevention of child abuse. He pointed out that, in real life, setting up and maintaining such programmes is associated with many difficulties: lack of adequate and secure funding, community and leadership level of denial, competing agendas, and community indifference. In principle, prevention of childhood violence should be much less costly than post-abuse and neglect interventions; it would also decrease the high level of human suffering. Many social engineering projects, however, have had economic difficulties. High initial costs and 'savings' that are unlikely to appear until much later easily discourage the funding politicians, who would like to see results not in ten to twenty years but in good time before the next election.

The conclusion is that programmes with direct government funding often have problems because politicians want rapid changes and might withdraw funds if results are not quickly visible. Programmes lacking success (Head Start and ICDS) have been operated top-down with insufficient community participation. Therefore, child violence prevention programmes need to be assigned to the civil society and to build on community mobilization to reduce the problems described by Plummer (2001).

Publicity about the consequences of childhood violence

Parents and the public are often ignorant about the medico-social health consequences of incompetent parenting. These were described in Chapters 8 and 9. What may be most unknown are the scientific findings that violence leads to specific changes in the brain's circulation, biochemistry and hormonal production. These in turn cause cell damage or destruction in parts of the brain. These cells cannot be repaired. This grim result suggests that much more effort must be made to prevent childhood abuse and neglect which now does irreversible harm to millions of young victims. Society reaps what it sows in the way it nurtures its children.

The US Parents and Teachers Against Violence in Education, in 2003, and the American Academy of Paediatrics in 2005 issued very strongly formulated recommendations to discourage parents from using physical punishment for children's education. In 2001, a large number of NGOs and private individuals launched the Global Initiative to end all corporal punishment of children. It is supported by several UN agencies, such as UNICEF, UNESCO and the High Commission of Human Rights.

The US Parents and Teachers Against Violence in Education (2003) state that:

> parents who fail to manage their children calmly, gently and patiently, but instead rely on physical punishment, tend to produce aggressive, assaultive children. The more severe and the earlier the mistreatment, the worse is the outcome. The lowest incidence of antisocial behaviour is always associated with children who are reared from infancy in attentive, supportive, non-violent, non-spanking families

Introduction of laws that forbid abuse of children

Sexual abuse is forbidden in all countries. The legal age limit for consensual sex varies; it is mostly 16–18 years. Consensual sex under the legal age is regarded as statutory rape, but in many countries, legal authorities – if reported – may choose not to prosecute those involved, especially if both partners are underage. In many developing countries, children as young as 12 marry, and among them the rules about sexual relations differ.

A growing number of countries, mainly in Europe, have introduced laws that forbid physical abuse at home and in schools.[35] Breaking the law will lead to fines or imprisonment for the adult. So far, it seems that cases are rarely brought to court. There are no regrets from the parents of those countries which have introduced this type of legislation. Some accused teachers have claimed that their physical aggression was self-defence, and it is clear that the violence generated by schoolchildren, especially teenagers, has increased in many countries. Many schools have introduced security guards and control of weapons, such as guns and knives, which some children bring with them to school. It is, however, important that the widespread teacher abuse be eliminated. To formulate rules about emotional abuse will require clear definitions of what is forbidden.

A study from Sweden confirms that legislation in combination with public education is highly effective (see Figure 14.1). Swedish law in 1979

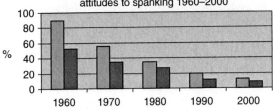

Figure 14.1 Effects of criminalization of corporal punishment in Sweden. Left columns show parental attitude levels (approving such punishment), and right columns the percentage of families applying corporal punishment (adapted from Daly, 2007)

forbade all physical punishment and any other humiliating treatment. In 1980, 51 per cent of all parents used such punishment during the previous year; in 2000, only 8 per cent did (Save the Children, Sweden, 2005).

The scarcity of legal consequences for the perpetrators depends (at least in the developing countries) on the failure to establish a proper, fully decentralized judicial system and keep it free from personal influence and corruption. In many countries, there is no easily available, affordable and accessible local 'judicial delivery system' that ensures that justice works for all with fairness and independence. Many developing countries still have the remnants of local mediation systems – for example, those traditionally maintained by local African chiefs, Arab sheiks and Indian maharajas, who used to preside over the community justice system. As complexities arrived with urbanization, industrialization, increased mobility of people and commercialization, the traditional system has lost much of its importance. Public judicial services are needed to fill this vacuum with a component of security and support to defend the abused children and punish the perpetrators.

Community-based action

The reasons for proposing a community-based approach for the child violence prevention programme (small-scale projects managed by local groups of concerned parents) are:

1. Small-size programmes in comparison with large government-managed ones are closer to the people and their needs; parents can

have a direct influence over what their children receive and will have ownership of the programme.

2. The existence of a core group of non-abusing parents in the community is important. Knowledge about them will spread quickly, especially through the children. Peer influence among them will help to make children reject abusive treatment.
3. No country will ever have enough professionals to deal with the large-scale child violence that exists in all societies. They must be complemented with community volunteers, who should be trained for their work.
4. Local programmes are less bureaucratized and have lower overhead costs (more cost-effective).
5. Scientific experience favours small-scale projects.
6. The risks of funding constraints are lower; the programme should be able to avoid seeing promises outrun delivery.
7. Supporting the civil society and mobilizing communities is a priority of today's governments that cannot afford to do everything. Most governments seek to reduce the number of persons employed by them and outsource functions to extra-governmental organizations or enterprises.

Experience of community mobilization

The UN Research Institute for Social Development (1994) defines community mobilization as the act of making something move: people are assembled, organized and made to perform certain functions. It focuses on the ability of the members of the movement to acquire resources and mobilize people in order to advance their goals (Kendall, 2005). It emerged in the 1970s and is viewed as rational: social institutions and social actors taking political action (Buechler, 1999).

The reasons to avoid too much top-down bureaucratic interference are described in several anthropological studies by Das et al. (2001). Such interference can be devastating, especially when several government agencies are involved:

> In small communities inhabiting increasingly uncertain worlds ... the effects of bureaucratic responses to human problems ... can and often do deepen and make more intractable the problems they seek to ameliorate.

There are many community mobilization initiatives functioning well, enabling local populations to escape from extreme poverty. Examples seen by the author include: Argentina, Benin, Botswana, Chad, Côte d'Ivoire, Guatemala, India, Indonesia, Iran, Mauritania, Mexico, Nepal, Palestine, Peru, the Philippines, the Republic of Korea, St Lucia, Thailand and Zimbabwe.

In 1992 India took a great step forward to encourage community initiatives and to mobilize local resources through a transfer of the authority to plan for, raise and spend locally collected taxes and to organize local elections (with quotas for women). The 1992 Constitutional Amendment encourages:

- more power in the hands of the rural people to determine their own destiny;
- enhancing the capabilities of the rural people to involve themselves in the planning from below;
- decentralizing the execution of all development activities with effective participation of peoples; and
- reorienting development administration based on the philosophy of popular participation.

The author has had twenty-five years of experience in the local management of the WHO's community-based rehabilitation programmes for persons with disabilities, which now exist in about 100 countries. A detailed description is published elsewhere (Helander, 1999). There are many culture-dependent challenges for community mobilization programmes. The roles and functions of the various stakeholders have to be defined: local administrators versus community leaders; the membership of the community committee and the roles of its leaders and institutions; managerial responsibility and methods of decision-making; inputs of resources, and so on. Details of a model for the preparation of a CDS programme appear in the Annex.

The action for the prevention of violence against children should preferably be taken by a community-based organization. Support by the government and local authorities should be sought. Community members should discover the fact that it is possible for them to transform the future of their children. To use all available, appropriate means to stop violence, abuse, maltreatment and neglect affecting children should be seen as a joint responsibility, because such acts have long-term consequences for us all. Bronfenbrenner (1990) sums up:

The effective functioning of child-rearing processes in the family and other child settings requires public policies and practices that provide place, time, stability, status, recognition, belief systems, customs, and actions in support of child-rearing activities not only on the part of parents, care-givers, teachers, and other professional personnel, but also relatives, friends, neighbours, co-workers, communities, and the major economic, social, and political institutions of the entire society.

15
Conclusion

Violence is a complex and not yet fully understood cultural phenomenon. It has ecological determinants as well as genetic roots. There is an 'archaeology' of human evil behaviour, which travels as a dominating theme through our past, leaving us with many disturbing questions about human nature. The better known historic evidence concerns past rulers and tyrants who used methods of intimidation, torture and execution, or threats of eternal condemnation. After their departure, they left traditions of Machiavellian prescriptions for their successors. We are now experiencing the era of terrorism: we fear threats – real or imagined – on a daily basis. We are also, finally, becoming aware of the less recognized evidence: the avalanche of domestic and community violence.

Violence is most often an expression of force in a situation of inequality: this is why children and other 'defenceless' people so frequently become victims. This is also why so many perpetrators escape justice. Violence, however, is also exhibited by frustrated and powerless people who are desperate for change; such violence is frequently misdirected towards innocent victims. Violence towards children is extremely common in all cultures and societies, and all economic, social and religious strata. The damage inflicted on individuals and on community life is massive and increasing. Still, even in our own time, it is insufficiently recognized as one of the most basic causes of many of our health and social problems. This short book can only serve to describe some of its contexts and why it is 'allowed' to occur.

The failure to prevent childhood violence is shared by all human ecology systems. The victims' trauma is aggravated by repression of facts, embarrassment, shame, secrecy and taboos. These are compounded by the victims' feelings that there is nobody who will help, and that not even the judicial system can be trusted to bring the perpetrators to justice. It is further enhanced by widespread public indifference, which appears to be related to the ignorance not just of the extent of the problem but also of its serious consequences. Among these is the organic (and at present irreparable) stress and neglect-related damage to the emotional and cognitive functions of the brain with impairments of its biochemistry, hormonal production, circulation and metabolism, leading to brain cell malfunction or destruction. Among the socio-medical sequels are the high population risks attributed to adverse childhood experiences: for chronic depression 41 per cent, suicide attempts 58 per cent, alcoholism 65 per cent, illicit drug use 50 per cent, injected drug use 68 per cent, sexual assault 62 per cent, domestic violence 52 per cent, and a doubling of the criminality rate.

Yet, there should be hope.

In terms of *micro- and meso-systems* much can be changed: parents should not remain the major problem but, through better preparation, be part of the solution. School education should not be limited to cognitive training, but also be a tool for learning and practising social and emotional skills, and empathy. Children should better know their rights and responsibilities.

In terms of *exo- and macro-systems* our communities and nations are ill-prepared for assisting the victims of childhood violence; perpetrators mostly escape justice. Primary violence prevention barely exists and is mainly concentrated on small groups of socially and economically marginal people. Social, technical and economic support to the families does exist, but it is far short of actual needs. Major efforts to deal with these shortcomings are essential.

The *global system* has great potential, but has largely failed: firstly, because most nations have not accepted the international law model created by the United Nations; and secondly, because international organizations have not succeeded in their ambitions to fulfil their priority development programmes. These have never included any action for the prevention of violence or assisting the victims.

To solve these problems a massive public education campaign is required in order to activate resources for violence prevention. We must be honest about the large-scale violence against children; we must open our media to the realities that are now hidden: people need to see what occurs in the life of the defenceless; they need to understand the pain of the victims.

World leaders have a choice: *either* countries, communities and families allow the continuation of a destructive and abusive child-rearing system which jeopardizes each nation's development and culture; *or* they create better conditions for their children to be raised in a positive social environment that builds progress, peace, humanity, productivity and creativity. The choice is between establishing and maintaining primary child violence prevention, or building more prisons for the perpetrators and more hospitals for the victims. Each violent act that is allowed to occur contributes to and authorizes the existing problem. Primary prevention is possible; future generations can largely be saved from childhood violence, but the change will not occur unless we generate a complete cultural change in the way most of our children are brought up. Because of the large extent of childhood violence, such change is unlikely to occur unless *communities* are mobilized. As explained in the previous chapter, it is a community responsibility to act using all available and appropriate means to stop violence, abuse, maltreatment and neglect of children because such acts have long-term consequences for us all. Most governments' present attempts to deal with social pathologies by providing more health care and more police avoid solving the root problems.

Primary prevention is not the only method for the reduction of child violence. Increased efforts are needed to develop further our scientific tools to improve the basic knowledge about the many causes and consequences of childhood violence. Such progress is urgently needed and should allow us to identify more effective methods to lessen the suffering of the victims.

Peace on earth is only possible if we can create a non-violent culture, the starting point of which is peace in our homes and communities – and in our own minds.

Annex: a Child Defence and Support Programme

There are large differences between countries, and what follows are simple guidelines that need adaptations.

The CDS programme is proposed to have:

- *a first line of defence and support* consisting of a **community level primary prevention programme**;
- *a second level of defence and support* directed towards solving the problems that remain in spite of the primary prevention, including those that are too complex to be dealt with at the community level. For the latter, a **referral system**, and if available, professional personnel are required.

A. The community level programme

Below follow suggestions for how the programme can be prepared and set up step by step.

Preparatory phase

Step 1

Finding out the present situation and the needs of the population. This may be done using a combination of two methods:

(a) community visits to meet families, children, teachers, health and social services, representatives of the judiciary and community leaders. The focus should be on seeing families at home and having separate meetings with the children and with the teachers;
(b) based on this information, conduct a national survey.

Step 2

Review existing services, their effectiveness and costs.
Review existing legislation and the experience of its effectiveness.
Review past and ongoing research in related subjects in the country.

Step 3

Based on the information, outline a detailed action plan. Formulate general objectives and set medium-term targets. Define the evaluation process, which should be done by an independent evaluator engaged at the start of the programme. Community evaluation should be included.

Step 4

(a) preparation of printed and audiovisual materials to be used in communities;
(b) training of personnel for community work. Two different persons are needed: one with skills for the family life preparation at pre-schools and schools, and the second for the community watch programme.

In developed countries, these may be recruited among teachers, social workers, psychologists and paediatric nurses. In the developing countries, one has to look for interested and suitable community facilitators. In some parts of the world they will be volunteers without remuneration; in others, some compensation, or a salary, will be needed. The community should contribute this compensation.

Step 5: Awareness-building (sensitization)

Awareness can be created in two ways:

(a) by media through national radio and television programmes and articles in newspapers. Their content should be carefully structured: people will be advised about the frequency and consequences of child violence, and how to prevent such abuse. Interviews with maltreated people should be included: they will describe their experience, their pain and frustrations and how they may or may not have overcome the haunting experience. Resilience as a mechanism should be included.
(b) by community visits. Trained persons (see above) can start building awareness through information/sensitization at community meetings. One approach is to invite a number of local leaders for information and discussion. Cases may be presented (e.g. by video) of maltreated persons, and the expected result of CDS explained.

People in the communities of the developing countries need to be informed that:

• child violence is common (although to a large extent hidden);
• child violence is followed by many consequences: difficult and aggressive behaviour, increased criminality, alcoholism, drug abuse, suicides, mental disorders and a doubling of many common diseases. In many persons who were abused as children, one will find damage to the brain, such damage cannot be repaired;
• there are simple methods of training and educating children at an early age that will transfer parenting skills and knowledge about child education that reduce problems when they become parents. Training can also be designed for parents who already have children;
• parents can form a community committee to set up the programme and ask for public support for it. Such support may, however, not be complete, thus voluntary efforts by the community will be needed. Members of the committee should abstain from corporal and psychological punishment of their children.

Step 6: Community organization

Each community will need a management structure to plan for the programme, supervise the programme's quality, mobilize resources, establish links with authorities and technical expertise at the district level, and evaluate the programme. Appropriate training should be provided for those who undertake the management. It is important that the community understands that once a CDS programme is started, it has to be maintained.

Initiation and maintenance phase

Step 7: Implementation

The programme starts with the training of the community members. These include, for example (in countries where professional staff are unavailable): community workers who, after training, are willing to undertake the home visiting programme, and schoolteachers trained for the family life preparation taught in the school.

It is important that the professionals (if available) regularly revisit the communities for technical guidance. There might be referrals for children with difficult problems (see below).

Step 8: Evaluation at the community level

It is important that communities thoroughly evaluate the outcome of the programme. A simple first tool is to count the number of children whose parents have changed their parental style. A more elaborate system is to evaluate:

- *relevance*: did the families and children feel that the programme is meeting their needs?
- *effectiveness*: did the children trained with CDS improve their knowledge, behaviour and attitudes?
- *efficiency*: have the resources provided by the community, and supplemented by the government, been used in the most efficient way?
- *sustainability*: are we as a community able to continue this programme using the existing resources?
- *impact*: have the attitudes of the community members who have taken part in CDS improved? Are the children participating happier, better behaved and are they listened to?

The community itself should take an active part in this evaluation; for the larger-scale national evaluation, an independent evaluator should be engaged.

B. The referral system

As indicated above, the community level programme will be supervised by professionals (or in developing countries persons with more advanced training and experience than the community worker). When problems cannot be solved at the community level because the interventions are complex or unusual, then the responsibility for the continued action will be taken over by the referral level. How to build up that level will vary, depending on the resources and culture of each nation.

The community will now decide what to do. Interested community members should meet and discuss their concerns, how the local administration can be carried out and whether they can use some of their time to guide the project.

A community may reject the programme. The reasons for rejection may be several, among them:

- they believe that there is no child violence in their community;
- nobody in the community has time or is willing to help.

Then the matter can be brought up at a later opportunity.

Once a community has decided to start a programme, there may be certain formalities: informing the authorities and obtaining formal permission. Other local stakeholders should be informed: teachers, health services, judicial authorities, local administrators and local politicians. Their co-operation should be sought. It should be made clear that the CDS will have no political or religious affiliation.

Notes

1. List of 152 countries from which information has been obtained ($v = 94$ working visits; $c = 90$ country courses held; $w = 132$ written (published or documented) information).

   Africa: Algeria (c), Angola (vcw), Benin (vcw), Botswana (vcw), Cameroon (w), Cape Verde (c), Chad (vcw), Congo (vw), Congo D.R. (c), Côte d'Ivoire (vcw), Egypt (vcw), Eritrea (c), Ethiopia (vcw), Gabon (vw), Gambia (vcw), Ghana (vcw), Kenya (vcw), Lesotho (cw), Liberia (w), Libya (w), Madagascar (c), Malawi (cw), Mauritania (vcw), Mauritius (vw), Mozambique (cw), Morocco (vw), Namibia (c), Nigeria (vcw), Rwanda (c), Senegal (vcw), Sierra Leone (w), Somalia (vcw), South Africa (vcw), Sudan (w), Swaziland (cw), Tanzania (vcw), Togo (vw), Uganda (w), Zambia (vcw), Zimbabwe (vcw). (40)

   America: Antigua (w), Argentina (vw), Aruba (c), Bahamas (vc), Barbados (vcw), Belize (w), Bolivia (vw), Brazil (vcw), Canada (vcw), Chile (vw), Colombia (cw), Costa Rica (w), Ecuador (vw), El Salvador (cw), Guatemala (vcw), Guyana (cw), Haiti (vw), Honduras (vc), Jamaica (w), Mexico (vcw), Nicaragua (w), Panama (vc), Peru (vw), Puerto Rico (w), St Lucia (vcw), Trinidad and Tobago (vw), United States (vcw), Uruguay (v), Venezuela (vw) (29)

   Asia: Afghanistan (cw), Bahrain (vw), Bangladesh (vw), Bhutan (c), Cambodia (cw), China (vcw), Hong Kong (vcw), India (vcw), Indonesia (vcw), Iran (vcw), Iraq (vcw), Israel (vw), Japan (vcw), Jordan (vcw), Korea (Republic of) (vcw), Korea PDR (w), Kuwait (cw), Laos (c), Lebanon (vcw), Malaysia (vcw), Mongolia (c), Myanmar (vcw), Nepal (vcw), Oman (vw), Pakistan (vw), Palestine (vcw), Papua New Guinea (cw), Philippines (vcw), Saudi Arabia (vw) Singapore (vw), Sri Lanka (vcw), Syria (v), Taiwan (vw), Thailand (vcw), United Arab Emirates (vcw), Vietnam (vwc), Yemen (cw) (37)

   Europe: Albania (w), Austria (vw), Belarus (cw), Belgium (vcw), Bosnia and Herzegovina (w), Bulgaria (cw), Croatia (w), Cyprus (vcw), Czech Republic (vw), Denmark (vw), Estonia (c), Finland (vcw), France (vcw), Germany (vcw), Greece (w), Hungary (w), Iceland (w), Ireland (w), Italy (vcw), Kazakhstan (w), Kyrgyzstan (w), Latvia (vcw), Lithuania (c), Macedonia (w), Moldova (cw), Montenegro (v), Netherlands (vw), Norway (vcw), Poland (vw), Portugal (vcw), Romania (vcw), Russian Federation (vcw), Serbia (vw), Slovenia (w), Spain (vw), Sweden (vcw), Switzerland (vw), Tajikistan (w), Turkey (w), Ukraine (w), United Kingdom (vcw) (41)

   Oceania: Australia (cw), Fiji (cw), New Zealand (w), Palau (w), Pitcairn (w) (5)

2. Sensitivity to initial meteorological conditions is known as the 'butterfly effect', based on a 1972 paper by Edward Lorenz at the American Association for the Advancement of Science in Washington, D.C. entitled 'Predictability: Does the Flap of a Butterfly's Wings in Brazil set off a Tornado in Texas?' The flapping wing represents a small change in the initial condition of the system, which causes a chain of events leading to large-scale phenomena. Had the

288

butterfly not flapped its wings, there would have been no tornado. Cutting a rose (meaning abusing a child) is seen here as a similar initial event causing large-scale human consequences, a 'tornado' in the lives of the victims.
3. Alice Miller describes in several books the childhood background of some tyrants. (The Childhood Trauma, lecture on 22 October 1998). From the age of 3 until 13 (when his father died), Hitler was severely beaten and humiliated almost every day by his father who used a rhinoceros whip. Once he was thrown out of the house and stood for four hours outside in the snow. Hitler himself described the conditions at home: 'a battle is carried on between the parents themselves, and almost every day, in forms which in vulgarity often leave nothing to be desired, then, if only very gradually, the results of such visual instruction must ultimately become apparent in the children. The character they will inevitably assume if the quarrel takes the form of brutal attacks by the father against the mother, of drunken beatings, is hard for anyone who does not know this milieu to imagine. At the age of six the pitiable little boy suspects the existence of things which can fill even an adult with nothing but horror.' Hitler's own father had suffered similar abuse ('poisonous pedagogy') at home (*Mein Kampf*, 1925). Hitler killed some 7–8 million defenceless people – many children – in the Holocaust. The Second World War resulted in the deaths of over 60 million people, and was the deadliest conflict in human history.

Mao Zedong grew up in similar circumstances; his authoritarian father was brutal and tyrannized the family. Mao was often beaten by his father, and humiliated in front of others. On rare occasions Mao admitted the full extent of the rage he felt for his own father, a very severe teacher who had tried through beatings to 'make a man' out of his son. He said that he would like to torment others as he had been tormented himself. For decades, he held power and was responsible for 70 million deaths in peacetime, more than any other twentieth-century leader.

Stalin grew up in Georgia; his father attempted to drown his frustration with liquor and whipped his son almost every day. His mother displayed psychotic traits, was completely incapable of defending her son, and was usually away from home either praying in church or running the priest's household. Stalin caused millions to suffer and die because even at the height of his power his actions were determined by an unconscious, infantile fear of powerlessness.

These three tyrants came from middle-class families. Miller's conclusions are: 'The same might be true of many other tyrants. They often drew on ideologies to disguise the truth and their own paranoia. And the masses chimed in enthusiastically because they were unaware of the real motives, including those in their own biographies. The infantile revenge fantasies of individuals would be of no account if society did not regularly show such naive eagerness in helping to make them come true. Mad tyrants would not have any power if society understood that it is their damaged brains which are constantly driving them to avoid dangers that no longer exist.'
4. This Pakistani law was changed in 2006 to allow for DNA testing and somewhat less strict requirements to prove rape.
5. In 1986 the author interviewed some eighty Somali women who were sexually mutilated.

6. This information is based on research of data from European and North American orphanages, for which admission and annual mortality rates are published.

7. The letters by Sigmund Freud to his friend and confessor Wilhelm Fliess (1887–1904, published in 1985) have been surrounded by controversy. In 1954, Marie Bonaparte, a well-known French psychoanalyst, with Freud's daughter Anna published *The Origins of Psycho-Analysis: Letters to Wilhelm Fliess, Drafts and Notes, 1887–1902*, by Sigmund Freud. Freud had wanted these letters destroyed. Anna Freud removed certain letters from her father which might cast doubt on his veracity. Not until 1985 (Anna Freud died in 1982) were these letters published in unedited form by Jeffrey M. Masson as *The Complete Letters of Sigmund Freud to Wilhelm Fliess 1887–1904* (Harvard University Press). Freud's suppression of the seduction theory was seen by some as displaying a lack of intellectual integrity; Masson explains it as the result of his attackers' viciousness and the surrounding culture of rabid anti-Semitism.

8. The Department of Health and Welfare, USA, at that time had official standards for institutions: Guidelines for Facilities for the Mentally Retarded (1972, 15 pages); and detailed rules by the Joint Commission for the Accreditation of Hospitals: Standards for Residential Facilities for the Mentally Retarded (1972, 159 pages). The professionals in charge of inspections and accreditation at Willowbrook knew that the institution was not following these standards, yet they continued year after year to close their eyes to the inhumane malpractices.

9. Report by Graça Machel, Expert of the Secretary-General of the United Nations (www.unicef.org/graca). The quote from Sierra Leone is from *The Economist*, 9 August 2003, the one from Uganda is from *The Economist*, 7 May 2005. A 2006 statement about widows by Mrs Machel reads, 'a common feature of widowhood is the violence perpetrated against them at the hands of near relatives and condoned by the inaction of governments. Many widows are hounded from their homes and denied access to essential resources such as shelter and land to grow food. They are also subject to degrading and life-threatening traditional practices. They have no status and often they are figures of shame and ridicule. This neglect of millions of widows has irrevocable long term implications for the future well-being and sustainable development of all our societies.'

10. K. Lalor (2004b) in 'Child sexual abuse in Tanzania and Kenya' recounts a survey, according to which most Tanzanian Members of Parliament believe that witchdoctors 'advise people looking for material wealth to have sexual intercourse with virgin girls or their sisters, their mothers and the like'.

11. Interview with the Nepalese Ambassador to India. Hindu Online, 'Victims of the Dark', 29 September 1996, describes the conditions among the prostitutes in Mumbai. In a raid carried out of 140 brothels, only 65 girls were above 18 and 238 were from Nepal.

12. The Hague Convention on Protection of Children and Co-operation in Respect of Intercountry Adoption was completed in 1993 under the auspices of the Hague Conference on Private International Law, an international organization begun in 1893.

13. Author's observations.

14. E. Helander (2005). In the small island of Pitcairn, with only forty-seven inhabitants, there has for many years been widespread child sexual abuse. Six men, including the mayor, were convicted and given long prison sentences in 2004.

15. E. Helander (1965), 'Health status of survivors from the Nazi concentration camps, 20 years afterwards', unpublished report. During the early months of 1945, the Swedish Red Cross evacuated about 30,000 mostly Jewish concentration camp victims from Nazi Germany to Sweden; many remained there. Some of them were children. In 1965, at the request of the Swedish Social Security Department, I examined a group of about eighty of them. They all had very pronounced symptoms of PTSD (this diagnosis was not established at that time) and co-morbid disorders. Although they had undergone psychiatric and rehabilitation treatment for twenty years, they all had been therapy-resistant. They were recommended for disability pensions.

16. Chilean government press release: 27 June 2006. The President announced that next year, 'treatment and rehabilitation of adolescents who abuse and are addicted to alcohol and drugs' would be included under the AUGE plan, covering a variety of treatment programmes in high-quality public and private facilities throughout the country. She also expressed concern about alcohol consumption, prevalent among 32 per cent of adolescents and 60 per cent of young people.

17. The following 80 UN States Parties had by October 2007 either not ratified the ICCPR, or if they had ratified it, refused to ratify the ICCPR optional protocol number 1: Afghanistan, Antigua and Barbuda, Bahamas, Bahrain, Bangladesh, Belize, Bhutan, Botswana, Brazil, Brunei Darussalam, Burundi, Cambodia, China, Comoros, Cuba, DPR Korea, Dominica, Egypt, Eritrea, Ethiopia, Fiji, Gabon, Grenada, Guinea-Bissau, Haiti, India, Indonesia, Iran, Iraq, Israel, Japan, Jordan, Kazakhstan, Kenya, Kiribati, Kuwait, Laos, Lebanon, Liberia, Malaysia, Marshall Islands, Mauritania, Micronesia, Moldova, Monaco, Morocco, Mozambique, Myanmar, Nauru, Nepal, Nigeria, Oman, Pakistan, Palau, Papua New Guinea, Qatar, Rwanda, Saint Kitts and Nevis, Saint Lucia, Samoa, Sao Tome and Principe, Saudi Arabia, Singapore, Solomon Islands, Sudan, Swaziland, Syria, Thailand, Timor-Leste, Tonga, Tunisia, Tuvalu, United Arab Emirates, United Kingdom, United Republic of Tanzania, United States of America, Vanuatu, Vietnam, Yemen, Zimbabwe.

18. The following 34 States Parties have not ratified the ICESCR: Antigua and Barbuda, Bahamas, Bahrain, Bhutan, Brunei Darussalam, Comoros, Cook Islands, Cuba, Fiji, Holy See, Kazakhstan, Kiribati, Malaysia, Maldives, Marshall Islands, Micronesia, Mozambique, Myanmar, Nauru, Niue, Oman, Pakistan, Palau, Papua New Guinea, Qatar, Saint Kitts and Nevis, Saint Lucia, Samoa, Saudi Arabia, Singapore, Tonga, Tuvalu, United Arab Emirates, Vanuatu.

19. A complete list of UN treaties is available on the internet. A Protocol is an additional legal instrument that complements and adds to a treaty. It is not automatically binding on those member states that have ratified the treaty; it has to be independently ratified.

20. The total non-UN treaties are several thousand; see the internet.

21. The status of ratification of CAT is annually published by the Office of the High Commissioner for Human Rights in Geneva, Switzerland. In June 2006,

42 states had not ratified the CAT, 10 had signed but not ratified, and 56 had not made the Declaration referred to in Article 22.1.

22. In 2006, the UN General Assembly elected forty-seven members to the Council. Six of these members came from countries which had not ratified the ICCPR and the ICESCR, three had not ratified the CAT and seventeen had not made the CAT Declaration in Article 22. *The Economist* writes in a leading article (14 January 2006): 'If the agreement [on reform of the Human Rights Commission] is stymied, the next-best solution will be to wind the existing commission up altogether. Human rights matter too much for the UN to continue to shunt the subject off to a cynical talking shop that has become the home to the worst violators. That just blackens the overall reputation of the UN.'

23. These declarations have been universally adopted:
    (a) World Medical Association: Declaration of Tokyo, October 1975;
    (b) The Hawaii Declaration by the World Psychiatric Association, adopted 1978;
    (c) The Second Hawaii Declaration, adopted at the General Assembly of the WPA in 1983;
    (d) United Nations Principles for the Protection of Persons with Mental Illness, adopted by the UN General Assembly in 1991, Resolution 46/119;
    (e) The Madrid Declaration by WPA in 1996;
    (f) World Health Organization: Guidelines for the Protection of Human Rights of Persons with Mental Disorders, 1996.

24. The texts of Chapters 12 and 13 are built on information from articles, books and newsletters published by the World Bank, the United Nations Development Programme, the International Labour Organization, UNESCO, UNICEF, World Food Programme and the World Health Organization during the period 1995–2007. They are available on the internet.

25. Many development programmes are sub-optimally designed and take a short-term perspective; large parts of the funds are either underutilized or squandered by capital or equipment destruction or by mismanagement. The evaluation procedures are open to critical questioning. Banerjee and He (2003), well-known economists at the Massachusetts Institute of Technology, claim that 'donor agencies are not particularly skilled at evaluating and comparing proposals for funding, neither do they make proper use of existing scientific evidence. The World Bank is not particularly effective either in dealing with countries that default or in promoting countries, projects and ideas that are likely to do well. We argue that this is probably related to the fact that the Bank does not make adequate use of scientific evidence in its decision-making and suggest ways to improve matters. Projects funded generously by the Bank do worse than those with smaller funding do. Policy makers may be forgiven if they resist the Bank's views on best practice.'

Lant Pritchett, a long-term World Bank employee and now Professor of the Practice of Economic Development at the Kennedy School of Government at Harvard University, wrote in a 2001 article: 'Nearly all World Bank discussions of policies and project design had the character of "ignorant armies clashing by the night" – there was heated debate amongst advocates of various activities but rarely any firm evidence presented and considered about the likely impact of the proposed actions. There was never any definitive evidence that would inform decisions of funding one broad set of activities versus another.'

26. Lant Pritchett, in 'It pays to be ignorant: a simple political economy of rigorous program evaluation', *Journal of Policy Reform*, 5(4), 2002, 'examines the systematic incentives to avoid rigorous evaluation. A model has been built in which advocates seek to mobilize public resources and choose between persuasion without rigorous evaluation and using rigorous evaluation. In many scenarios, advocates will choose not to perform a rigorous evaluation because it will be used against them politically.'

Korten and Siv (1989) state that 'The introduction of a new data source [related to an ongoing development project] is seldom sufficient in itself to improve decision-making in a development organization. It is the sad reality that most development agencies do not have the capacity to use nor an interest in using field data – even if they have it. Such data may actually complicate the design and construction process because ... the data challenge the viability of standardized solutions and highlight the need for actions that may delay project completion and require changes in the budget. Responding to such data may result in reprimands from superiors who are not evaluated in terms of the performance of the resulting [project] ... but rather in terms of budget expenditures, schedules and facilities constructed ... we may need a new more committed generation of doers rather than of file-keepers and speechwriters.'

27. The overhead costs incurred by the donors include fund-raising, administration and personnel at headquarters and at country and field offices, preparations, meetings, planning in detail, travel, information and publications, evaluation, accounting and auditing. Some amounts are passed on to multilateral agencies and their overhead costs are high. Other grants are transferred to non-governmental organizations; again, it is common to see expensive administrations. Giving away money directly to the poor would not incur much administrative cost, but to provide services, assist in setting up health and education programmes, roads, ports, and so on lead to high overheads. These costs may be estimated at about 50 per cent of the gross donor amounts.

28. The recipient governments have to cover their administrative costs; they are required to prepare complicated 'logical framework plans'; prove that they have paid attention to the 'conditionalities'; dispense and co-ordinate the use of the funds; account for these; and audit the funds. There are costs for travel and attending meetings in the donor's home country. Many ministerial cars, computers and other office equipment are bought using the foreign donations. In addition, there is the corruption factor.

29. The Swedish International Development Agency (SIDA), in August 2004, asked the government of Mozambique to return US$500,000 granted to the Ministry of Education. The funds had been inappropriately used for – among other things – sending the Minister's relatives abroad on 'fellowships', paying for dentistry (while they were abroad), and expensive restaurants. A Portuguese NGO intending to start a programme in the same country was requested by the Minister for an 'envelope' of US$25,000 in cash to get permission to start. It is interesting to see that Mozambique was still in January 2005 included by UN (MDG publication *Investing in Development*, p. 17) in the list of 'well governed countries'. Its World Bank Governance dimension

for corruption was, in 2004, 24.6. In this publication, the World Bank states that a distinct cause of poor governance is 'genuinely corrupt leadership', and 'in such countries there is little hope for major reductions in poverty'. SIDA, Sweden, took an internationally well-known reverend to court in South Africa for fraud and corruption. He had received large funds for development work. The reverend was convicted.

30. A purchasing power parity (PPP) *exchange rate* equalizes the purchasing power of different *currencies* in their home countries for a given basket of goods. It is often used to compare the *standards of living* between countries, rather than a per capita *gross domestic products* comparison at market exchange rates. One example is that a dinner with Indian food will cost you much less in Calcutta than in London. The PPP has been widely used, e.g. by the World Bank, but has been criticized (see below).

The UN *Statistical Yearbook* writes about its own economic data in 2003: 'Much work needs to be done in this [comparability and reliability of data] area and, for this reason, some tables can only serve as a first source of data, which require further adjustment before being used for more in-depth analytical studies ... there are many limitations, for a variety of reasons ... One common cause of non-comparability of economic data is the different valuations of statistical aggregates, such as national income, wages and salaries, output of industries and so forth. Comparison of these and similar series originally expressed in a common currency, for example United States dollars, through the use of exchange rates is not always satisfactory owing to frequent wide valuations in market rates and differences between official rates and rates which could be indicated by unofficial markets or purchasing power parities. For this reason data ... are subject to certain distortions and can be used as only a rough approximation of the relative amounts involved.'

Deaton (2000), a well-known US economist asks whether 'the poverty estimates as constructed by the World Bank can bear the burden placed on them. One specific difficulty is the use of purchasing power parity (PPP) exchange rates, whose revision induces large changes in poverty estimates for the same countries in the same years. Another area of dispute is the discrepancy in many countries between national accounts statistics, which are used to compute growth rates, and survey estimates, which are used to compute poverty estimates. To a considerable extent, the failure of world poverty to diminish in the face of world growth is the failure of household survey data to be consistent with national income data. The details of survey design are also important. In India, changing the reference period for reporting consumption removes around 200 million people, a sixth of the world total, if not from poverty, at least from the poverty counts.'

When the 1996 method was used in Thailand that country saw its poverty rate suddenly decrease to 0.1 per cent, the lowest in the world (UNDP, 1997). The same question marks are due when UNDP estimated the proportion of extremely poor people in Uganda at 37 per cent in 2002 and at 82 per cent in 2003; in Pakistan that proportion was quoted as being 31 per cent in 2002 and 13 per cent in 2003. Publishing poverty research results of this quality creates scepticism as to the reliability of the poverty measurements of the Millennium Programme.

Reddy and Pogge (2005) state that 'The World Bank's approach to estimating the extent, distribution and trend of global income poverty is neither meaningful nor reliable. The Bank uses an arbitrary international poverty line that is not adequately anchored in any specification of the real requirements of human beings. Moreover, it employs a concept of purchasing power equivalence that is neither well defined nor appropriate for poverty assessment. These difficulties are inherent in the Bank's "money-metric" approach and cannot be credibly overcome without dispensing with this approach altogether. In addition, the Bank extrapolates incorrectly from limited data and thereby creates an appearance of precision that masks the high probable error of its estimates. It is difficult to judge the nature and extent of the errors in global poverty estimates that these three flaws produce. However, there is reason to believe that the Bank's approach may have led it to understate the extent of global income poverty and to infer without adequate justification that global income poverty has steeply declined in the recent period.'

31. The official numbers of the populations of many developing countries are sometimes not very exact. For example, the UN Population Division, in 2002, published the 2005 projected population for Oman as 3,020,000. However, in 2003, a census was carried out showing that the population was 2,341,000 with a projection for 2005 of 2,425,000, thus the UN had overestimated the population by some 600,000, or 25 per cent of the real population. The UN, for the period 2000–5, estimated the annual growth at 68,000; instead, the Oman national census found the annual growth to be 42,000, so the UN estimate was 62 per cent above the real.

32. UNICEF (2002) estimates that some 131 million children are born each year in the world. However, the same organization also tells us that we do not even know how many children there are in the world, or how many are born each year. Still details are produced about the numbers we do not know: 'In 2002, one third of the children in the world were not registered. The distributions for the different regions of un-registered children were in: Sub-Saharan Africa 78%, Central Asia 44%, East Asia and the Pacific 35%, Middle East and Northern Africa 19%, Americas 8% and Europe 3%.' 'In Bolivia, about 778,000 (9.4% of total population) are not legally registered, and do not have birth certificates to prove their identity. 62% of these are children and adolescents.'

33. No developing country has reliable and complete data about mortality. WHO (Lopez et al., 2006) report that only 64 of its 192 member states, mostly high-income countries, have complete mortality data; for 77 there are no recent data, or no data at all. 'Ideal systems for cause-of-death-reporting operate only in 29 countries. In the remaining countries, mortality statistics suffer from one or more of the following problems: incomplete registration of births and deaths, lay reporting of the cause of death, poor coverage and incorrect reporting of ages. For the majority of the world's populations – there are no "proper" mortality diagnoses.' Neither are the data about length of life built on good quality data. Death, in developing countries, may be attributed to 'old age', 'evil spirits', 'visitation from God', 'magic', real or imagined 'poisoning', 'fever', or 'malaria' (undiagnosed, so it could be something else). 'The sum of deaths claimed by different WHO programmes exceeded the total number of deaths in the world' (Lopez et al., 2006).

34. The literacy rate is not always well known. Few poor people have books at home, or pens and paper for writing; literacy skills acquired in primary school may soon be lost. Some data submitted to UNESCO regarding education have been collected with the help of payments to the responsible official in the Ministry of Education to have the information 'produced' and delivered on time. Numbers about school attendance, doubling of classes, drop-out and literacy rates are often produced on the basis of guesstimates.
35. Corporal punishment, according to available information, is forbidden in Austria, Bulgaria, Croatia, Cyprus, Denmark, Finland, Germany, Greece, Hungary, Iceland, Israel, Latvia, Norway, Romania, Sweden, the Netherlands and Ukraine. In the following countries such punishment is forbidden in schools: American Samoa, Belgium, China, Cyprus, Fiji, France, Ireland, Italy, Japan, Kenya, Luxembourg, Namibia, New Zealand, Poland, Portugal, Russia, South Africa, Switzerland, Thailand, Trinidad and Tobago, Turkey, United Kingdom, Zambia and Zimbabwe.

Bibliography

Ackerman, P. et al. (1998), 'Prevalence of posttraumatic stress disorder and other psychiatric diagnoses in three groups of abused children (sexual, physical, and both)'. *Child Abuse Negl*, 22: 759.

Adams, J. A. et al. (2007), 'Guidelines for medical care of children who may have been sexually abused'. *J. Pediatr Adolesc Gynecol*, 20: 163.

Adedoyin, M. and Adegoke, A. A. (1995), 'Teenage prostitution – child abuse, a survey of the situation'. *African J. Medical Science*, 24: 27.

Afifi, T. et al. (2006), 'Physical punishment, childhood abuse and psychiatric disorders'. *Child Abuse Negl*, 30: 1093.

African Network for the Prevention and Protection against Child Abuse and Neglect (2000), 'Awareness and views regarding child abuse and child rights in selected communities in Kenya'. Nairobi, Kenya.

Agathonos-Georgopoulou, H. and Brown, K. (1997), 'The prediction of child maltreatment in Greek families'. *Child Abuse Negl*, 21: 721.

Aghion, P., Caroli, E. and Garcia-Peñalosa, C. (1999), 'Inequality and economic growth: the perspective of the new growth theories'. *Journal of Economic Literature*, 37: 1615.

Agrawal H. R. et al. (2004), 'Attachment studies with borderline patients: a review'. *Harv Rev Psychiatry*, 12: 94.

Ahmad, K. (2004), 'Health and money in Afghanistan'. *The Lancet*, 364: 1301.

Ahmand, J. et al. (1992), 'An epidemic of Neisseria Gonorrhea in a Somalia orphanage'. *Int J. of STD AIDS*, 3: 52.

Alami, K. and Kadri, N. (2004), 'Moroccan women with a history of child sexual abuse and its long-term repercussions: a population-based epidemiological study'. *Arch Women's Mental Health*, 7: 237.

Alexander, K.W. et al. (2005), 'Traumatic impact predicts long-term memory for documented child sexual abuse'. *Psychol Sci*, 16: 33.

Allahbadia, G. (2002), 'The 50 million missing women'. *J. Assist Reprod Genet*, 19: 411.

Al-Mahroos, F. (2007), 'Child abuse and neglect in the Arab peninsula'. *Saudi Med J.*, 28: 241.

Al-Mahroos, F. et al. (2005), 'Child abuse: Bahrain's experience'. *Child Abuse Negl*, 29: 187.

Al-Moosa, A. et al. (2003), 'Pediatricians' knowledge, attitudes and experience regarding child maltreatment in Kuwait'. *Child Abuse Negl*, 27: 1161.

American Academy of Child and Adolescent Psychiatry (2004), 'Facts for families: conduct disorder' (adaptation). Internet.

American Academy of Pediatrics (2001), 'Assessment of maltreatment of children with disabilities'. Committee on Child Abuse and Neglect, and Committee on Children With Disabilities. *Pediatrics*, 108: 508.

American Academy of Pediatrics (2005). Internet.

American Psychiatric Association (2004), 'Practice guidelines for the treatment of patients with acute stress disorder (ASD) and post-traumatic stress disorder (PTSD)'. Published by APA, November 2004. Internet.

Ammerman, R. et al. (1989), 'Abuse and neglect in psychiatrically hospitalized multihandicapped children'. *Child Abuse Negl*, 13: 335.

Amoako, J. (1976), 'Expert meeting on social services'. United Nations, Geneva.

Anda, R. F. et al. (2004), 'Childhood abuse, household dysfunction, and indicators of impaired adult worker performance'. *The Permanente Journal*, 8, 1: 30.

Anderson, C. and Bushman, B. (2001), 'Effects of violent video games on aggressive behaviour, aggressive cognition, aggressive affect, physiological arousal, and prosocial behaviour: a meta-analytic review of the scientific literature'. *Psychological Science*, 12: 353.

Anderson, C. et al. (2002), 'Abnormal T2 relaxation time in the cerebellar vermis of the sexually abused in childhood: potential role of the vermis in stress-enhanced risk for drug abuse'. *Psychoneuro-endocrinology*, 27: 231.

Andrews, G. et al. (2003), 'Child sexual abuse', in M. Ezzati et al. (eds), *Comparative Quantification of Health Risks: Global and Regional Burden of Disease Attributable to Selected Major Risk Factors*. Geneva: World Health Organization, p. 1851.

Annerén, G. (2002), personal information.

Antisocial Personality Disorder Forum (2006), *Encyclopedia of Mental Disorders*. Thomson Corporation.

Arkes, H. (1972), *Bureaucracy, the Marshall Plan, and the National Interest*. Princeton, NJ: Princeton University Press.

Arnold, F. et al. (1998), 'Son preference, family building and child mortality in India'. *Popul Studies*, 52: 301.

Arszman, A. and Shapiro, R. (2000), Report. Children's Hospital Medical Center, Cincinnati, Ohio, US.

Artemis (2000), 'The Artemis programme for girls and women against sexual abuse'. *Cluj Napoca*, Romania.

Asbury, E. (2003), 'Personality Theory: Marilyn Monroe'. Internet.

Aston, M. (1999), 'Project MATCH, unseen colossus'. *Drug and Alcohol*, 1: 15.

Atlantic Monthly Affairs (1996), 'In a Chinese orphanage'. April.

Aulard, F. (1883), *Les Orateurs de la Legislative et de la Convention and Les Portraits littéraires a la fin du XVIII siècle, pendant la Révolution*. Bibliothèque Nationale de France, Paris.

Bader, S. et al. (2007) 'Female sexual abuse and criminal justice intervention: a comparison of child protective service and criminal justice samples'. *Child Abuse Negl*. 17 December (Epub ahead of print).

Baker, C. et al. (2005), 'Violence and PTSD in Mexico: gender and regional differences'. *Soc Psychiatry Epidem*, 40: 519.

Baker, R. and Mednick, B. (1985), *Influences on Human Development: a Longitudinal Perspective*. Dordrecht: Kluwer.

Balvig, F. (1999), *RisikoUngdom–Ungdomsundersøgelse 1999*. Copenhagen: Det Kriminalpræventive Råd.

Banerjee, A. and He, R. (2003), 'Making aid work: the World Bank of the future'. BREAD Working Paper No. 013.

Barak, G. (2003), *Violence and Nonviolence: Pathways to Understanding*. Thousand Oaks, CA: Sage.

Barclay, G. and Tavares, C. (2003), *International Comparisons of Justice Statistics*. London: Home Office.

Barlow, J. et al. (2006), 'Individual and group-based parenting programmes for the treatment of physical child abuse and neglect'. *Cochrane Database of Systematic Reviews*, Issue 4.

Barnes, D. and Bell, C. (2003), 'Paradoxes of black suicide: preventing suicide'. *The National Journal*, 2: 2.

Barnet, B. et al. (2002), 'The effect of volunteer home visitation for adolescent mothers on parenting and mental health outcomes: a randomized trial'. *Arch Pediatr Adolesc Med*, 156: 1216.

Barraclough, S. (2002), 'Development policy review', in *Toward Integrated and Sustainable Development?* Geneva: UNRISD.

Barthauer, L. and Leventhal, J. (1999), 'Prevalence and effects of sexual abuse in a poor rural community in El Salvador'. *Child Abuse Negl*, 23: 1117.

Bastian, P. (1994), 'Family care in the United Kingdom', in M. Gottesman (ed.), *Recent Changes and New Trends in Extrafamiliar Child Care*. London: FICE.

Baumrind, D. (1973), 'The development of instrumental competence through socialization', in A. D. Pick (ed.), *Minnesota Symposia on Child Psychology* (Vol. 7, pp. 3–46). Minneapolis: University of Minnesota Press.

Baumrind, D. (1991), 'The influence of parenting style on adolescent competence and substance use'. *Journal of Early Adolescence*, 1: 56.

Beck, J. and Shaw, D. (2005), 'The influence of perinatal complications and environmental adversity on boys' antisocial behaviour'. *J. Child Psychol Psychiatry*, 46: 35.

Becker-Weidman, A. (2006), 'Treatment for children with trauma-attachment disorders: dyadic developmental psychotherapy'. *Child and Adolescent Social Work Journal*, 23: 2.

Belfield, C. R. (2006), *Economic Analysis of Pre-kindergarten: an Overview of the Evidence*. Queens College, City University of New York.

Bem, D. J. (1972), 'Self-perception theory', in L. Berkowitz (ed.), *Advances in Experimental Social Psychology*, Vol. 6: 1. New York: Academic Press.

Benbenitshty, R. et al. (2002), 'Maltreatment of primary school students by educational staff in Israel'. *Child Abuse Negl*, 26: 1291.

Bendixen, M., Muus, K. and Shei, B. (1994), 'The impact of child sexual abuse: a study of a random sample of Norwegian students'. *Child Abuse Negl*, 18: 837.

Berkowitz, C. (1998), 'Medical consequences of child sexual abuse'. *Child Abuse Negl*, 22: 541.

Bernal, M., Klinnert, M. and Schultz, L. (1980), 'Outcome evaluation of behavioural parent training and client-centered parent counselling for children with conduct problems'. *Journal of Applied Behaviour Analysis*, 13: 677.

Berrien, F. et al. (1995), 'Child abuse prevalence in Russian urban populations: a preliminary report'. *Child Abuse Negl*, 19: 261.

Besley, T. and Cord, L. (eds) (2007), *Delivering on the Promise of Pro-poor Growth*. New York: Palgrave Macmillan and the World Bank.

Bhardwaj, R. et al. (2006), 'Neurocortical neurogenesis is restricted to development'. *Proc Nat Acad Sci USA*, 103: 125–64.

Bifulco, A. et al. (2002), 'Exploring psychological abuse in childhood: II. Association with other abuse and adult clinical depression'. *Bull Menninger Clin*, 66: 241.

Biji, R. et al. (1998), 'Prevalence of psychiatric disorder in the general population: results of the Netherlands mental health survey and incidence study'. *Soc Psychiatry Epidemiol*, 33: 587.

Bilir, S., Ari, M. and Donmez, N. (1986), 'Physical abuse in 16,000 children with 2–4 years of age'. *J. Child Development & Education*, 1: 7.

Birbaumer, N. et al. (2005), 'Deficient fear conditioning in psychopathy: a functional magnetic resonance imaging study'. *Arch Gen Psychiatry*, 62: 799.

Bloch, S. (1997), 'Psychiatry: an impossible profession?' *Aust NZ J. Psychiatry*, 31: 173. For a further detailed review, see: *Acta Psychiatrica Scand*, Suppl. 399, vol. 101, 'Ethics, law and human rights in psychiatric care', 2000.

BMA, Ahmedabad (1997), 'Disability household survey'. Report.

Bochenek, M. and Dalgadoi, F. (2006), 'Children in custody in Brazil'. *The Lancet*, 367: 696.

Bode, C., Odelola, M. and Odiacho, R. (2001), 'Abuse and neglect in the surgically ill child'. *West Afr J. Med*, 20: 86.

Bödvarsdóttir, I. and Elklit, A. (2007), 'Victimization and PTSD-like states in an Icelandic youth probability sample'. *BMC Psychiatry*, 7: 51.

Boney-McCoy, S. and Finkelhor, D. (1996), 'Is youth victimization related to trauma symptoms and depression after controlling for prior symptoms and family relationships? A longitudinal, prospective study'. *Journal of Consulting and Clinical Psychology*, 64: 1406.

Boris, B. et al. (1998), 'Attachment disorders in infancy and early childhood: a preliminary investigation of diagnostic criteria'. *American Journal of Psychiatry*, February.

Bourguignon, F. (2004), 'The poverty-growth-inequality triangle'. Paper presented at the Indian Council for Research on International Economic Relations, New Delhi, 4 February.

Bouvier, P. et al. (1999), 'Typology and correlates of sexual abuse in children and youth'. *Child Abuse Negl*, 23: 8.

Bowlby, J. (1951), *Maternal Care and Mental Health*. Geneva, WHO Monograph. Series: 2.

Brandt, I., Sticker, E. and Lentze, M. (2003), 'Catch-up growth of head circumference of very low birth weight, small for gestational age preterm infants and mental development to adulthood'. *J. Pediatr*, 142: 459.

Bremner, J. et al. (2003), 'Assessment of the hypothalamic-pituitary-adrenal axis over a 24-hour diurnal period and in response to neuroendocrine challenges in women with and without childhood sexual abuse and posttraumatic stress disorder'. *Biological Psychiatry*, 54: 710.

Bremner, J. et al. (2005), 'Positron emission topographic imaging of neural correlates of fear acquisition and extinction paradigm in women with childhood sexual-abuse-related post-traumatic stress disorder'. *Psychol Med*, 435: 791.

Brennan, K. and Shaver, P. (1998), 'Attachment styles and personality disorders: their connections to each other and to parental divorce, parental death, and perceptions of parental care giving'. *Journal of Personality*, 66: 835.

Brestan, E. and Eyberg, S. (1998), 'Effective psychosocial treatments of conduct-disordered children and adolescents: 29 years, 82 studies, and 5,272 kids'. *Journal of Clinical Child Psychology*, 27: 180.

Brian, M., Borne, A. and Noten, T. (2004), *Joint East West Research on Trafficking in Children for Sexual Purposes in Europe: the Sending Countries*. Europe: ECPAT.

Bridget, F. (1998), National Institute of Alcohol Abuse and Alcoholism's Epidemi-ologic Bulletin No. 39, 'The impact of a family history of alcoholism on the relationship between age at onset of alcohol use and DSM-IV alcohol depen-dence. Results from the National Longitudinal Alcohol Epidemiologic Survey'. *Alcohol Health and Research World*, 22, 2.

Briere, J. and Runtz, M. (1989), 'University males' sexual interest in children: predicting potential indices of "pedophilia" in a nonforensic sample'. *Child Abuse Negl*, 13: 65.

Briggs, L. and Joyce, P. (1997), 'What determines post-traumatic stress disorder symptomatology for survivors of childhood sexual abuse?' *Child Abuse Negl*, 21: 575.

British Crime Survey (2005), Government of United Kingdom, London.

Brodzinsky, D., Schechter, M. and Henig, R. (eds) (1992), *On Being Adopted*. New York: Doubleday.

Bronfenbrenner, U. (1979), *The Ecology of Human Development*. Cambridge, MA: Harvard University Press.

Bronfenbrenner, U. (1990), *Rebuilding the Nest: a New Commitment to the American Family*. Family Service America.

Bronfenbrenner, U. (2004), *Making Human Beings Human: Bioecological Perspectives on Human Development*. London: Sage Publications.

Brown, L. et al. (2006) 'Sexual violence in Lesotho'. *Stud Fam Plann*, 37: 269.

Brown, R. et al. (1998), 'Recommended practices: parent education and support. Internet.

Buechler, S. (1999), *Social Movements in Advanced Capitalism*. Oxford: Oxford University Press.

Buitelaar, J. et al. (2003), 'Prenatal stress and cognitive development and temperament in infants'. *Neurobiol Aging*, 24, Suppl.1: 561.

Burnside, C. and Dollar, D. (2000), 'Aid policies and growth'. *American Economic Review*, 90: 847.

Butchart, A. and Poznyak, V. (2005), *Child Maltreatment and Alcohol Fact Sheet*. Geneva: World Health Organization.

Cáceres, F., Marin, B. and Hudes, E. (2000), 'Sexual coercion among youth and young adults in Lima, Peru'. *Journal of Adolescent Health*, 27: 361.

Caldwell, H. and Young, W. (2006), 'Oxytocin and vasopressin: genetics and behavioural implications', in R. Lim (ed.), *Handbook of Neurochemistry and Molecular Neurobiology*, 3rd edition. New York: Springer, p. 573.

Caldwell, R. (1992), *The Costs of Child Abuse vs. Child Abuse Prevention: Michigan's Experience*. Lansing, MO: Children's Trust Fund.

Canada Department of Health (1995), National Clearinghouse on Family Vio-lence, Ottawa.

Canadian Psychiatric Journal (February 2001), 'The neuropsychopharmacology of criminality and aggression'.

Canter, D. and Kirby, S. (1995), 'Prior convictions of child molesters'. *Sci Justice*, 35: 73.

Cantor, J. et al. (2008), 'Cerebral white matter deficiencies in pedophile men'. *J. Psychiatr Res*, 42: 167.

Carey, G. (2002), 'Criminality linked to early abuse and genes'. *Science*, 297: 851.

Carlson, E. A. (1998), 'A prospective longitudinal study of attachment disorgani-zation/disorientation'. *Child Development*, 69: 1107.

Cawson, P. et al. (2000), *Child Maltreatment in the United Kingdom: a Study of the Prevalence of Child Abuse and Neglect*. London: National Society for the Prevention of Cruelty to Children.

Centers for Disease Control and Prevention (2002), Task Force on Community Preventive Services CDC, Atlanta, GA.

Chadwick, D. (1999), 'The message'. *Child Abuse Negl*, 23: 957.

Chakravarthy, C. (1990), 'Community workers estimate of drinking and alcohol-related problems in rural areas'. *Indian J. Psychological Medicine*, 13: 49.

Chalk, R. and King, P. (eds) (1998), *Violence in Families: Assessing Prevention and Treatment Programmes*. Washington: National Academies Press.

Chamberlain, A. et al. (1984), 'Issues in fertility control for mentally retarded female adolescents, I: sexual activity, sexual abuse and contraception'. *Pediatrics*, 7: 445.

Chambers, R. (1995), 'Poverty and livelihoods. Whose reality counts?' Policy paper commissioned by UNDP.

Chan, C. (1995), 'Gender issues in market socialism', in L. Wong and S. MacPherson (eds), *Social Change and Social Policy in Contemporary China*. Aldershot: Avebury, p. 188.

Chen, J., Han, P. and Dunne, M. (2004), 'Child sexual abuse: a study among 892 female students of a medical school'. *Zhonghua Er Ke Za Zhi*, 42: 39.

Chianu, E. (2000), 'Two deaths, one blind eye, one imprisonment: child abuse in guise of corporal punishment in Nigerian schools'. *Child Abuse Negl*, 24: 1005.

Christopher, M. and Winters, K. (1998), 'Diagnosis and assessment of alcohol use disorders among adolescents', *Alcohol Health and Research World*, 22, 2.

Chung, T., Martin, C. and Winters, K. (2005), 'Diagnosis, course, and assessment of alcohol abuse and dependence in adolescents'. *Recent Dev Alcohol*, 17: 5.

Cicchetti, D. and Rogosh, F. (2001), 'The impact of child maltreatments and psychopathology on neuroendocrine functioning'. *Dev Psychopathol*, 13: 783.

Cicchetti, D. et al. (1990), 'An organizational perspective on attachment beyond infancy', in M. Greenberg, D. Cicchetti and E. Cummings (eds), *Attachment in the Preschool Years*. Chicago: University of Chicago Press.

Clemmons, J. C. et al. (2003), 'Co-occurring forms of child maltreatment and adult adjustment reported by Latina college students'. *Child Abuse Negl*, 27: 751.

Cloitre, M. (1998), 'Sexual re-victimization: risk factors and prevention', in V. M. Follette, J. I. Ruzek and F. R. Abueg (eds), *Cognitive-Behavioural Therapies for Trauma*. New York: Guilford Press.

Coale, A. and Banister, J. (1994), 'Five decades of missing females in China'. *Demography*, 31: 459.

Cohen, R. A. et al. (2006), 'Early life stress and morphometry of the adult anterior cingulate cortex and caudate nuclei'. *Biological Psychiatry*, 59: 975.

Coker, A. and Richter, D. (1998), 'Violence against women in Sierra Leone: frequency and correlates of intimate partner violence and forced sexual intercourse'. *African J. Reproductive Health*, 2: 61.

Collier, A. et al. (1999), 'Culture-specific views of child maltreatment and parenting styles in a Pacific-island community'. *Child Abuse Negl*, 23: 229.

Collin-Vézina, D. and Cyr, M. (2003), 'La transmission de la violence sexuelle: description du phénomène et pistes de compréhension'. *Child Abuse Negl*, 27: 489.

Collings, S. J. (1991), 'Childhood sexual abuse in a sample of South African university males: prevalence and risk factors'. *South African Journal of Psychology*, 21: 153.

Collings, S. J. (1995), 'The long-term effects of contact and noncontact forms of child sexual abuse in a sample of university men'. *Child Abuse Negl*, 19: 1.

Collins Cobuild English Dictionary (2002), London: HarperCollins.

Colucci-D'Amato, L. et al. (2006), 'The end of the central dogma of neurobiology: stem cells and neurogenesis in adult CNS'. *Neurol Sci*, 27: 266.

Colwell Report (1976), *Children at Risk: Joint Report of the County Secretary and Director of Social Services*. Lewes, East Sussex County Council.

Conradie, H. (2003), 'Are we failing to deliver the best interest of the child?' Department of Criminology, University of South Africa. Internet publication.

Courtois, R., Mullet, E. and Malvy, D. (2001), 'Survey on sexual behaviour by Congolese and French high-school students in an AIDS context'. *Santé*, 11: 49.

Cowen, T. (1985), 'The Marshall Plan: myths and realities', in D. Bandow (ed.), *US Aid to the Developing World: a Free Market Agenda*. Washington: Heritage Fund, p. 61.

Crandell, L. and Hobson, R. (1999), 'Individual differences in young children's IQ: a social development perspective'. *J. Child Psychol Psychiatry*, 40: 455.

Croll, E. (2001), *Endangered Daughters: Discrimination and Development in Asia*. London: Routledge.

Cross, T. et al. (2003), 'Prosecution of child abuse: a meta-analysis of rates of criminal justice decisions'. *Trauma Violence Abuse*, 4: 323.

Csorba, R. et al. (2006), 'Female child sexual abuse within the family in a Hungarian county'. *Gynecological and Obstetric Investigation*, 6: 188.

Daly, M. (ed.) (2007), *Parenting in Contemporary Europe: a Positive Approach*. Council of Europe.

Darling, N. (1999), *Parenting Style and Its Correlates*. Clearinghouse on Elementary and Early Childhood Education.

Daro, D. (1988), *Confronting Child Abuse*. New York: Free Press.

Das, V., Kleinman, A., Ramphele, M. and Reynolds, P. (2000), *Violence and Subjectivity*. California: University of California Press.

Das, V., Kleinman, A., Lock, M. and Ramphele, M. (2001), *Remaking a World: Violence, Social Suffering and Recovery*. California: University of California Press.

Davis, E. et al. (2007), 'Prenatal exposure to maternal depression and cortisol influences infant temperament'. *J. Am Acad Child Adolsc Psychiatry*, 46: 737.

Deaton, A. (2000), 'Counting the world's poor: problems and possible solutions'. Document for the World Bank. Princeton University Research Programme in Development Studies.

De Bellis, M. et al. (2002), 'Brain structures in pediatric maltreatment-related post-traumatic stress disorder: a sociodemographically matched study'. *Biological Psychiatry*, 52: 1066.

De Keseredy, W. and Perry, B. (eds) (2006), *A Critical Perspective on Violence in Advancing Critical Criminology: Theory and Application*. Lanham, MD: Lexington Books.

Deres, S. and Kulik-Rechberger, B. (2001), 'Child abuse as a problem of the family physician'. *Przegl Lek* (Poland), 58: 87.

Derogates, L. (1977), 'SCL-90-R, administration, scoring procedures manual-I for the revised version'. Johns Hopkins University School of Medicine.

De Weerth, C., van Hees, Y. and Buitelaar, J. (2003), 'Prenatal maternal cortisol levels and infant behavior during the first 5 months'. *Early Hum Dev*, 74: 139.

De Weid, D. et al. (1991), 'Interactive effects of neurohypophyseal neuropeptides with receptor antagonist on passive avoidance behaviour: mediation by a cerebral neurohypophyseal receptor?' *Proc Natl Acad Sci, USA*, 88: 1494.

Diagnostic and Statistical Manual-IV (DSM-IV) (1993), 4th edition. American Psychiatric Association.

Dick, D. et al. (2006), 'The role of GABRA2 in risk for conduct disorder and alcohol and drug dependence across developmental stages'. *Addiction Biology*, 11: 386.

Dietz, T. (2000), 'Disciplining children: characteristics associated with the use of corporal punishment'. *Child Abuse Negl*, 24: 1529.

Documentation Française (2002), 'Les violences contre les femmes en France. Une enquête nationale', INSEE, Paris.

Doren, D. (1998), 'Recidivism base rates, predictions of sex offender recidivism, and the "sexual predator" commitment laws'. *Behavioural Sciences and the Law*, 16: 97.

Douglas, E. and Straus, M. (2006), 'University students in 19 countries and their relation to corporal punishment experienced as a child'. *European Journal of Criminology*, 3: 293.

Doyle, C. (2006), *Working With Abused Children*, 3rd edition. Basingstoke: Palgrave Macmillan.

Driessen, M. et al. (2000), 'Magnetic resonance imaging volumes of the hippocampus and the amygdala in women with borderline personality disorder and early traumatization'. *Arch Gen Psychiatry*, 57: 1115.

'DSM-IV criteria for conduct disorder' (1994), American Psychiatric Association.

Dube, S. et al. (2001), 'Childhood abuse, household dysfunction and the risk of attempted suicide throughout the life span: findings from the Adverse Childhood Experiences Study'. *Journal of the American Medical Association*, 286: 3089.

Dube, S. et al. (2003a), 'Childhood abuse, neglect, and household dysfunction and the risk of illicit drug use: the Adverse Childhood Experiences Study'. *Pediatrics*, 111: 564.

Dube, S. et al. (2003b), 'The impact of adverse childhood experiences on health problems: evidence from four birth cohorts dating back to 1900'. *Preventive Medicine*, 3: 267.

Dube, S. et al. (2006), 'Adverse childhood experiences and the association with ever using alcohol and initiating alcohol use during adolescence'. *Journal of Adolescent Health*, 38: 444.

Duggan, M. (2001), 'More guns, more crime'. *Journal of Political Economy*, 109: 1086.

Dunne, M. et al. (2003), 'Is child sexual abuse declining? Evidence from a population-based survey of men and women in Australia'. *Child Abuse Negl*, 27: 141.

Dunsieth, N. W. Jr et al. (2004), 'Psychiatric and legal features of 113 men convicted of sexual offenses'. *J. Clin Psychiatry*, 65: 293.

Dwairy, M. and Menshar, K. (2006), 'Parenting style, individuation, and mental health of Egyptian adolescents'. *Journal of Adolescence*, 29: 103.

Easterlin, R. (1995), 'Will raising the incomes of all increase the happiness of all?' *J. Econ Behaviour & Organization*, 27: 35.

Easterlin, R. (2003), 'Explaining happiness'. *Proc National Academy of Sciences*, 100: 1176.

Easterly, W. (2005), 'A modest proposal'. *Washington Post*, 13 March.

Easterly, W., Levine, R. and Roodman, D. (2004), 'Aid policies and growth: comment'. *American Economic Review*, 94: 774.

Economist (The) (2007), 'Missing the barefoot doctors'. 11 October.

ECPAT Focal Point against Sexual Exploitation of Children (2005), available at: www.ecpat.net/ecpat1/index2.htm

ECPAT International: Experts Meeting on Violence in Cyberspace, East Asia and Pacific Regional Consultation. 12–15 June 2005.

Edwards, V. (2003), 'Relationship between multiple forms of childhood maltreatment and adult mental health in community respondents: results from the Adverse Childhood Experiences Study'. *Am J. Psychiatry*, 160: 1453.

Egeland, B., Carlson, E. and Sroufe, L. A. (1993), 'Resilience as process'. *Development and Psychopathology*, 5: 517.

Einstein, A. (1950), *Out of My Later Years*. London: Thames and Hudson.

Eisner, M. (2003), *Long-term Historical Trends in Violent Crime*. Chicago: University of Chicago Press.

Elal, G. et al. (2000), 'A comparative study of child sexual abuse among university students'. 16th Annual Meeting of Traumatic Stress Studies, San Antonio.

Elbedour, S. et al. (2006), 'The scope of sexual, physical and psychological abuse in a Bedouin-Arab community of female adolescents: the interplay of racism, urbanization, polygamy, family honor, and the social marginalization of women'. *Child Abuse Negl*, 30: 577.

Elias, M. et al. (1986), 'Impact of a preventive social problem solving intervention on children's coping with middle-school stressors'. *Am J. Community Psychol*, 14: 259.

Eliot, L. (2001), *Early Intelligence: How the Brain and Mind Develop in the First Five Years of Life*. Harmondsworth: Penguin.

Elklit, A. (2002), 'Victimization and PTSD in a Danish national youth probability sample'. *J. Am Acad Child Adolesc Psychiatry*, 41: 174.

Elliott, D. et al. (1989), *Multiple Problem Youth: Delinquency, Substance Abuse and Mental Health Problems*. New York: Springer-Verlag.

Ellsberg, M. (2000) 'Candies in hell: women's experience of violence in Nicaragua'. *Social Science & Med*, 51: 1595.

Encyclopaedia Britannica (2003), 'Ethics'.

English, D., Widom, C. and Brandford, C. (2002), 'Childhood victimization and delinquency, adult criminality, and violent criminal behaviour: a replication and extension'. US Department of Justice, Washington, DC.

Ertem, I. et al. (2000), 'Intergenerational continuity of child physical abuse: how good is the evidence?' *Lancet*, 356: 814.

Eskin, M., Kayak-Demir, H. and Demir, S. (2005), 'Same-sex orientation, childhood sexual abuse, and suicidal behaviour in university students in Turkey'. *Arch Sex Behav*, 34: 185.

Etkin, A. and Wager, T. (2007), 'Functional neuroimaging of anxiety: a meta-analysis of emotional processing in PTSD, social anxiety disorder, and social phobia'. *Am J Psychiatry*, 164: 1476.

European Forum for Child Welfare (1998), 'Are children protected against violence in Europe?' European Union.

Fabricius, Brink O. and Charles, A. (1998), 'Domestic violence'. *Ugeskr Laeger*, 160L: 431.

Fagan, P. et al. (2002), 'Paedophilia'. *JAMA*, 288: 2458.

Famularo, R. et al. (1996), 'Psychiatric co-morbidity in childhood post traumatic stress disorder'. *Child Abuse Negl*, 20: 953.

Farley, M., Lynne, J. and Cotton, A. (2005), 'Prostitution in Vancouver: violence and the colonization of First Nations women'. *Transcult Psychiatry*, 42: 24.

Farrington, D. (1989), 'Early predictors of adolescent aggression and adult violence'. *Violence and Victims*, 79.

Federal Court of the Eastern District of New York (1972), *New York ARC v. Rockefeller*.

Felitti, V. (2002), 'Belastungen in der Kindheit und Gesundheit im Erwachsenenalter: die Verwandlung von Gold in Blei'. *Z. Psychsom Med Psychother*, 48: 359.

Felitti, V. (2003), 'The relationship of adverse childhood experiences to adult health status'. Snowbird Conference, Division of Child Protection and Family Health, Pediatrics Department, University of Utah, Salt Lake City.

Felitti, V. et al. (1991), 'Long-term medical consequences of incest, rape, and molestation'. *Southern Med J.*, 84: 328.

Felitti, V. J. et al. (1998), 'Relationship of childhood abuse and household dysfunction to many of the leading causes of death in adults'. *Am J. Prev Med*, 14: 245.

Fergusson, D. and Lynskey, M. (1997), 'Physical punishment/maltreatment during childhood and adjustment in young adulthood'. *Child Abuse Negl*, 21: 617.

Fergusson, D., Lynskey, M. and Horwood, J. (1996), 'Childhood sexual abuse and psychiatric disorders in young adulthood: I. Prevalence of sexual abuse and factors associated with sexual abuse'. *J. Am Academy Child Psychiatry*, 34: 1355.

Ferrari, A. (2002), 'The impact of culture upon child rearing practices and definitions of maltreatment'. *Child Abuse Negl*, 26: 793.

Fikree, F. and Pasha, O. (2004), 'Role of gender in health disparity: the South Asian context'. *British Med J.*, 328: 823.

Fine, M. (1980), *Handbook on Parent Education*. New York: Academic Press.

Finkelhor, D. (1994), 'The international epidemiology of child sexual abuse'. *Child Abuse Negl*, 18: 409.

Finkelhor, D. and Browne, A. (1986), 'Impact of sexual abuse'. *Psych Bull*, 99: 66.

Finkelhor, D. and Jones, L. (2004), 'Sexual abuse decline in the 1990s: evidence for possible causes'. *Juvenile Justice Bulletin*, Washington, DC.

Finkelhor, D., Ormrod, R. K. and Turner, H. A. (2007), 'Poly-victimization: a neglected component in child victimization'. *Child Abuse Negl*, 31: 3.

Finkelhor, D. et al. (1990), 'Sexual abuse in a national survey of adult men and women'. *Child Abuse Negl*, 14: 19.

Finkelhor, D. et al. (2005), 'The victimization of children and youth: a comprehensive, national survey'. *Child Maltreat*, 10: 5.

Fischer, D. and McDonald, W. (1998), 'Characteristics of intrafamilial and extrafamilial child sexual abuse'. *Child Abuse Negl*, 22: 915.

Fitzgerald, J., Gottschalk, P. and Moffitt, R. (1998), 'An analysis of sample attention in panel data: the Michigan Panel study of income dynamics'.

Technical Working Paper 0220, National Bureau of Economic Research, Inc. (website).

Fleck, F. (2004), 'Children are the main victims of trafficking in Africa'. *British Med J.*, 328: 1036.

Flisher, A. et al. (1997), 'Psychosocial characteristics of physically abused children and adolescents'. *J. Am Acad Child Adolesc Psychiatry*, 36: 123.

Forjuoh, S. (1995), 'Pattern of international burns to children in Ghana'. *Child Abuse Negl*, 19: 837.

Frank, D. et al. (1996), 'Infants and young children in orphanages: one view from pediatrics and child psychiatry'. *Pediatrics*, 97: 569.

Freund, K., Watson, R. and Dickey, R. (1990), 'Does sexual abuse in childhood cause pedophilia? An exploratory study'. *Arch Sex Behav*, 19: 557.

Friedman, M. et al. (2005), 'Thyroid hormone alterations among women with posttraumatic stress disorder due to childhood sexual abuse'. *Biol Psychiatry*, 15: 1186.

Friedrich, W. (1998), 'Behavioural manifestations of child sexual abuse'. *Child Abuse Negl*, 22: 523.

Fries, A. B. W. et al. (2005), 'Early experience in humans is associated with changes in neuropeptide critical for regulating social behaviour'. *Proc National Academy for Science of USA*, 102: 17237.

Frisk, V., Amsel, R. and Whyte, H. (2002), 'The importance of head growth patterns in predicting the cognitive abilities and literacy skills of small-for-gestational-age children'. *Dev Neuropsychol*, 22: 565.

Gadour, A. (2006), 'Libyan children's views on the importance of school factors which contributed to their emotional and behavioural difficulties'. *School Psychology International*, 27: 171.

Galli, V. et al. (1999), 'The psychiatric diagnoses of twenty-two adolescents who have sexually molested other children'. *Compr Psychiatry*, 40: 85.

Garbarino, J. (1995) *Raising Children in a Socially Toxic Environment*. San Francisco: Jossey-Bass Publishers.

Garbarino, J. (1996), 'CAN reflections on 20 years of searching'. *Child Abuse Negl*, 20: 157.

Garbarino, J. (1998), 'Supporting parents in a socially toxic environment'. Parenthood in America. General Library System. University of Wisconsin-Madison. Internet.

Gardner, J. et al. (2003), 'Perceptions and experience of violence among secondary school students in Jamaica'. *Rev Panam Salud Publica*, 14: 97.

Garmezy, N. and Masten, A. S. (1994), 'Chronic adversities', in M. Rutter, E. Taylor and L. Hersow (eds), *Child and Adolescent Psychiatry*, 3rd edn. Oxford: Blackwell, p. 191.

Gershoff, E. (2002), 'Corporal punishment by parents and associated child behaviours and experiences: a meta-analytic and theoretical review'. *Psychological Bulletin*, 128, 4.

Giddens, A. (2001), *Sociology*. Cambridge: Polity Press.

Glass, N. (1999), 'Maternal filicide in Hungary faces stiffer penalties'. *Lancet*, 13 February.

Global Health Watch (2005–6), *An Alternative World Health Report*. People's Health Movement Bangalore, Medact, London, Global Equity Gauge Alliance, Durban. London: Zed Books.

Global Initiative to End all Corporal Punishment of Children (2006), 'Global summary of the legal status of corporal punishment of children'. Internet.

Glynn, L. et al. (2007), 'Postnatal maternal cortisol levels predict temperament in healthy breastfed infants'. *Early Hum Dev*, 27 February.

Goldberg, D. (1972), *Detection of Psychiatric Illness by Questionnaire*. Oxford: Oxford University Press.

Goldman, J. and Padayachi, U. (1997), 'The prevalence and nature of child sexual abuse in Queensland, Australia'. *Child Abuse Negl*, 21: 489.

Goldstein, R. et al. (2006), 'Lack of remorse in antisocial personality disorder'. *Comprehensive Psychiatry*, 47: 289.

Gonçales, H., Ferreira, S. and Marques, M. (1999), 'Evaluating a support program for child victims of domestic violence'. *Rev Saude Publica*, 33: 547.

Gonzales-Heydrich, J. et al. (2001), 'Corticotropin releasing hormone increases apparent potency of adrenocorticotropic hormone stimulation of cortisol secretion'. *Medical Hypotheses*, 57: 544.

Gordon, M. (2005), *Roots of Empathy: Changing the World Child by Child*. Toronto: Thomas Allen Publishers.

Gordon, R. (ed.) (2007), *Languages of the World*, 15th edition. Dallas, TX: Ethnologue.

Gorey, K. and Leslie, D. (1997), 'Prevalence of child sexual abuse'. *Child Abuse Negl*, 21: 391.

Gould, E. and Gross, C. (2002), 'Neurogenesis in adult mammals: some progress and problems'. *J. Neuroscience*, 22: 619.

Gould, M. and O'Brien, T. (1995), 'Child maltreatment in Colorado: the value of prevention and the cost of failure to prevent'. Colorado Children's Trust Fund, Denver, USA.

Govindshenoy, M. and Spencer, N. (2007), 'Abuse of the disabled child: a systematic review of population-based studies'. *Child Care Health Dev*, 33: 552.

Gray, S., Akol, H. and Sundal, M. (2008), 'Mixed-longitudinal growth in infancy and early childhood of Karimojong children in three communities in Moroto District, Uganda'. Department of Anthropology, University of Kansas Lawrence, Kansas.

Greenwood, P. (2005). *Diverting Children from a Life of Crime: Measuring Costs and Benefits*. Online book.

Gujarat study (1997), Disability Household Survey conducted by BMA, Ahmedabad, India.

Gupta, A. (2001), 'Governing population: the integrated child development services program in India', in Thomas Blom Hansen and Finn Stepputat (eds), *States of Imagination: Ethnographic Explorations of the Postcolonial State*. Durham: Duke University Press, p. 65.

Gupta, P. C. et al. (2003), 'Alcohol consumption among middle-aged and elderly men: a community study from Western India'. *Alcohol and Alcoholism*, 28: 327.

Hadi, A. (2000), 'Child abuse among working children in rural Bangladesh: prevalence and determinants'. *Public Health*, 114: 38.

Hageman, I., Andersen, H. and Jorgensen, M. (2001), 'Post-traumatic stress disorder: a review of psychobiology and pharmacotherapy'. *Acta Psychiatr Scand*, 104: 411.

Hahm, H. and Guterman, N. (2001), 'The emerging problem of physical child abuse in South Korea'. *Child Maltreatment*, 6: 169.

Haines, M. (2006) *Historical Statistics of the United States*. Millennial Edition. Editor in Chief with Susan B. Carter, Scott Sigmund Gartner, Alan L. Olmstead, Richard Sutch, and Gavin Wright. New York: Cambridge University Press.

Haj-Yahia, M. and Abdo-Kaloti, R. (2003), 'The rates and correlates of the exposure of Palestinian adolescents to family violence: toward an integrative-holistic approach'. *Child Abuse Negl*, 27: 781.

Haj-Yahia, M. and Tamish, S. (2001), 'The rates of child sexual abuse and its psychological consequences as revealed by a study among Palestinian university students'. *Child Abuse Negl*, 25: 1303.

Hakimi, M. et al. (2001), 'Silence for the sake of harmony: domestic violence and women's health in central Java'. Yogyakarta, Gadjah Mada University.

Hall, D. and Williams, J. (2008), 'Safeguarding, child protection and mental health'. *Arch Dis Child*, 93, 1, January: 11–13.

Halperin, D. et al. (1999), 'Prevalence of child sexual abuse among adolescents in Geneva: results of a cross sectional survey'. *British Medical Journal*, 312: 1326–9.

Hardy, L. (2007), 'Attachment theory and reactive attachment disorder: theoretical perspectives and treatment implications'. *J. Child Psychiatry Nursing*, 20: 2.

Harris, G. T. et al. (2007), 'Coercive and precocious sexuality as a fundamental aspect of psychopathy'. *J. Personal Disord*, 21: 1.

Hart, S. and Hare, R. (1996), 'Psychopathy and antisocial personality disorder'. *Current Opinion in Psychiatry*, 9: 1292.

Hawkins, J. D. et al. (2000), 'Predictors of youth violence'. *Juvenile Justice Bulletin*, US Department of Justice.

Hay, S. et al. (2004). 'The global distribution and population at risk of malaria: past, present, and future'. *Lancet Infect Dis*, 4: 327.

Head Start Office (2006), Washington, DC.

Heckman, J. (2006), 'Skill formation and the economics of investing in disadvantaged children'. *Science*, 312 (5782): 1900–2.

Heckman, J. (2007), 'The economics, technology and neuroscience of human capability formation'. Discussion paper no. 2875, German Institute for the study of Labour, Bonn (IZA).

Heckman, J., Knudsen, E., Cameron, J. and Shonkoff, J. (2006a), 'Economic, neurobiological, and behavioral perspectives on building America's future workforce'. *Proceedings of the National Academy of Sciences*, 103(27): 10155–62.

Heckman, J., Stixrud, J. and Urzua, S. (2006b), 'The effects of cognitive and noncognitive abilities on labor market outcomes and social behavior'. *Journal of Labor Economics*, 24(3): 411–82.

Heise, L. (1994), 'Gender-based abuse: the global epidemic'. *Cad Saúde Pública*, 10, supl. 1, Rio de Janeiro.

Heise, L., Ellsberg, M. and Gottemoeller, M. (2002), 'A global overview of gender-based violence'. *Int J. Gynecol & Obstet*, 78: 5.

Helander, B. (1988), *Family Health Management in the Gansaxdheere District of the Bay Region*. Somalia. UNICEF, Mogadishu, Somalia.

Helander, E. (1999), *Prejudice and Dignity*, 2nd edition. New York: United Nations Development Programme.

Helander, E. (2002–7), personal observations.

Helander, E. (2007), 'The origins of community-based rehabilitation'. *Asia Pacific Rehabilitation Journal*, 18: 2.

Helander, E., Mendis, P., Nelson, G. and Goerdt, A. (1991), *Training in the Community of People with Disabilities*, 4th edition. Geneva: World Health Organization.

Hesketh, T., Hong, Z. and Lynch, M. (2000), 'Child abuse in China: the views and experiences of child health professionals'. *Child Abuse Negl*, 24: 867.

Higgins, J. et al. (2006). 'Child abuse prevention: what works? The effectiveness of home visiting programs for preventing child maltreatment'. *Research Brief* no. 2.

Himelein, M. and McElrath, J. (1996), 'Resilient child sexual abuse survivors: cognitive coping and illusion'. *Child Abuse Negl*, 20: 747.

Hirschi, T. (1969), *Causes of Delinquency*. Edison, NJ: Transaction Publishers.

Holla, R. and Gupta, A. (2005), 'Child abuse – where do we stand?' *Indian Pediatrics*, 42: 1251.

Holmes, W. and Sammel, M. (2005), 'Brief communication: physical abuse of boys and possible associations with poor adult outcomes'. *Ann Intern Med*, 18: 581.

Holmes, W. and Slap, G. (1998), 'Sexual abuse of boys'. *JAMA*, 280: 1855.

Holzer, P. et al. (2006), 'The effectiveness of parent education and home visiting child maltreatment prevention programs'. *Child Abuse Prevention Issues*, 24, Autumn.

Hong, K. et al. (2004), 'Influence of parenting self-efficacy and belief in corporal punishment on physical abuse of children in Korea'. *Korean J. Child Health Nurs*, 10: 479.

Howard, P., Marumo, L. and Coetzee, D. (1991), 'Child abuse in Alexandria: a clinic-based study and a community programme'. *South African Medical Journal*, 80: 393.

Huang, C. et al. (2004), 'A comparative analysis of abandoned street children and formerly abandoned street children in La Paz, Bolivia'. *Arch Disease in Childhood*, 89: 821.

Hubbard, J. et al. (1995), 'Co-morbidity of psychiatric diagnosis with post-traumatic stress disorder in survivors of childhood trauma'. *J. Am Academy Child and Adolescent Psychiatry*, 34: 1167.

Hughes, D. (2003), 'Psychological intervention for the spectrum of attachment disorders and intrafamilial trauma'. *Attachment & Human Development*, 5: 271.

Hughes, J. (2007), 'Review of medical reports on pedophilia'. *Clinical Pediatrics*, 46: 667.

Huizink, A. (2003), 'Stress during pregnancy is associated with developmental outcome in infancy'. *J. Child Psychol Psychiatry*, 44: 810.

Hull, A. (2002), 'Neuroimaging findings in post-traumatic stress disorder'. *British J. Psychiatry*, 181: 102.

Human Development Reports (1995–2006), New York: United Nations Development Programme.

Human Rights Watch (1996a), 'Chinese orphanages: a follow-up'. March.

Human Rights Watch Children's Rights Project (1996b).

Human Rights Watch (2004), internet report.

Human Rights Watch (2006), 'Discrimination and exploitative forms of labour. India'.

Human Rights Watch and Amnesty International (2005). 'The rest of their lives: life without parole for child offenders in the United States'.

Iglehart, J. (2007), 'The fate of SCHIP – Surrogate marker for health care ideology?' *New England Journal of Medicine*, 357: 2104.

Ikedar, Y. (1995), 'Child abuse and child abuse studies in Japan'. *Acta Paediatric. Japan*, 37: 240.

Innocenti Report Card, No. 5 (2003), *A League Table of Child Maltreatment Deaths in Rich Nations*. UNICEF.

International Labour Organization (2001), International Programme for the Elimination of Child Labour, Tanzania.

International Labour Organization (2006), *The End of Child Labour: Within Reach*.

International Work Group for Indigenous Affairs (2004), 'Indigenous issues'. Copenhagen: International Work Group for Indigenous Affairs.

Irazuzta, J. et al. (1997), 'Outcome and cost of child abuse'. *Child Abuse Negl*, 21: 751.

Isaranurug, S. et al. (2002), 'Violence against children by parents'. *J. Med Assoc Thai*, 85: 875.

Jaffe, P. et al. (1992), 'An evaluation of a secondary school primary prevention program on violence in intimate relationships'. *Violence and Victims*, 7: 129.

Japan Society of Legal Medicine (1995), Planning and Development Committee. *Nippon Hoigaku Zasshi*, 56: 276 (in Japanese).

Jensen, J. et al. (1991), 'Growth hormone response patterns in sexually or physically abused boys'. *J. American Academy of Child and Adolescent Psychiatry*, 30: 784.

Jewkes, R. and Abrahams, N. (2002), 'The epidemiology of rape and sexual coercion in South Africa'. *Social Science & Medicine*, 55: 1231.

Jirapramukpitak, T. et al. (2005), 'The experience of abuse and mental health in the young Thai population'. *Soc Psychiatry Epidemiol*, 40: 955.

Johnson, F. and Ambihaipahar, U. (1999), 'Child abuse in Papua New Guinea'. *Med Law*, 18: 61.

Johnson, J. G. et al. (2006), 'Parenting behaviors associated with risk for offspring personality disorder during adulthood'. *Arch Gen Psychiatry*, 63: 579.

Jones, L. and Finkelhor, D. (2003), 'Putting together evidence on declining trends in sexual abuse: a complex puzzle'. *Child Abuse Negl*, 27: 133.

Jubilee Action (2000), 'Brazilian street children'. Internet.

Jumaian, A. (2001), 'Prevalence and long-term impact of child sexual abuse among a sample of male college students in Jordan'. *East Mediterr Health Journal*, 7: 435.

Jung, M. H. (2004), 'A study on the sexual harassment among university students'. *Korean J. Child Health Nurs*, 10: 291.

Kacker, S. (2007), 'Study on child abuse, India'. Ministry of Woman and Child Development, New Delhi, India.

Kafka, M. and Hennen, J. (2002), 'A DSM-IV Axis 1 co-morbidity study of males (n = 120) with paraphilias and paraphilia-related disorders'. *Sex Abuse*, 14: 349.

Kandel, E. and Mednick, S. (1991), 'Perinatal complications predict violent offending'. *Criminology*, 29: 519.

Kassim, M., Cheah, I. and Shafie, H. (1995), 'Childhood deaths from physical abuse'. *Child Abuse Negl*, 19: 847.

Kaufman, J. et al. (2004), 'Social supports and serotonin transporter gene moderate depression in maltreated children'. *Proc Nat Acad Sci USA*, 101: 17325.

Kaufman, J. et al. (2007), 'Brain-derived neurotrophic factor-5-HTTLPR gene interactions and environmental modifiers of depression in children'. *Biol Psychiatry*, 61, 9 (May): 1112–13.

Kaufmann, D. and Kraay, A. (2007), 'On measuring governance: framing issues for debate'. Issues paper for 11 January 2007 Roundtable on Measuring Governance, the World Bank.

Kawsar, M. et al. (2004), 'Prevalence of sexually transmitted infections and mental health needs of female child and adolescent survivors of rape and sexual assault attending a specialist clinic'. *Sex Transm Infect*, 80: 138.

Keenan, T. and Ward, T. (2000), 'A theory of mind perspective on cognitive, affective, and intimacy deficits in child sexual offenders'. *Sex Abuse*, 12: 49.

Keidel, A. (2007), 'The limits of a smaller, poorer China'. *Financial Times*, 17 November.

Keily, M. et al. (2001), 'The timing of child physical maltreatment: a cross-domain growth analysis of impact on adolescent externalizing and internalizing problems'. *Dev Psychopathol*, 13: 891.

Kempe, C. et al. (1962), 'The battered child syndrome'. *JAMA*, 181: 4.

Kendall, D. (2005), *Sociology in Our Times*. Andover: Thomson Wadsworth.

Kendall-Tackett, K., Williams, L. and Finkelhor, D. (1993), 'Impact of sexual abuse on children: a review and synthesis of recent empirical studies'. *Psychological Bulletin*, 113: 164.

Kernic, M. et al. (2003), 'Behavioural problems among children whose mothers are abused by an intimate partner'. *Child Abuse Negl*, 27: 1231.

Kessler, R. et al. (1994), 'Lifetime and 12-month prevalence of DSM-III psychiatric disorders in the United States'. *Arch Gen Psychiatry*, 51: 8.

Kessler, R. C. et al. (1995), 'Posttraumatic stress disorders in the National Co-morbidity Survey'. *Arch Gen Psychiatry*, 52: 1048.

Kessler, R. et al. (2003), 'The epidemiology of major depressive disorder'. *JAMA*, 289: 3095.

Ketsela, T. and Kebede, D. (1997), 'Physical punishment of elementary schoolchildren in urban and rural communities in Ethiopia'. *Ethiop Med Journal*, 35: 23.

Khamis, V. (2000), 'Child psychological maltreatment in Palestinian families'. *Child Abuse Negl*, 24: 1047.

Khor, G. (2003), 'Update on the prevalence of malnutrition among children in Asia'. *Nepal Med Coll J.*, 5: 113.

Khuory-Kassabri, M. (2006), 'Student victimization by educational staff in Israel'. *Child Abuse Negl*, 30: 691.

Kiehl, K. et al. (2004), 'Temporal lobe abnormalities in semantic processing by criminal psychopaths as revealed by functional magnetic resonance imaging'. *Psychiatry Res*, 130: 297.

Kiehl, K. et al. (2006), 'Brain potentials implicate temporal lobe abnormalities in criminal psychopaths'. *J. Abnorm Psychol*, 115: 443.

Kim, D. et al. (2000), 'Children's experience of violence in China and Korea: a transcultural study'. *Child Abuse Negl*, 24: 1163.

Kim-Cohen, J. et al. (2003), 'Prior juvenile diagnoses in adults with mental disorder: development follow-back of a prospective longitudinal cohort'. *Arch Gen Psychiatry*, 60: 709.

Kim-Cohen, J. et al. (2005), 'Maternal depression and children's antisocial behavior: nature and nurture effects'. *Arch Gen Psychiatry*, 62: 173.

Kim-Cohen, J. et al. (2006), 'MAOA, maltreatment, and gene–environment interaction predicting children's mental health: new evidence and a meta-analysis'. *Molecular Psychiatry*, 11: 903.

Kleinman, A., Das, V. and Locke, M. (eds) (1997), *Social Suffering*. California: University of California Press.

Kleinman, A., Das, V. and Locke, M. (eds) (2001), *Remaking a World*. California: University of California Press.

Knapp, J. (1998), 'The impact of children witnessing violence'. *Pediatric Clinics of North America*, 45: 3.

Knudsen, E. et al. (2006), 'Economic, neurobiological and behavioural perspectives on building America's future workforce'. Working Paper 12298. Cambridge, MA: National Bureau of Economic Research.

Knutson, J. et al. (2005), 'Care neglect, supervisory neglect, and harsh parenting in the development of children's aggression: a replica and extension'. *Child Maltreatment*, 10: 92.

Koenen, K. et al. (2003), 'Domestic violence is associated with environmental suppression of IQ in young children'. *Dev Psychopathol*, 15: 297.

Korten, F. and Siv, R. (1989), *Transforming a Bureaucracy: the Experience of the Philippine National Irrigation Administration*. Hartford, CT: Kumaria Press.

Kostrzewa, W. (1990), 'Marshall Plan for Middle and Eastern Europe'. *World Economy*, 13: 27.

Kouno, A. and Johnson, C. (1995), 'Child abuse and neglect in Japan: coin-operated-locker-babies'. *Child Abuse Negl*, 19: 25.

Krantz, G. and Östergren, P. (2000), 'The association between violence victimization and common symptoms in Swedish women'. *J. Epidemiol Community Health*, 54: 815.

Kumpulainen, K. et al. (2000), 'The persistence of psychiatric deviance from the age of 8 to the age of 15 years'. *Soc Psychiatry Psychiatr Epidemiol*, 35: 5.

Labadarios, D. et al. (2005), 'The National Food Consumption Survey (NFCS): South Africa, 1999'. *Public Health Nutr*, 8: 533.

Lagace-Seguin, D. and d'Entremont, M. (2006), 'Less than optimal parenting strategies predict maternal low-level depression beyond that of child transgressions'. *Early Child Development and Care*, 176: 343.

Laime, A. (1997), 'Health care allocation and selective neglect in rural Peru'. *Social Science & Medicine*, 44: 1711.

Lakew, Z. (2001), 'Alleged cases of sexual assault reported to two Addis Ababa hospitals'. *East Afr Med Journal*, 78: 80.

Lalor, K. (2004a), 'Child sexual abuse in sub-Saharan Africa: a literature review'. *Child Abuse Negl*, 28: 439.

Lalor, K. (2004b), 'Child sexual abuse in Tanzania and Kenya'. *Child Abuse Negl*, 28: 833.

Lampe, A. (2002), 'The prevalence of childhood sexual abuse, physical abuse and emotional neglect in Europe'. *Z Psychosom Med Psychotherapy*, 48: 370.

Lange, C. et al. (2005), 'Reduced glucose metabolism in temporo-parietal cortices of women with borderline personality disorder'. *Psychiatry Res*, 1439: 115.

Langhinrichsen-Rohling, J. (2005), 'Top 10 greatest "hits": important findings and future directions in intimate partner violence research'. *J. Interpersonal Violence*, 10: 100.

LaPierre, D., Braun, C. and Hodgins, S. (1995), 'Ventral frontal deficits in psychopathy: neuropsychological test findings'. *Neuropsychologia*, 33: 139.

Lavely, W. (2001), *First Impressions of the 2000 Census of China*. Sociology Department and Center for Studies in Demography and Ecology, University of Washington.

Laws, D. R. and Marshall, W. L. (1990). 'A conditioning theory of the etiology and maintenance of deviant sexual preference and behaviour', in H. E. Barbaree, W. L. Marshall and D. R. Laws (eds), *Handbook of Sexual Assault: Theories and Treatment of the Offender* (pp. 209–29). New York: Plenum.

Leach, P. (1999), *The Physical Punishment of Children: Some Input from Recent Research*. London: NSPCC.

Leiva Plaza, B. et al. (2001), 'The impact of malnutrition on brain development, intelligence and school work performance'. *Arch Latinoam Nutr*, 51: 64.

Lema, V. (1997), 'Sexual abuse of minors: emerging medical and social problems in Malawi'. *East African Medical Journal*, 74: 743.

Leserman, J. and Drossman, D. (2007), 'Relationship of abuse history to functional gastrointestinal disorders and symptoms: some possible mediating mechanisms'. *Trauma Violence Abuse*, 8: 331.

Levy, K. (2005), 'The implications of attachment theory and research for understanding borderline personality disorder'. *Dev Psychopathol*, 17: 959.

Li, Y. et al. (2001), 'Child behaviour problems: prevalence and correlates in rural minority areas of China'. *Pediatr Int*, 43: 651.

Lie, N. (1999), *Deprivation in Orphanages*. Iaşi, Romania: Cantes Publishing House.

Liu, J. et al. (2003), 'Malnutrition at age 3 years and lower cognitive ability at age 11 years: independence from psychosocial adversity'. *Arch Pediatr Adolesc Med*, 157: 593.

Locke, John [1692] (1989), *Some Thoughts Concerning Education*. Oxford: Clarendon Press.

Loeber, R. (1991), 'Antisocial behaviour: more enduring than changeable?' *J. Am Acad Child Adolesc Psychiatry*, 30: 393.

Lombardo, L. (2001), *Introduction to Alice Miller, 'The truth will set you free'*. New York: Farrar, Straus and Giroux.

Lopez, A., Begg, S. and Bos, E. (2006), *Demographic and Epidemiological Characteristics of Major Regions*. Global Burden of Disease and Risk Factors: 17. New York: Oxford University Press.

Lopez, F. et al. (1995), 'Prevalencia y consecuuencias del abuso sexual al menor en España'. *Child Abuse Negl*, 19: 1039.

Louvain Unversity, Belgium (2004), Database on international disasters.

Lundqvist, G., Svedin, C. and Hansson, K. (2004), 'Childhood sexual abuse: women's health when starting in group therapy'. *Nord J. Psychiatry*, 58: 25.

Luo, T. (1996), 'Marrying my rapist? Cultural traumas among Chinese rape survivors'. Paper presented at the 91st American Sociological Association Meeting, New York.

Luo, T. (1998), 'Sexual trauma among Chinese survivors'. *Child Abuse Negl*, 22: 1013.

Luster, T. and Youatt, J. (1989), 'The effects of pre-parenthood education on high school students'. Paper presented at the Biennial Meeting of the Society for Research in Child Development, Kansas City, Kansas, 27 April.

Machado, C. et al. (2007), 'Child and partner abuse: self-reported prevalence and attitudes in the north of Portugal'. *Child Abuse Negl*, 31: 657.

Mackenzie, G. et al. (1993), 'The incidence of child sexual abuse in Northern Ireland'. *International Journal of Epidemiology*, 22: 299.

Macmillan, H. et al. (1997), 'Prevalence of child physical and sexual abuse in the community: results from the Ontario health supplement'. *JAMA*, 278: 1311.

Macmillan, H. et al. (2003), 'Reported contact with child protection services among those reporting child physical and sexual abuse: results from a community survey'. *Child Abuse Negl*, 27: 1397.

MacPhail, R. (1990), *Environmental Modulation of Neurobehavioural Toxicity: Behavioural Measures of Neurotoxicity*. National Academy's Commission on Behavioural and Social Sciences and Education, Washington, DC.

Madu, S. (2001), 'Prevalence of child psychological, physical, emotional, and ritualistic abuse among high school students in Mpumalanga Province, South Africa'. *Psychol Rep*, 89: 431.

Madu, S. and Peltzer, K. (2001), 'Prevalence and patterns of child sexual abuse and victim perpetrator relationship among secondary school students in the Northern Province'. *Arch Sex Behav*, 30: 311.

Maes, M., Van West, D., Westerberg, H. et al. (2001a), 'Lower baseline plasma and prolactin together with increased body temperature and higher MCPP-induced cortisol responses in men with paedophilia'. *Neuropsychopharmacology*, 24: 37.

Maes, M., De Vos, N. and Van Hunsel, F. (2001b), 'Paedophilia is accompanied by increased plasma concentration of catecholamines, in particular epinephrine'. *Psychiatry Res*, 103: 43.

Maguin, E. and Loeber, R. (1996), 'Academic performance and delinquency', in M. Tonry (ed.), *Crime and Justice: a Review of Research*, Vol. 20. Chicago: University of Chicago Press, p. 145.

Maguin, E. et al. (1995), 'Risk factors measured at three ages for violence at age 17–18'. Paper presented at the American Society of Criminology, September, Boston, MA.

Mahlangu, T. and Sibindi, F. (1995), 'Child sexual abuse in Matabeleland, Zimbabwe'. *Social Science & Medicine*, 41: 1693.

Marsa, F. et al. (2004), 'Attachment styles and psychological profiles of child sex offenders in Ireland'. *J. Interpers Violence*, 19: 228.

Martsolf, D. (2004), 'Childhood maltreatment and mental and physical health in Haitian adults'. *J. Nurs Scholarship*, 36: 293.

Mash, E. and Johnston, C. (1983) 'Parental perceptions of child behaviour problems, parenting self-esteem, and mothers' reported stress in younger and older hyperactive and normal children'. *J Consult Clin Psychol*, 51: 86.

Masten, S. (1997) 'Resilience in children-at-risk'. *Carei*, University of Minnesota, 5: 1.

Matasha, E. et al. (1998), 'Sexual and reproductive health among primary and secondary school pupils in Mwanza, Tanzania: need for intervention'. *AIDS Care*, 10: 571.

Matchinda, B. (1999), 'The impact of the home background on the decision of children to run away: the case of Yaoundé City in Cameroon'. *Child Abuse Negl*, 23: 245.

Mathew, S. et al. (2004), 'Dorsolateral prefrontal cortical pathology in generalized anxiety disorder: a proton magnetic resonance spectroscopic imaging study'. *Am J. Psychiatry*, 161: 1119.

Mathoma, A. et al. (2006), 'Knowledge and perceptions of parents regarding child sexual abuse in Botswana and Swaziland', *J. Pediatric Nursing*, 2: 67.

Maunder, R. and Hunter, J. (2001), 'Attachment and psychosomatic medicine: development contributions to stress and disease'. *Psychosomatic Medicine*, 63: 556.

May, P. M. et al. (2000), 'Epidemiology of foetal alcohol syndrome in a South African community in the Western Cape Province'. *Am J. Public Health*, 90: 1905.

May, P. et al. (2006), 'Epidemiology of FASD in a province in Italy: prevalence and characteristics of children in a random sample of schools'. *Alcoholism: Clinical and Experimental Research*, 30: 1562.

McClure, E. B. et al. (2007), 'Abnormal attention modulation of fear circuit function in pediatric generalized anxiety disorder'. *Arch Gen Psychiatry*, 64: 97.

McCormick, K. (1992), 'The attitudes of primary care physicians and pediatricians towards corporal punishment'. *J. American Medical Association*, 267: 161.

McCrann, D. et al. (2006), 'Childhood sexual abuse among university students in Tanzania'. *Child Abuse Negl*, 30: 1343.

McDermott, D. (2002), 'From theory to practice: some successful methods of parent education'. Prepare tomorrow's parents.org.

McFarlane, J. et al. (2003), 'Behaviors of children who are exposed and not exposed to intimate partner violence: an analysis of 330 black, white, and Hispanic children'. *Pediatrics*, 112: 202.

McGee, H. et al. (2003), *The SAVI Report: Sexual Abuse and Violence in Ireland*. Dublin Rape Crisis Centre: Liffey Press.

McGloin, J. and Widom, C. (2001), 'Resilience among abused and neglected children grown up'. *Dev Psychopathol*, 13: 1021.

McGuigan, W. and Pratt, C. (2001), 'The predictive impact of domestic violence on three types of child maltreatment'. *Child Abuse Negl*, 25: 869.

Mednick, S. (1971), 'Birth defects and schizophrenia'. *Psychology Today*, 4: 48.

Mehta, D. and Chatterji, R. (2001), 'Boundaries, names, alterities: a case study of a "communal riot" in Dharavi, Bombay', in A. Kleinman, V. Das and M. Locke (eds), *Remaking a World*. California: University of California Press, p. 201.

Melchert, P. (1998), 'Family of origin history, psychological distress, quality of childhood memory, and content of first and recovered childhood memories'. *Child Abuse Negl*, 22: 1203.

Menick, D. (2000), 'Les contours psychosociaux de l'Infanticide en Afrique Noire: Le Cas du Sénégal'. *Child Abuse Negl*, 24: 1557.

Menick, D. and Ngoh, F. (2003), 'Seroprevalence of HIV infection in sexually abused children in Cameroon'. *Med Trop*, 63: 155.

Merton, R. K. (1968), *Theory and Social Structure*. London: Collier-Macmillan.

Mezey, G. et al. (2005), 'Domestic violence, lifetime trauma and psychological health of childbearing women'. *BJOG*, 112: 197.

Miles, G. (2000), ' "Children don't do sex for pleasure": Sri Lankan children's views on sex and sexual exploitation'. *Child Abuse Negl*, 24: 995.

Milgram, S. (1974), *Obedience to Authority*. New York: Harper & Row.

Miringhoff, M. (1996), *A Very Different Country*. The Fordham Institute for Innovation in Social Policy Social Report, May.

Miringhoff, M. et al. (1999), *The Social Health of the Nation: How America is Really Doing*. Oxford: Oxford University Press.

Mitchell, K. J., Ybarra, M. and Finkelhor, D. (2007), 'The relative importance of online victimization in understanding depression, delinquency, and substance use'. *Child Maltreat*, 12: 314.

Mitchell, S. and Rosa, P. (1979), 'Boyhood behaviour problems as a precursor to criminality: a fifteen-year follow-up study'. *J. Child Psychology and Psychiatry*, 22: 19.

Mocan, H. and Tekin, E. (2006), 'Guns and juvenile crime'. *Journal of Law and Economics*, October: 507.

Moffitt, T. (2001), 'Adolescence-limited and life-course-persistent antisocial behaviour: a developmental taxonomy', in A. Piquero and P. Mazerolle (eds), *Life-course Criminology: Contemporary and Classic Readings*. Belmont, CA: Wadsworth.

Moffitt, T. (2005), 'The new look of behavioral genetics in developmental psychopathology: gene–environment interplay in antisocial behaviors'. *Psychol Bull*, 131: 533.

Morris, I. et al. (1997), 'Physical and sexual abuse of children in the West Midlands'. *Child Abuse Negl*, 21: 285.

Mulder, R. T. et al. (1998), 'Relationship between dissociation, childhood sexual abuse, childhood physical abuse, and mental illness in a general population sample'. *Am J. Psychiatry*, 155: 806.

Muller, R., Hunter, J. and Stollak, G. (1995), 'The intergenerational transmission of corporal punishment: a comparison of social learning and temperament models'. *Child Abuse Negl*, 19: 1323.

Mulugeta, E., Kassaye, M. and Berhane, Y. (1998), 'Prevalence and outcomes of sexual violence among high school students'. *Ethiopian Medical Journal*, 36: 167.

Nader, K. et al. (1993), 'A preliminary study of PTSD and grief among the children of Kuwait following the Gulf Crisis'. *British J. Clinical Psychology*, 32: 407.

Nakamura, Y. (2002), 'Child abuse and neglect in Japan'. *Pediatrics International*, 44: 580.

Nathanielsz, P. (1999), *Life in the Womb: the Origin of Health and Disease*. Portland, OR: Promethean Press.

National Centre on Sexual Behaviour of Youth (2003), 'Adolescent sex offenders'. Available at www.ncsby.org.

National Clearinghouse on Child Abuse and Neglect Information (2000). US Department of Health and Human Services.

National Survey on Drug Use and Health. Report, 13 February 2004. Bethesda, MD: Department of Health and Human Services.

Naveillan, P. and Vargas, S. (1989). 'The prevalence of alcoholism in Chile over three decades (1952–1982)'. *Rev Saúde Pública*, 23: 128.

Nelson, E. and Zimmermann, C. (1996), Household Survey on Domestic Violence in Cambodia. Phnom Penh, Ministry of Women's Affairs and Project Against Domestic Violence.

Neumann, D. A. et al. (1996), 'The long-term sequelae of childhood sexual abuse in women: a meta-analytic review'. *Child Maltreatment*, 1: 6.

Neumark-Sztainer, D. et al. (1997), 'Psychosocial correlates of health compromising behaviours among adolescents'. *Health Education Research*, 12: 37.

Newport, D. et al. (2004), 'Pituitary-adrenal responses to standard and low-dose dexamethasone suppression tests in adult survivors of child abuse'. *Biol Psychiatry*, 55: 10.

Newton, C. (2001), 'Child abuse: an overview'. TherapistFinder.net Mental Health Journal (http://www.therapistfinder.net/Child-Abuse/).

New York State Office of Mental Health (1989), Official Report on Child Abuse at Western New York Children's Psychiatric Center.

Ngwudike, B. (2005). 'Program for International Student Assessment (PISA) 2000: analysis of questionnaire data from United States students'. ERIC Online.

Nhundu, T. and Shumba, A. (2001), 'The nature and frequency of reported cases of teacher perpetrated child sexual abuse in rural primary schools in Zimbabwe'. *Child Abuse Negl*, 25: 1517.

Nicholson, S. et al. (2005), 'Alcohol consumption and increased mortality in Russian men and women: a cohort study based on the mortality of relatives'. *Bull World Health Organization*, 83: 812.

Niederberger, J. (2002), 'The perpetrator's strategy as a crucial variable: a representative study of sexual abuse of girls and its sequelae in Switzerland'. *Child Abuse Negl*, 26: 55.

Niederhofer, H. and Reiter, A. (2004), 'Prenatal maternal stress, prenatal foetal movements and perinatal temperament factors influence behaviour and school marks at the age of 6'. *Foetal Diagn Ther*, 19: 160.

Niksić, D. and Kurspahić-Mujcić, A. (2007), 'The presence of health-risk behaviour in Roma family'. *Bosn J. Basic Med Sci*, 7: 144.

Nutt, D. and Malizia, A. (2004), 'Structural and functional brain changes in posttraumatic stress disorder'. *J. Clin Psychiatry*, 65, supp. 1: 11.

O'Brien, M. and Nutt, D. (1998), 'Loss of consciousness and post-traumatic stress disorder', *Br J. Psychiatry*, 173: 102.

OECD publication, comments by Sylvia Allegretto, internet, 23 June 2004.

OECD (2007), Reports on Official Development Aid (ODA).

OEEC (October 1948), Report to the Economic Cooperation Administration on the First Annual Programme. Paris: 21.

Office of the United Nations High Commissioner for Human Rights (2006), 'Summary of status of ratifications', June. Internet.

Official report, Government of Oman, 2004.

Olds, D. et al. (1997), 'Long-term effects of home visitation on maternal life course and child abuse and neglect'. *JAMA*, 278, 8: 637.

Olds, D. et al. (2002). 'Home visiting by nurses and by paraprofessionals: a randomised controlled trial'. *Paediatrics*, 110: 486.

Olsson, A. et al. (2000), 'Sexual abuse during childhood and adolescence among Nicaraguan men and women: a population-based anonymous survey'. *Child Abuse Negl*, 24: 1579.

Orhon, F. et al. (2006), 'Attitudes of Turkish parents, pediatric residents, and medical students toward child disciplinary practices'. *Child Abuse Negl*, 30: 1081.

Ovediran, K. and Isiugo-Abanihe, U. (2005) 'Perceptions of Nigerian women on domestic violence: evidence from 2003 Nigeria Demographic and Health Survey'. *Afr J. Reprod Health*, 9: 38.

Owen, M. (1996), *A World of Widows*. London: Zed Books.

Paintal, S. (2007), 'A position paper for the Association for Childhood Education International'. Olney, Maryland. Internet.

Pan, J. P. et al. (2005), 'Study on the current situation and influential factors of child neglect among 3–6 year-olds in the urban areas of China'. *Zhonghua Liu Xing Bing Xue Za Zhi*, 26: 258.

Park, H. and Comstock, G. (1994), 'The effects of television violence on antisocial behaviour: a meta-analysis'. *Communication Research*, 21: 516.

Parry, H. (2002), 'Alcohol use in South Africa: findings from the South African Community Epidemiology Network on Drug Use (SACENDU) project'. Alcohol Research Documentation, Inc.

Paúl, J., Milner, J. and Múgica, P. (1995), 'Childhood maltreatment, childhood social support, and child abuse potential in a Basque sample'. *Child Abuse Negl*, 19: 907.

Pedersen, W. and Hegna, K. (2003), 'Children and adolescents who sell sex: a community study'. *Social Science & Medicine*, 56: 135.

Pederson, C. et al. (2004), 'Hippocampus volume and memory performance in a community based on samples of women with post-traumatic stress disorder secondary to child abuse'. *J. Trauma Stress*, 17: 37.

Pelo, J. (2000), 'Large families'. Internet.

Pereda, N. and Forns, M. (2007), 'Prevalence and characteristics of child sexual abuse among Spanish university students'. *Child Abuse Negl*, 31: 417.

Perera, S. (2001) 'Spirit possessions and avenging ghosts: stories of supernatural activity as narratives of terror and mechanism of coping and remembering', in A. Kleinman, V. Das and M. Locke (eds), *Remaking a World*. California: University of California Press.

Perez-Albeniz, A. (2003), 'Dispositional empathy in high- and low-risk parents for child physical abuse'. *Child Abuse Negl*, 27: 769.

Perry, B. D. (2002), 'Childhood experience and the expression of genetic potential: what childhood neglect tells us about nature and nurture'. *Brain and Mind*, 3: 79.

Perry, J. (2006), 'Seven institutionalized children and their adaptation in late adulthood: the children of Duplessis'. *Psychiatry*, 69: 283.

Petersen, I. et al. (2005), 'Sexual violence and youth in South Africa: the need for community-based preventive interventions'. *Child Abuse Negl*, 29: 1233.

Petersilia, J. (1997), 'Persons with mental retardation in the California criminal justice system: prevalence, processing, and programs'. Proposal for 1998 CPS Research Program.

Pfeifer, C., Wetzels, P. and Enzmann, D. (1999), *Innerfamiliäre Gewalt gegen Kinder and Jugendliche und ihre Auswirkung*. Hannover: Kriminilogisches Forschungsinstitut Niedersachsen.

Pico-Alfonso, M. A. et al. (2004), 'Changes in cortisol and dehydroepiandrosterone in women victims of physical and psychological intimate partner violence'. *Biol Psychiatry*, 56: 233.

Pitman, R. et al. (2002), 'Pilot study of secondary prevention of posttraumatic stress disorder with propranolol'. *Biol Psychiatry*, 51: 189.

Pluchino, S. et al. (2007), 'Rationale for the use of neural stem/precursor cells in immune-mediated demyelinating disorders'. *J. Neurol*, 254, supp. 1: 123.

Plummer, C. (2001), 'Prevention of sexual abuse: a survey of 87 programs'. *Violence Vict*, 15: 575.

Popma, A. and Raine, A. (2006), 'Will future forensic assessment be neurobiologic?' *Child Adolesc Psychiatr Clin N Am*, 15: 429.

Premi, M. K. (2001), 'The missing girl child'. *Economic and Political Weekly*, 26 May.

Protestantse Stichting voor Verantwoorde Gezinsvorming (1981), *Pedophilia*. PSVG Booklet, The Netherlands.

Qasem, F. S. et al. (1998), 'Attitudes of Kuwaiti parents toward physical punishment of children'. *Child Abuse Negl*, 22: 1189.

Qin, L. Z. et al. (2008), 'Risk factors for emotional abuse in 844 adolescents'. *Zhongguo Dang Dai Er Ke Za Zhi*, 10: 228.

Rahman, H. (1995), 'Child domestic workers: is servitude the only option?' *Shoishib*, Dhaka, Bangladesh.

Rahman, L. (2003), 'Alcohol prohibition and addictive consumption in India'. London School of Economics.

Räikkönen, K. and Keltikangas-Järvinen, L. (1992), 'Mothers with hostile, type A predisposing child-rearing practices'. *J. Genetic Psychol*, 153: 343.

Raine, A. et al. (1990), 'Relationships between central and autonomic measures of arousal at age 15 years and criminality at age 24 years'. *Arch Gen Psychiatry*, 47: 1003.

Raine, A. et al. (2003), 'Corpus callosum abnormalities in psychopathic antisocial individuals'. *Arch Gen Psychiatry*, 60, 11.

Rajani, R. (1998), 'Child sexual abuse in Tanzania: much noise, little justice'. *Sex Health Exch*, 1: 13.

Rajani, R. and Kudrati, M. (1996), 'The varieties of sexual experience of the street children in Mwanza, Tanzania', in S. Zeidenstein and K. Moore (eds), *Learning About Sexuality: a Practical Beginning*. New York: The Population Council, p. 323.

Rapp, J., Carrington, F. and Nicholson, G. (1986), *School Crime and Violence: Victim's Rights*. Malibu, CA: Pepperdine University Press.

Rarboch, J. (1996), 'Incidence of sexual abuse'. *Cas Lek Cesk*, 135: 270.

Ravallion, M. (1997), 'Can high-inequality developing countries escape absolute poverty?' *Economics Letters*, 56: 51.

Ravallion, M. (2004), 'Pro-poor growth: a primer'. Policy Research Working Paper 3242, World Bank, Washington, DC.

Ravamudan (2003), 'Born to die'. www.rediff.com/news/2001oct/24spec.htm

Rebellon, C. and Van Gundy, K. (2005), 'Can control theory explain the link between parental and physical abuse and delinquency?' *J. Research in Crime and Delinquency*, 42: 247.

Reddington, F. and Wallace, D. (eds) (2004), 'Impacting juvenile justice and transition from prison to community initiative'. *Journal of the Institute of Justice and International Studies*, Central Missouri State University, Warrensburg, MO.

Reddy, S. and Pogge, T. (2005), 'How not to count the poor'. Columbia University Department of Economics, Social Science Research Network, internet.

Reed, D. and Reed, E. (1997), 'Children of incarcerated parents', *Social Justice*, 24.

Rekart, M. (2005), 'Sex work harm reduction'. *Lancet*, 366: 2123.

Report of the Special Rapporteur on violence against women on the mission to the United States of America on the issue of violence against women in state and federal prisons (E/CN.4/1999/68/Add.2).

Reports, World Economic Indicators, publications and newsletters from the World Bank (1995–2005); Human Development Reports 1995–2006, United Nations Development Programme, New York.

Reports from OECD, Paris.

Reynolds, B. and Weiss, S. (1992), 'Generation of neurons and astrocytes from isolated cells of the adult mammalian central nervous system'. *Science*, 255: 1707.

Richards, M. and Wadsworth, M. (2004), 'Long-term effects of early adversity on cognitive function'. *Arch Dis Childhood*, 89: 92.

Riis, L., Bodelsen, H. and Knudsen, F. (1998), 'Incidence of child neglect and child abuse in the region of Copenhagen'. *Ugeskrift for Laeger*, 160: 5358.

Rinne, T. et al. (2002), 'Hyper-responsiveness of hypothalamic-pituitary-adrenal axis and combined dexamethasone/corticotropin-releasing hormone challenge in female borderline personality disorder subjects with a history of sustained childhood abuse'. *Biological Psychiatry*, 52: 1102.

Rivera, G. (1972), *Willowbrook: a Report on How it is and Why it Does Not Have to Be That Way*. New York: Vintage Books.

Robin, R. et al. (1997), 'Prevalence, characteristics, and impact of childhood sexual abuse in a southwestern American Indian tribe'. *Child Abuse Negl*, 2: 769.

Robins, L. et al. (1988), 'The Composite International Diagnostic Interview'. *Arch Gen Psychiatry*, 45: 1069.

Rogers, R. et al. (1999), 'Dissociable deficits in the decision-making cognition of chronic amphetamine abusers, opiate abusers, patients with focal damage to prefrontal cortex, and tryptophan-depleted normal volunteers: evidence for monoaminergic mechanisms'. *Neuropsychopharmacology*, 20: 322.

Rogerson, A., Hewitt, A. and Waldenberg, D. (2004), *The International Aid System 2005–2010: Forces For and Against Change*. Overseas Development Institute, London.

Rosen, L. and Martin, L. (1996), 'Impact of childhood abuse history on psychological symptoms among male and female soldiers in the US Army'. *Child Abuse Negl*, 29: 1149.

Rothman, D. and Rothman, S. (1984), *The Willowbrook Wars*. New York: Harper & Row.

Rotoru, T. (Co-ord) (1996), *Expunereao minorilor la abuz şi neglijare in judeful Cluij* (Child abuse and neglect in the district of Cluij). Romania, Cluij: Ed. Comprex.

Roxell, L. (2007), 'Prison networks'. Swedish study of interaction between prisoners, in Swedish. Institute of Criminology, University of Stockholm, Sweden.

Rozenblatt, C. (2002), Adapted from chart, United Nations Environment Programme, Nairobi, Kenya.

Rutter, M. (2006), *Genes and Behaviour: Nature–Nurture Interplay Explained*. Oxford: Blackwell.

Rwenge, M. (2000), 'Sexual risk behaviours among young people in Bamenda, Cameroon'. *International Family Planning Perspectives*, 28: 118.

Sabu, M. (1997), 'Female maternal filicide in Tamil Nadu, India: from recognition back to denial'. *Repr Health Matters*, 124: 124.

Sadler, B. L., Chadwick, D. L. and Hensler, D. (1999), 'The summary chapter – the national call for action: moving ahead'. *Child Abuse Negl*, 23: 1011.

Sameroff, A. et al. (1987), 'Intelligence quotient scores of 4-year-old children: social-environmental risk factors'. *Pediatrics*, 79: 343.

Santos, D. et al. (2006), 'Mental disorders prevalence among female care-givers of children in a cohort study in Salvador, Brazil'. *Revista Brasileira Psiquiatria*, 28: 2.

Sariola, H. and Utella, A. (1994), 'The prevalence of child sexual abuse in Finland'. *Child Abuse Negl*, 18: 827.

Save the Children, Sweden (2005), study reported on its website.

Schein, M. et al. (2000), 'The prevalence of history of child sexual abuse among adults visiting family practitioners in Israel'. *Child Abuse Negl*, 24: 667.

Scher, C. et al. (2004), 'Prevalence and demographic correlates of childhood maltreatment in an adult community sample'. *Child Abuse Negl*, 28: 167.

Schiltz, K. et al. (2007), 'Brain pathology in pedophilic offenders: evidence of volume reduction in the right amygdala and related diencephalic structures'. *Arch Gen Psychiatry*, 64: 737.

Schmal, C. et al. (2004), 'A positron emission tomographic study of memories of childhood abuse in borderline personality disorder'. *Biological Psychiatry*, 55: 759.

Schneider, R., Baumrind, N. and Kimerling, R. (2007), 'Exposure to child abuse and risk for mental health problems in women'. *Violence Vict*, 22: 620.

Schore, A. (1994), *Affect Regulation and the Origin of the Self: the Neurobiology of Emotional Development*. Hills Day, NJ: Lawrence Erlbaum Assoc.

Schumacher, E. F. (1973), *Small is Beautiful: Economics as if People Mattered*. Republished in 1999 with commentaries. Hartley & Marks Publishers.

Schweinhart, L. (2005), 'High-quality preschool program found to improve adult status'. High/Scope Research Foundation.

Scott, S. (2007), 'Multiple traumatic experiences and the development of post-traumatic stress disorder'. *J. Interpers Violence*, 22: 932.

Segal, U. (1995), 'Child abuse by the middle class? A study of professionals in India'. *Child Abuse Negl*, 19: 217.

Sen, S. and Nair, P. (2004), 'Trafficking women and children in India'. Institute of Social Sciences, National Human Rights Commission and UNIFEM, New Delhi.

Shaaban, S. et al. (2005), 'Early detection of protein energy malnutrition in Sharkia Governorate, Egypt'. *J. Egypt Public Health Assoc*, 80: 665.

Shaffer, D. et al. (1994), The NIMH Diagnostic Interview Schedule for Children', Version 2.3 (DISC-2.3): description.

Shaw, B. and Krause, N. (2002), 'Exposure to physical violence during childhood, aging and health'. *J. Aging & Health*, 14: 467.

Shaw, C. and McKay, H. (1972), *Juvenile Delinquency in Urban Areas*. Chicago: University of Chicago Press.

Sheikhattari, P., Stephenson, R. et al. (2006), 'Child maltreatment among schoolchildren in the Kurdistan Province, Iran'. *Child Abuse Negl*, 30: 575.

Shim, Y.-H. (1992), 'Sexual violence against women in Korea: a victimization survey of Seoul women'. Paper presented at the Conference on International Perspectives: Crime, Justice and Public Order. St Petersburg, Russia, 21–27 June.

Shin, L. et al. (1999), 'Regional cerebral blood flow during script-driven imagery in childhood sexual abuse-related PTSD: a PET investigation'. *Am J. Psychiatry*, 156: 575.

Shin, L., Rauch, S. and Pitman, R. (2006) 'Amygdala, medial prefrontal cortex, and hippocampal function in PTSD'. *Ann NY Acad Sci*, 1071: 67.

Sickmund, M. (2004), 'Juveniles in correction'. Department of Justice, Washington.

Silverman, A. et al. (1996), 'The long-term sequelae of child and adolescent abuse: a longitudinal community study'. *Child Abuse Negl*, 20: 709.

Sing, H., Yiing, W. and Nurani, H. (1996), 'Prevalence of childhood sexual abuse among Malaysian paramedical students'. *Child Abuse Negl*, 20: 487.

Skute, D. et al. (1998), 'Risk factors for development of sexually abusive behaviour in sexually victimised adolescent boys: cross sectional study'. *British Medical Journal*, 31: 175.

Slaby, R., Wilson-Brewer, R. and Dash, K. (1995), 'Aggressors, victims and bystanders: thinking and acting to prevent violence'. Education Development Center, Newton, MA, USA.

Sloan, E. et al. (2007), 'Insecure attachment is associated with the alpha-EEG anomaly during sleep'. *Biopsychosoc Med*, 1: 20.

Smiljanich, K. and Briere, J. (1996) 'Self-reported sexual interest in children: sex differences and psychosocial correlates in a university sample'. *Violence Vict*, 11: 39.

Smith, C. and Thornberry, T. (1995), 'The relationship between childhood maltreatment and adolescent involvement on delinquency'. *Criminology*, 22: 451.

Smith, C. et al. (1994), 'National extension parent education model of critical parenting practices'. Manhattan, Kansas: Kansas Co-operative Extension Service.

Sobsey, D. (2000), 'Abuse and children with a disability'. Congress of the British Association for the Study and Prevention of Child Abuse and Neglect (internet).

Sobsey, D. and Doe, T. (1991), 'Patterns of sexual abuse and assault'. *Sexuality and Disability*, 9: 243.

Sobsey, D. and Varnhagen, C. (1990), 'Sexual abuse, assault and exploitation of individuals with disabilities', in C. Bagley and R. Thompson (eds), *Child Sexual Abuse: Critical Perspectives on Prevention, Assessment and Treatment*. Toronto: Wall and Emerson.

Sobsey, D. et al. (eds) (1995), *Violence and Disability: an Annotated Bibliography*. Baltimore, MD: Paul H. Brookes.

Soderstrom, H. et al. (2000), 'Reduced regional cerebral blood flow in non-psychotic violent offenders'. *Psychiatry Research*, 98: 29.

Somavia, J. (2004), Press conference, 11 August, by the Director-General of the International Labour Organization.

Southall, D. et al. (1997), 'When mothers try to kill their children: lessons for child protection'. *Pediatrics*, 100: 7.

Speltz, A (2002), 'Description, history, and critique of corrective attachment therapy'. *The APSAC Advisor*, 14: 4.

Sperry, D. and Gilbert, B. (2005), 'Child peer abuse: preliminary data on outcomes and disclosure experiences'. *Child Abuse Negl*, 29: 889.

Sri Lanka Ministry of Social Welfare, Colombo (2003), National policy on disability for Sri Lanka.

Stattin, H. and Magnusson, D. (1989), 'The role of early aggressive behaviour in the frequency, seriousness and type of later crime'. *J. Consulting and Clinical Psychology*, 57: 710.

Stein, M. et al. (1996), 'Childhood physical and sexual abuse in patients with anxiety disorders and in a community sample'. *Am J. Psychiatry*, 153: 275.

Stewart, W. et al. (2003), 'Cost of productive work time among US workers with depression'. *JAMA*, 289: 3135.

Stiglitz, J. E. (2002), *Globalization and its Discontents*. Harmondsworth: Penguin Books.

Stirpe, T. et al. (2006), 'Sexual offenders' state-of-mind regarding childhood attachment: a controlled investigation'. *Sex Abuse*, 18: 289.

Stoltz, J. A. et al. (2007) 'Associations between childhood maltreatment and sex work in a cohort of drug-using youth'. *Soc Sci Med*, 65: 1214.

Stouthammer-Loeber, M. et al. (2001), 'Maltreatment of boys and the development of disruptive and delinquent behaviour'. *Dev Psychopathol*, 14: 941.

Strange, B., Hurleman, R. and Dolan, R. (2003), 'An emotion-induced retrograde amnesia in humans is amygdala- and β-adrenergic-dependent'. *Proc Nat Acad Sciences*, 100: 13626.

Strathearn, L. et al. (2000), 'Childhood neglect and cognitive development in extremely low birth weight infants: a prospective study'. *Paediatrics*, 108: 142.

Straus, M. and Gelles, R. (1986), 'Societal change and change in family violence from 1975 to 1985 as revealed by two national surveys'. *Journal of Marriage and the Family*, 48: 466.

Straus, M. and Savage, S. (2005), 'Neglectful behaviour by parents in the life history of university students in 17 countries and its relation to violence against dating partners'. *Child Maltreat*, 10: 124.

Straus, M. and Stewart, J. (1999), 'Corporal punishment by American parents: national data on prevalence, chronicity, severity, and duration in relation to child and family characteristics'. *Clin Child Fam Psychol Rev*, 2: 55.

Straus, M. et al. (1997), 'Spanking by parents and subsequent antisocial behavior of children'. *Arch Pediatr Adolesc Med*, 151: 761.

Street children (2006), Internet sources: Pangea: Street Children Worldwide Resource Library; Street Kids International; Florida State University School of Criminology and Criminal Justice; Defence for Children International; National Coalition for the Homeless: Who is Homeless? www.nationalhomeless.org

Substance Abuse and Mental Health Services Administration (1999), 'Summary findings from the 1998 National Household Survey on Drug Abuse'. Bethesda, MD: Department of Health and Human Services.

Sukjumbe, R. and Bwibo, N. (1993), 'Child battering in Nairobi, Kenya'. *East African Medical Journal*, 70: 682.

Sullivan, P. et al. (1991), 'Patterns of physical and sexual abuse of communicatively handicapped children'. *Annals of Otology, Rhinology, and Laryngology*, 100: 188.

Sullivan, P. and Knutson, J. (2000a), 'Maltreatment and disabilities: a population-based epidemiological study'. *Child Abuse Negl*, 24: 1257.

Sullivan, P. and Knutson, J. (2000b), 'The prevalence of disabilities and maltreatment among runaway children'. *Child Abuse Negl*, 24: 1275.

Swanston, H. et al. (2003), 'Nine years after child sexual abuse'. *Child Abuse Negl*, 27: 967.

Swedin, C. and Back, C. (2003), 'Varför berättar de inte? O matt utnyttjas I barnpornografi'. Save the Children, Stockholm, Sweden.

Sylvestre, A., Payette, H. and Tribble, D. S. (2002), 'The prevalence of communication problems in neglected children under three years of age'. *Can J. Public Health*, 93: 349.

Takayanagi, Y. et al. (2005), 'Pervasive social deficits, but normal parturition, in oxytocin receptor-deficient mice'. *Proc Natl Acad Sci USA*, 102: 16096.

Tang, C. (1998), 'The rate of physical abuse in Chinese families: a community survey in Hong Kong'. *Child Abuse Negl*, 22: 381.

Tang, K. (2002), 'Childhood experience of sexual abuse among Hong Kong Chinese college students'. *Child Abuse Negl*, 26: 23.

Tardieu, A. (1860), *Étude médico-légale sur les sérvices et mauvais traitements exercés sur des enfants*. Paris: Librairie J. B. Baillière et fils.

Tardieu, A. (1868), *Étude médico-légale sur l'infaticide*. Paris: Librairie J. B. Baillière et fils.

Tarimura, M., Matsui, I. and Kobayashi, N. (1995), 'Analysis of child abuse cases admitted in pediatric service in Japan'. *Acta Pediatric Japan*, 37(2): 248–61.

Taylor, G. (1997), *Curriculum Strategies: Social Skills Intervention for Young African American Males*. Westport, CT: Praeger.

Taylor, R. R. and Jason, L. (2001), 'Sexual abuse, chronic fatigue and chronic fatigue syndrome: a community-based study'. *J. Nerv Ment Dis*, 189: 709.

Taylor, S. E. et al. (2006), 'Neural responses to emotional stimuli are associated with childhood family stress'. *Biol Psychiatry*, 60: 296.

Tebbutt, J. et al. (1997), 'Five years after child sexual abuse: persisting dysfunction and problems of prediction'. *J. Am Acad Child Adolesc Psychiatry*, 36: 330.

Terry, K. J. and Tallon, J. (2005), 'Child sexual abuse: a review of the literature'. John Jay College of Criminal Justice, New York.

Tharinger, D., Horton, C. and Millea, S. (1990), 'Sexual abuse and exploitation of children and adults with mental retardation and other handicaps'. *Child Abuse Negl*, 14: 371.

Thomas, M. (2001), 'Getting debt relief right'. *Foreign Affairs*, September/October.

Thomasson, E. (2006), 'Pedophile party legal in the Netherlands', Reuters, 20 July.

Thompson, R. (2007), 'Mothers' violence victimization and child behaviour problems: examining the link'. *Am J. Orthopsychiatry*, 77: 306.

Thompson, R. et al. (2006), 'Intimate partner violence: prevalence, types, and chronicity in adult women'. *Am J. Prev Med*, 30: 447.

Thurber, C. (2003), 'Do as I do: the circle of parenting and socialization'. *Camping Magazine*, September.

Ticoll, M. (1992), 'Violence and people with disabilities: a review of the literature', Roeher Institute, Toronto.

Tiihonen, J. et al. (2000), 'Amygdaloid volume loss in psychopathy'. Society for Neuroscience Abstracts, 2017.

Tomison, A. (1998), 'Valuing parent education: a cornerstone of child abuse prevention'. Issues paper no. 10. See www.aifs.org.au

Torella, A. and Zuppinger, K. (1994), 'The abused and neglected child in Switzerland'. *Schweiz Med Wochenschr*, 124: 2331–40.

Touwen, B. et al. (1980), 'Obstetrical condition and neonatal neurological morbidity: an analysis with the help of the optimality concept'. *Early Human Development*, 4/3: 207.

Treatment for Children with Trauma-Attachment Disorders (2005), 'Dyadic Developmental Psychotherapy'. *Child and Adolescent Social Work Journal*, 12.

Trocmé, N. and Lindsey, D. (1996), 'What can child homicide rates tell us about the effectiveness of child welfare services?' *Child Abuse Negl*, 20: 174.

Trocmé, N. et al. (2002), 'Canadian incidence study of reported child abuse and neglect'. Ottawa, Canada.

Tuin-Batstra, L. van der (2004), 'Difficult birth, difficult life?' Doctoral dissertation, University of Groningen, Netherlands.

Tyler, K. A. et al. (2004), 'Risk factors for sexual victimization among male and female homeless and runaway youth'. *J. Interpers Violence*, 19: 503.

UNCTAD (2007), *Handbook of Statistics*.

UNICEF (2002), State of the Children Report, New York.

UNICEF, UNAIDS and USAID (2005), *Children on the Brink*. A Joint Report on Orphan Estimates and Program Strategies.

United Nations Department of Economic and Social Affairs, Division of Population, New York (2000), adapted from chart by Céline Rozenblatt, United Nations Environment Programme.

United Nations General Assembly Resolution 40/33, 29 November 1985.

United Nations General Assembly Resolution 45/113, 14 December 1990.

United Nations General Assembly, 11 August 2000, 'Questions of torture and other cruel, inhuman or degrading treatment or punishment'. Note by the Secretary-General.

United Nations High Commissioner for Refugees (2007), '2006 global trends'.

United Nations Human Rights document. Fact Sheet No. 4: 'Combating torture'.

United Nations Millennium Development Declaration. September 2000.

United Nations Millennium Programme (2005), 'Investing in development: a practical plan to achieve the United Nations Development Programme (UNDP)', Human Development Reports 1995–2006, New York.

United Nations Population Division, 2007, New York.

United Nations Research Institute for Social Development (1994), 'A voice for the excluded'. Geneva.

United Nations Secretary-General (2005), Report. *In Larger Freedom*. New York.

Universal Declaration of Human Rights. Adopted and proclaimed by General Assembly Resolution 217 A (III) of 10 December 1948.

University of California (2006), Internet report.

University of Stockholm (2003), Children and Residential Care, Department of Social Work.

US Accountability Office (2007), Report from the US Census Bureau.

US Census Bureau, International database.

US Department of Health and Human Services (1997), 'Child maltreatment', Washington, DC.

US Department of Health and Human Services (2001), 'Child welfare outcomes 2000'. Annual report.

US Department of Health and Human Services (2003), 'Strengthening Head Start: what the evidence shows'. Washington, DC.

US Department of Health and Human Services (2004), National Survey on Drug Use and Health. Washington, DC.

US Department of Health and Human Services (2005), 'Child maltreatment'.

US Department of Health and Human Services (2007), 'Administration on children, Youth and Families'.

US Department of State (2000), Report on Nigeria.

US Department of State (2003), Report on Pakistan.

US Department of State (2004), Human Rights Reports on Pakistan and Ecuador.

US Department of State (2005), 'Trafficking in persons report'. Office to Monitor and Combat Trafficking in Persons.

US Justice Department (2003a), United States Crime Index Rates, Washington, DC.

US Justice Department (2003b), 'The commercial sexual exploitation of children in the US, Canada and Mexico'. Washington, DC.

US Justice Department, Bureau of Statistics (2002).

US Justice Department, Bureau of Statistics, and Juvenile Justice Bulletin (2002), Report on missing children: Crimes against juveniles, children as victims, battered child syndrome.

United States Parents and Teachers Against Violence in Education (PTAVE) (2003), internet.

Vahíp, I. and Doğanavşargil, Ö. (2006), 'Domestic violence and female patients'. *Türk Psikiyatri Dergisi*, 17: 107.

Valenti-Hein, D. and Schwartz, L. (1995), 'The sexual abuse interview for those with developmental disabilities'. James Stanfield Company. Santa Barbara, California.

Vargas, N. et al. (1995), 'Parental attitude and practice regarding physical punishment of schoolchildren in Santiago, Chile'. *Child Abuse Negl*, 19: 1077.

Varhade, Y. (1998), 'International advocacy and the role of the United Nations and civil society'. Ambedkar Centre for Justice and Peace. Presidential address, Conference: 3.

Vianna, M. et al. (2004), 'Pharmacological studies of the molecular basis of memory extinction'. Department of Biochemistry, Universidade Federal de Rio Grande do Sul, Porto Alegre, Brazil.

Viding, E. et al. (2005), 'Evidence for substantial genetic risk for psychopathy'. *J. Child Psychology and Psychiatr*, 592.

Vieth, V. (2004), 'When parental discipline is a crime'. *The American Prosecutors Institute*, 12: 10.

Viklund Olofsson, M. (2005), Star of Hope International. Stockholm.

Vonk, R. et al. (1993), 'Growth of under five-year-old-children in Kyeni, Kenya'. *Trop Geogr Med*, 45: 175.

Walmsley, R. (2006), The Research Development and Statistics Directorate. Home Office, UK, London.

Walsh, C. A. et al. (2007), 'Child abuse and chronic pain in a community survey of women'. *J. Interpers Violence*, 22: 1536.

Ward, T. and Keenan, T. (1999), 'Child molesters' implicit theories'. *J. Interpersonal Violence*, 14: 821.

Waterhouse Inquiry (2000), 'Lost in care'. Report of the tribunal of inquiry into the abuse of children in care. London: HMSO.

Wattendorf, D. and Muenke, M. (2005), 'Foetal alcohol spectrum disorders'. *American Family Physician*, 72: 279.

Watts, C. et al. (1998), 'Withholding sex and forced sex: dimensions of violence against Zimbabwean women'. *Reproductive Health Matters*, 9: 57.

Webster-Stratton, C. (1994). 'Advancing videotape parent training: a comparison study'. *J. Consult Clin Pychol*, 62: 583.

Weinrott, M. R. (ed.) (1998), 'Juvenile sexual aggression: a critical review'. University of Boulder, CO, Centre for the Study and Prevention of Violence.

Welbourne, A. et al. (1983), 'A comparison of the sexual learning experiences of visually impaired and sighted women'. *J. Visual Impairment and Blindness*, 77: 256.

Wells, L. and Rankin, J. (1988), 'Direct parental controls and delinquency'. *Criminology*, 26: 263.

Wetzels, P. and Pfeiffer, C. (1995), 'Sexuelle Gewalt gegen Frauen im öffentlichen and privaten Raum'. Forschungsbericht des Kriminologischen Forschungsinstituts Niedersachsen e.V.

Whiting, B. and Whiting, J. (1975), *Children of Six Cultures: a Psycho-cultural Analysis*. Cambridge, MA: Harvard University Press.

Wicksteed, J. (1936) *The Challenge of Childhood*. London: Chapman & Hall Ltd.

Widom, C. (2000), 'Understanding the consequences for childhood victimization', in M. D. Robert and M. Reese (eds), *Treatment of Child Abuse*. Baltimore: Johns Hopkins University Press.

Widom, C. S., DuMont, K. and Czaja, S. J. (2007), 'A prospective investigation of major depressive disorder and co-morbidity in abused and neglected children grown up'. *Arch Gen Psychiatry*, 64: 49.

Widom, S. P. et al. (2004), 'The case for prospective longitudinal studies in child maltreatment research: commentary on Dube et al. (2004)'. *Child Abuse Negl*, 28: 715.

Wignaraja, P. (1996), *Poverty Eradication: Lessons from China and South Korea in the 1950s and 1960s*. ISSJ 148/1996. UNESCO Paris, Oxford: Blackwell Publishers.

Wikipedia (2007), World Population. Internet.

Witanowska, J. et al. (2002), 'Problem of violence in the family in the opinion of health service workers'. *Wiad Lek*, 55, Supp. 1: 958.

Wolthuis, A. and Blank, M. (2001), 'Trafficking in children for sexual purposes from Eastern Europe to Western Europe'. ECPAT, Europe.

Wood, W. et al. (1991), 'Effects of media violence on viewers' aggression in unconstrained social interaction'. *Psychological Bulletin*, 109: 307.

Woods, B. (1996), *The Dying Rooms*. Internet and an ABC film.

Worku, D. et al. (2006), 'Child sexual abuse and its outcomes among high school children in southwest Ethiopia'. *Tropical Doctor*, 36: 137.

World Bank (1995–2007), Global Economic Prospects and the Developing Countries. Washington, DC.

World Bank (2007), Governance Matters VI: Governance Indicators for 1996–2006.

World Bank Development reports and World Economic Indicators; other publications, and newsletters by the World Bank.

World Health Organization (1992), 'Psychosocial consequences of disasters'. Geneva.

World Health Organization (1995), Working Group on Female Circumcision. Geneva, Switzerland.

World Health Organization (2001a), 'Years living with a disability'. Geneva. Switzerland.

World Health Organization (2001b), 'International classification of functioning, disability and health', Geneva.

World Health Organization (2002), 'Violence and health'. Geneva, Switzerland.

World Health Organization (2003), 'Health behaviour in school-aged children'. Geneva, Switzerland.

World Health Organization (2004a), 'The economic dimensions of interpersonal violence'. Geneva, Switzerland.

World Health Organization (2004b), 'Preventing violence'. Geneva, Switzerland.

World Health Organization (2005) 'Make every mother and child count'. Geneva, Switzerland.

World Health Organization (2007a), 'Integrated management of pregnancy and childbirth'. WHO MPS 07/05.

World Health Organization (2007b), *World Health Statistics*.

World Health Organization Health Report (2001), *Mental Health: New Understanding, New Hope*.

World Health Organization and UNICEF (2000), 'Report on water supply and assessment'.

Wyatt, G. et al. (1999), 'The prevalence and circumstances of child sexual abuse: changes across a decade'. *Child Abuse Negl*, 23: 45.

Yacoub, M. et al. (1995), 'Early child health in Lahore'. *Acta Pediatrica*, 84: 269.

Yanowitz, K., Monte, E. and Tribble, J. (2003), 'Teachers' beliefs about the effects of child abuse'. *Child Abuse Negl*, 27: 438.

Yiming, C. and Fung, D. (2003), 'Child sexual abuse in Singapore with special reference to medico-legal implications: a review of 38 cases'. *Med Sci Law*, 43: 260.

Yoo, H. et al. (2006), 'Parental attachment and its impact on the development of psychiatric manifestations in school-aged children'. *Psychopathology*, 39: 165.

Youssef, R., Sattia, M. and Kamel, M. (1998a), 'Children experiencing violence, I: parental use of corporal punishment'. *Child Abuse Negl*, 22: 959.

Youssef, R., Sattia, M. and Kamel, M. (1998b), 'Children experiencing violence, II: prevalence and determinants of corporal punishment in schools'. *Child Abuse Negl*, 22: 975.

Ystgaard, M. et al. (2004), 'Is there a specific relationship between childhood sexual and physical abuse and repeated suicidal behaviour?' *Child Abuse Negl*, 28: 863.

Zeira, A. et al. (2002), 'Sexual harassment in Jewish and Arab public schools in Israel'. *Child Abuse Negl*, 26: 149.

Zigler, E. (1979), 'Controlling child abuse in America. An effort doomed to failure?' in R. Bourne and E. Newberger (eds), *Critical Perspectives on Child Abuse*. Lexington, MA: Lexington Books, pp. 171–213.

Zingraff, M. et al. (1993), 'Child maltreatment and youthful problem behaviour'. *Criminology*, 321: 173.

Zingraff, M. et al. (2005), 'Corrélats de la déinquance autodéclarée: Une analyse de l'Enquête longitudinale nationale sur les enfants et les jeunes'. Ministère de la Justice, Canada.

Index